Eugene Braunwald and the Rise of
Modern Medicine

Eugene Braunwald and the Rise of Modern Medicine

Thomas H. Lee

Harvard University Press
Cambridge, Massachusetts
London, England
2013

Book design by Dean Bornstein

Library of Congress Cataloging-in-Publication Data

Lee, Thomas H., 1953–
  Eugene Braunwald and the rise of modern medicine / Thomas H. Lee
  p. cm.
  Includes bibliographical references and index.
  ISBN 978-0-674-72497-6 (alk. paper)
  I. Title.
  [DNLM: 1. Braunwald, Eugene, 1929– 2. Cardiology—Austria—
Biography.   3. Cardiology—United States—Biography.   4. Cardiology—
history—Austria.   5. Cardiology—history—United States.   6. History,
20th Century—Austria—Biography.   7. History, 20th Century—United
States—Biography. WZ 100]
  616.1'20092—dc23
  [B]   2012050701

To
Soheyla
and our daughters,
Simin, Sabrina, and Ariana—
four additional wondrous results of
twentieth-century patterns of immigration to America

Contents

Preface

In the second half of the twentieth century, knowledge in medicine exploded. Research produced major advances in our understanding of the causes of illness, and the number of therapeutic interventions that could actually change the course of diseases dramatically increased. Rigorous comparison of the outcomes that might be expected with various treatment strategies became possible and even expected. Evidence from research began to matter to doctors and to patients.

This progress and these changes were particularly apparent in cardiovascular medicine. In 1950, heart attacks were "bolts from the blue"—unpredictable, unpreventable, and untreatable—but in the decades that followed, mortality from myocardial infarction fell from 30–40 percent to 5–8 percent. Throughout cardiology and the rest of medicine, untreatable diseases became treatable, and some even became curable. Progress helped to drive fatalism out of medicine.

Inevitably, the culture of medicine also evolved. In the 1970s, when I was in medical school, the tutor on my medicine rotation used to say, "Never open a book in front of a patient." He told his students that if we did not know something (such as the dosage of a drug we were about to prescribe), we should excuse ourselves, leave the room, and look up the information out of sight of the patient. Then we should return to the room and continue as if we had known everything all along.

That tutor was not a charlatan; he was a brilliant and caring physician who believed that patients' trust in their doctors was critical to the therapeutic relationship. And, he said, critical to preserving that trust was fulfilling patients' expectations that the physician had everything (at this point, he would tap the side of his head) "right up here." That belief lives on among some physicians even today.

My fellow students and I tried to follow his example. The best way to *act* as if you had everything "right up here" was to *actually* know everything, and many of us tried. We would buy each new edition of *Harrison's Principles of Internal Medicine* and try to read the entire two thousand pages.

It was probably impossible to know "everything" in 1979, and it became increasingly impossible as the century continued. Researchers like Eugene Braunwald were producing too much new knowledge, too many new tests, too many new treatments. In *Chaos and Organization in Healthcare* (2009), James Mongan and I described how this flood of progress had been superimposed on a woefully unprepared, fragmented healthcare delivery system. The results were chaos, inefficiency, safety challenges, and disappointing quality. We argued that the solution to these challenges was better organization of the health delivery system, and we explored policies that might hasten the development of such organization.

When I began working on this book, I did not realize that it would in many ways be a "prequel" to that other work—that it would describe how the explosion in knowledge that was overwhelming the healthcare system had come to pass. My initial goal was simply to tell a good story and describe the life of a remarkable person.

This is the story of that person, Eugene Braunwald, whom I first met in 1979 when I came to Boston's Peter Bent Brigham Hospital for my internal medicine and cardiology training. Braunwald was chairman of the Department of Medicine during the first seventeen years of my career. I was never part of Braunwald's research teams, but I attended many of his teaching conferences and, from time to time, sought his advice on career decisions.

The advice that he gave was always good—thoughtful, savvy,

forward looking. He would tell me how he had always focused his career on trying to answer important questions (such as reducing mortality from myocardial infarction), and tried to ensure that his work was always connected to his big-picture goals. He said he had been fortunate to do his work at institutions that were on the upswing, and described some of the steps he had taken to make sure they progressed. I did not follow his advice in every instance, but I always thought very carefully before deviating from it. With my friends in academic medicine, I spent hours in conversation trying to analyze how he thought and how he had planned his career—wondering, in short, what made Braunwald Braunwald.

This book began with a chance 2009 conversation—described at the beginning of Chapter 13—during which I politely asked him how he was doing. He said that he was in the "Still Years," and made a self-effacing, slightly wistful joke about how many people seemed surprised that he was "still" so deeply engaged in education and research at the age of eighty. That comment opened a door for me, and I asked for his cooperation with a project that I had been contemplating for about twenty-five years: a description of the evolution of medicine in the past half-century as viewed through the lens of his life and career.

To my surprise and delight, he agreed. Over the next couple of years, we had two-hour interviews every two to four weeks. My research was supplemented by interviews with his friends and colleagues, most notably Burton Sobel, Donald Seldin, Jean Wilson, Jonathan Uhr, Joseph Goldstein, William Roberts, Milford Parker, Gerald Austen, Lawrence Cohn, Marshall Wolf, and Joseph Dorsey. I am extremely grateful to them for giving so generously of their time. (In this book, I sometimes describe conversations that include the words of people who are deceased. These quotes are all derived from my interviews with the other parties to the conversations.)

I am also indebted to Beverly Merz for her help with editing and organizing the manuscript. Hank Grasso, Barbara Harkins, and their colleagues in the Office of NIH History at the National Institutes of Health aided my work in numerous ways and provided photographs of Braunwald and his colleagues from their archives. Additional thanks go to Jerry and Sheridan Kassirer, who read excerpts of the manuscript and offered thoughtful comments and encouragement; to Alana Ju, my resourceful research assistant; to Laura Cushing-Kidney, my superb administrative assistant at Partners HealthCare System; and to Amanda Urban, who furnished wise advice on writing and publication strategies. Leigh Weiss and Anna Tarasova performed the brilliant social-network analysis of publications by Braunwald and other leading researchers that is described in the appendix. I am also grateful to my colleagues at Partners who have always believed that stepping back to consider broad perspectives was an important component of my "day job."

Finally, my deepest debt is to my wife, Soheyla Gharib, who has understood from the outset that the story of Eugene Braunwald and the emergence of modern medicine is hugely important, and that our shared intellectual lives would not be complete without its telling. She knows (better than me) the advances that have occurred in medicine during our careers, and sees in Braunwald's life a journey analogous to those of her parents, my parents, and other immigrants who came to America and sought safety and the opportunity to make some broader contribution. Her enthusiasm, love, and support made this book possible.

Eugene Braunwald and the Rise of
Modern Medicine

Introduction

The Window

One afternoon in 1965, Eugene Braunwald stood on the sidewalk of a quiet street in Vienna, one block off the Schottenring, the main thoroughfare in the city's First District. Looking up, he could see the windows of the living room on the second floor of Number 4 Zelinkagasse. He had lived in that spacious apartment with his parents and younger brother until 1938, when Germany had annexed Austria. Braunwald had been only eight years old that spring, but he could remember the crowds cheering the arrival of Nazi soldiers and then of Adolf Hitler himself. He remembered watching from those windows one night as his father had been forced onto a truck with other Jewish men from the neighborhood. And he remembered how his family had fled from their home soon thereafter, leaving all their possessions behind.

In the decades that followed that hasty departure, Braunwald would become a professor at Harvard Medical School and chairman of the Department of Medicine at Peter Bent Brigham Hospital in Boston. He would become the most prolific and arguably the most influential cardiology researcher in the world. He would visit Vienna for many medical meetings, but that day in 1965 marked the first time he returned to his boyhood home.

As Braunwald stood outside 4 Zelinkagasse, hundreds of cardiology researchers were gathered nearby at a medical research meeting. They all knew of Braunwald, who at age thirty-five was no longer the "boy wonder" of cardiology, but the key leader of cardiovascular research at the U.S. National Institutes of Health (NIH). At the conference, researchers pointed him out to one another and when he asked a question or made a comment, they sought meaning in every word. But no one recognized him as he stood on the street of his earliest memories.

Braunwald crossed that street, and knocked on the door. A middle-aged woman answered, and Braunwald explained that he had lived there long ago. Would she mind if he came in and looked around? She opened the door and let him in.

Braunwald was quiet as he walked around his boyhood home. Much had changed, of course, but the ceilings remained high and the woodwork elegant. Each room released a flood of memories. The dining room, in particular, held a trove of recollections: the long discussions about opera over dinner; the quick lunches when his father would dash home from their clothing business next door; and, in the spring of 1938, the SS officer who had sipped coffee at their dining table while dissolving the Braunwald family business.

Until that spring, Braunwald's family had been poised for the kind of progress measured in generations. Neither of his parents had gone to college, but their wholesale textile business was thriving. Because the Braunwald business was prominent, a correspondingly prominent SS officer had been sent to close it down and sell off the assets. In the midst of this business "liquidation," William Braunwald had been arrested one night, and his family had watched him being driven away, presumably to be taken to a work camp. Instead, he had been released the next day when his wife, Claire, made an ingenious argument to the SS officer overseeing the business liquidation.

After that narrow escape, Braunwald's parents knew that they had to leave Vienna, and do so as rapidly as possible. On July 30, 1938, they had packed some lunches as if they were all going on a picnic—this, in fact, is what his mother had told her two young sons. They had boarded a trolley, then a taxi, then a train, and eventually had crossed into Switzerland and made their way to London. After fifteen months in England and the start of World War II, they had arrived in New York City on the day after Thanksgiving, 1939.

Now, twenty-six years later, Braunwald was back in his boyhood home for the first time since that escape. He walked to the living-room window through which he had watched his father being taken away that night in the spring of 1938. He stood there in silence for several minutes, reflecting on all that had happened in the intervening years.

The last time Braunwald had been in this house, survival had been uncertain for him and his family. They had not known that they would make it out of Vienna and to the United States, or that young Eugene would become his family's first college graduate when he was nineteen, and a physician a few years after that. Medical schools had strict quotas limiting the number of Jewish enrollees at the time, and Braunwald would be the very last student admitted to New York University's medical school in his entrance year (1948)—but he would graduate at the top of his class.

At the age of thirty-one, he would become chief of cardiology at the National Heart Institute, the part of the NIH known today as the National Heart, Lung, and Blood Institute. He would play a critical role in research that helped reduce the death rate from heart attacks, from more than 30 percent to 5–8 percent. He would start a textbook, *Heart Disease,* which would quickly become the bible of cardiovascular medicine. And in 1995 the University of Vienna would invite him to come "home" to receive an honorary doctorate.

But the life of Eugene Braunwald is more than the tale of one individual. His story and those of some of his contemporaries call to mind the famous opening lines of Oscar Handlin's history *The Uprooted: The Epic Story of the Great Migrations That Made the*

American People. Like Braunwald, Handlin grew up in Brooklyn, and eventually became a Harvard professor. In his Pulitzer Prize-winning history, Handlin wrote: "Once I thought to write a history of the immigrants in America. Then I discovered that the immigrants *were* American history."[1]

Similarly, Braunwald's life and accomplishments are inextricably intertwined with the post–World War II history of medicine, and especially of cardiology. He was part of the wave of immigrants who injected energy and ambition into American academic medicine. His generation created a tremendous surge in knowledge through their research at the National Institutes of Health, and then at American medical schools and teaching hospitals. And they changed the way in which students and trainees learned medicine and the institutions through which healthcare was delivered.

The work of Braunwald and his contemporaries led to a new aggressiveness in medicine. At the beginning of Braunwald's era, patients with myocardial infarction would be put in a bed in a quiet room, and their physicians could only hope for the best. A few decades later, physicians would use drugs, devices, and operations to attack the heart attack itself. Similar revolutions occurred with diseases affecting other organs throughout the body.

Braunwald has often said that he was lucky to be in the right place at the right time with the right people, and this luck enabled him to make contributions to medical progress—but the fact is that, over six decades, he was *repeatedly* in the right place at the right time with the right people. He became interested in and worked on cardiovascular hemodynamics when he was a medical student in 1951, just as modern cardiac catheterization was being developed. He went to the National Heart Institute in 1955, when it was small enough for someone in his mid-twenties to be a creative force, discover new conditions, and describe principles of management of cardiovascular disorders that continue to guide treatment today. His research with colleagues on heart failure and myocardial infarction contributed to ongoing and remarkable progress—sometimes in small steps, sometimes in large ones.

If his judgment in picking the "right time" to work on a medical problem was impeccable, he was effective in making wherever he happened to be the "right place." He led the creation of a new and vibrant Department of Medicine at the University of California, San Diego, and then took an old one to greatness at Boston's Peter Bent Brigham Hospital. Over the decades, he adapted his approach to research. After starting his career in intimate laboratories with just a few colleagues, he saw that many big questions in medicine could be addressed only through big studies—often randomized trials involving tens of thousands of patients in multiple countries. In performing such research, he not only produced new information, but helped to shape the evolution of medicine's culture.

Eugene Braunwald would not claim credit for the explosion of knowledge that has characterized American medicine since World War II, or the changes in healthcare that have resulted. While he was a major force in cardiology research, thousands of others made important contributions to advances in his areas and the rest of medicine. Nonetheless, as a key leader of institutions with broad academic and patient care portfolios, and as a textbook author and editor, he was involved directly or indirectly in the work of colleagues who were advancing knowledge in almost every specialty.

Over six decades, he became a key participant, someone who was a driver of and witness to the evolution of medicine in his times. When he entered medicine, it was very much an art characterized by fatalism and focused on observation, diagnosis, and relief of symptoms. As his career progressed, medicine was becoming more of a scientific discipline imbued with optimism that diseases could be predicted and the future could be changed. Braunwald endured and learned difficult lessons from controversies that reflected medical research's growing pains. The "story lines" in which he was an important player include specific cardiovascular conditions (such as coronary artery disease, valvular heart disease, and heart failure), but also the nature of medical research, medical education, and healthcare delivery.

His life provides a window through which these histories can be viewed.

Flight from Europe

1929–1939

When Eugene Braunwald was born in Vienna, on August 15, 1929, it was one of the great cultural centers of the world. It had lost much of its political significance with the collapse of the Austro-Hungarian Empire in 1918, but the city was the home of important musicians, artists, and intellectuals, including Sigmund Freud (1856–1939), Karl Kraus (1874–1936), Arthur Schnitzler (1862–1931), and Robert Musil (1880–1942). A major reason for Vienna's vibrancy was that, for Jewish families like that of Eugene Braunwald, it was perhaps the most welcoming city in eastern Europe.

The family of Eugene Braunwald's father, William (né Wilhelm), had lived in Vienna for at least five generations—an extraordinary period of stability for a Jewish family in central Europe. It was long enough for William to consider himself "Viennese to the core." His son Eugene would later say, "He certainly felt that he was at home in Vienna—more than I ever felt at home anywhere." That feeling of comfort in Vienna would make the events of 1938 all the more painful for the Braunwald family.

Vienna had a long history of cycles of anti-Semitism; during better times, it served as a haven for Jewish refugees. In the fourteenth century, it was among the few European cities that did not blame the Jews for the Black Death epidemic (1348–1349), and the Judenplatz in the center of the city became the site of one of the largest synagogues in Europe. But during worse times, Jews were expelled from the city and their businesses and homes were seized. In 1420,

Duke Albrecht V initiated a wave of imprisonments and executions of Jews and destroyed the Judenplatz synagogue. The synagogue's stones were used to build the University of Vienna.

Just a few decades later, the Hapsburg emperors allowed Jews to return, and awarded them special protection. That led to a second round of immigration into the city—Jewish families fleeing pogroms and persecution in the east. In 1624, Rabbi Yom-Tov Lipmann Heller became the rabbi of Vienna, and won the right for Jews to establish a Jewish community in what is today the heart of the city.

In 1670, however, the Holy Roman Emperor Leopold I expelled Jews once again and destroyed their synagogues. The Jewish district of Vienna was renamed Leopoldstadt in his honor by the non-Jews who remained behind. This new round of expulsions was brief: because of the economic repercussions, the emperor invited wealthier Jews to return. Even after Jews returned to Vienna, the name Leopoldstadt persisted for the area (Vienna's Second District), where so many of them lived.

There were other periods during which anti-Semitism surged and waned, but a prolonged period of relative calm began in 1848—a period sometimes called the Jewish Renaissance of Vienna. Jews were granted civil rights, including full citizenship in 1867, and this brought another large influx of immigrants from the eastern part of the Austro-Hungarian Empire. Jewish immigrants from the east flocked to Leopoldstadt, in part because the Nordbahnhof train station was in such close proximity.

Encouraged by the atmosphere of economic, religious, and social freedom, Vienna's Jewish population grew from 6,200 in 1860 to 40,200 in 1870, and to 147,000 in 1900. In the 1920s, Leopoldstadt's population was 38.5 percent Jewish, and the district was nicknamed Mazzesinsel ("Matzoh Island").

By 1938, the Jewish population of Vienna had peaked at 185,000, and Jews had become increasingly central to the cultural and scientific life of Austria. The Salzburg Festival was directed by Max Reinhardt; the Vienna Opera was conducted by Bruno Walter; two of the most popular writers in the German language were Stefan Zweig and Franz Werfel; and in 1929 Elias Canetti was giving up chemistry and starting to write the works that would win the 1981 Nobel Prize in Literature. Two of the three Austrians who won the Nobel Prize in Physiology or Medicine in the 1930s were Jewish: Karl Landsteiner and Otto Loewi. Half of the practicing physicians and medical faculty at the University of Vienna were Jewish. The first Jewish museum in the world was founded in Vienna in 1895, and several important synagogues were built in the district.

Then, in 1938, came the *Anschluss*—the annexation of Austria by Nazi Germany. None of those museums, synagogues, or other Jewish institutions survived the *Kristallnacht* pogroms of November 1938. After *Kristallnacht,* the Jewish population was increasingly isolated and terrorized, and was ultimately deported to concentration camps. Only about 800 survived the war in hiding in Vienna. The once-vibrant Viennese Jewish life came to an end.

~

Prior to that period of tragedy, during the rapid growth of Vienna's Jewish community in the nineteenth century, the ancestors of William Braunwald arrived in the city from somewhere in eastern Europe. William's father, Samuel, worked in the textile business, but the family was poor. William did not complete his high-school education; he took a job as a runner at the Vienna Stock Exchange. Eventually, he, too, joined the textile business, buying fabric from factories, then preparing it for sale to merchants. He started his own wholesale business and became quite successful, even wealthy. But his circumstances were still quite limited when he met and married a young Jewish woman named Claire (née Klara) Wallach.

Claire had been born in 1905 in Podvolochiska, a small village in a mountainous area that throughout history shifted back and forth between Poland and Ukraine. Before World War I, Podvolochiska was part of the Austrian Empire; between the wars, it was part of Poland; after World War II, it became part of the Soviet Union; today it is part of Ukraine.

Podvolochiska was an unstable home for Jewish families, and the threat of a pogrom forced Claire Wallach's family to flee in 1917. Her father, Isaac, had had a series of strokes at an early age, so when they left Podvolochiska, his family laid him amid their possessions in the back of a wagon pulled by a mule. Claire and the rest of the family walked the 440 miles to Vienna behind the wagon. She was twelve years old, the youngest of the family's six children who survived infancy.

Life in Vienna may have been safer for the Wallach family, but it was not easy and was far from happy. Isaac Wallach died shortly after they arrived, and the family struggled to survive financially. Claire received very little education, a lack that would remain a source of deep regret throughout her life.

The combination of intellectual appetite and limited economic circumstances brought Claire together with her future husband, then an apprentice in the textile business. "Somehow," Eugene Braunwald would comment later, "these two uneducated people with no culture in their homes, totally independently, had become opera buffs." Neither could afford to buy tickets for seats, but for a minimal fee they could get into the standing-room area of the Vienna State Opera.

William Braunwald would later tell Eugene how they noticed each other there at several performances. "When my father would tell this story, he would describe how he finally got the nerve to ask this beautiful girl out for a cup of coffee," Eugene Braunwald recalled. "Then my father would point to me and say, 'This is the result.'"

William and Claire married, and William's business began to take off. By the 1930s, the family was living in a spacious thirteen-room apartment on the second floor of 4 Zelinkagasse. They had initially lived in Vienna's Fourth District, but when Eugene's brother, Jack (né Hans), was born, they moved to these larger quarters in the old city of Vienna, just over a mile from the opera and close to other sites of cultural activity in the First District. William's business was right next door, so he would frequently come home for lunch. Claire often sent young Eugene to bring a cup of tea to his father. The family had two meals together every day, and Braunwald remembers long conversations about history, economics, politics, and music.

William and Claire were determined that their two children would have the education they themselves had been denied, as well as opportunities to appreciate music. They began taking Eugene to the opera when he was just six or seven. "I was the apple of their eye," he recalls. "I felt totally secure. I had private piano lessons, I had an English tutor, and I went to a very good school. . . . My mother would take me to the park, and I would be in my 'Lord Fauntleroy' outfit, including the white gloves. The University of Vienna was just two or three blocks away. We would take a walk, and she would point to the university and say, 'You are going to be a professor here.'"

The first signs of the trouble that lay ahead came in July 1934, when a band of Austrian Nazis disguised as policemen assassinated the Austrian chancellor, Engelbert Dollfuss. Dollfuss had outlawed the Nazi Party in 1933, and subsequently the Communist Party as well, in an effort to consolidate his own power. The assas-

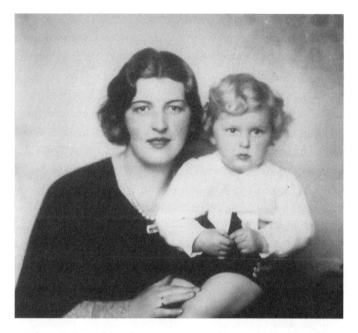

1. Claire Braunwald and young Eugene. *Photo courtesy of Eugene Braunwald.*

sination was part of a failed coup d'état, after which the Austrian Nazi Party went further underground. But Dollfuss himself had begun a drive toward authoritarianism in Austria, and this aided Hitler's move to unite all German-speaking people into a "Greater Germany."

Braunwald's years of innocence ended abruptly with the *Anschluss,* in March 1938. Of the 120,000 people living in Linz, almost 100,000 turned out to greet Hitler. The crowd that cheered his arrival in Vienna was just as enthusiastic. Theodor Cardinal Innitzer, the archbishop of Vienna, along with other Catholic leaders, signed a declaration endorsing the *Anschluss;* on Hitler's birthday, in April 1938, Innitzer ordered all the Catholic churches in the city to fly the Nazi flag and ring their bells.

In the weeks that followed, Jews were harassed and beaten, and sometimes forced to scrub the sidewalks with toothbrushes. Jews' apartments were pillaged, and their businesses seized. In May 1938, the Nazis enacted the Nuremberg Race Laws, and Jews lost nearly all of their civil liberties. They were unable to attend university, were excluded from most professions, and were forced to wear yellow badges.

Even Germans were shocked by the viciousness of attacks on Jews in Austria. The screenwriter Carl Zuckmayer, who had moved to Vienna in 1936 to escape Hitler, described it in those early days as a city transformed "into a nightmare painting of Hieronymus Bosch. . . . What was unleashed upon Vienna had nothing to do with seizure of power in Germany. . . . What was unleashed upon Vienna was a torrent of envy, jealousy, bitterness, blind, malignant craving for revenge."[1]

"It was idyllic, it was idyllic—and then it was awful," Braunwald said of his life as a young boy during this transition. "I don't consider myself a child of the Holocaust. I consider myself a child of a dreadful annexation of a country with extreme discrimination— someone who came very close to the cliff but did not go over. I never missed a meal throughout the whole period. I was very, very lucky.

"But it was dreadful. My parents were frightened. Within three days, I couldn't go back to school. I remember crying to my mother, 'But I love school, and my teacher likes me, and my friends are there! Why can't I go to school?' Both of them tried to explain something that was impossible to explain to a child.

"Within a few days of the annexation, there were signs on park benches banning use by Jews. My parents were whispering to each other. They were no longer going to the opera or the symphony. There were meetings with my mother's siblings. One uncle ended up in a concentration camp and died. But of a larger family of about thirty people, he was the only one."

William Braunwald's successful business made him a special target in the weeks after the Nazis took control of Vienna. Jewish businesses were liquidated under the oversight of appointed government officers, who would receive a large proportion (as much as half) of the proceeds. Braunwald's business was of such value that it was given as a prize to a prominent SS officer named Pavlik. Braunwald's recollection was that this SS officer had been one of the Austrian Nazi members of SS Regiment 89 who had assassinated Chancellor Dollfuss.

Young Eugene got to know Pavlik because the officer would frequently come to the apartment, where Claire served him lunch or coffee. Pavlik was cold and businesslike, but always polite. He wanted the breakup of the Braunwald business to be rapid and complete, but also to yield as great a financial return as possible.

That business liquidation was interrupted in mid-May 1938, with the arrest of Braunwald's father, William, who was just thirty-four years old at the time. Braunwald later recalled the event as beginning with "the proverbial knock on the door in the middle of the night."[2] Braunwald's parents awakened their two boys at around 3:00 A.M., and Braunwald remembered that his mother was hysterical. "They're taking your father away!" she screamed. William had only a few minutes to get dressed, hug his wife and sons, and say goodbye. Eugene's recollection was that he was remarkably stoic, though deathly pale. The family ran to a window of their second-floor living room, and looked down to see him being loaded onto an open truck with fifteen to twenty other men. They were other Jewish men from the neighborhood who were likewise being arrested and taken to the railroad station.

Eugene, his brother, and their mother knew what this meant. They wept through the rest of the night, fearing and expecting the worst. In the morning, Pavlik arrived as usual and saw that William was missing. "Where is the Jew?" he asked. Claire reported that he had been taken away, presumably to be sent to a work camp. The SS officer shrugged and said, "It was bound to happen sooner or later." And then he sat down to read the newspaper, as he had on every other day, drinking the coffee that Claire had prepared.

Next came a moment that Eugene and his mother were to review again and again in the years that followed—a moment that he would later say taught him just how resourceful people under enormous pressure can be. His mother told Pavlik that the arrest was a tragedy for the family, but a problem for him as well. After all, she pointed out, William was the only person who fully understood the business, and now no one would really know how to sell it off. The SS officer would receive just a fraction of its value.

Pavlik paused; the argument made sense. He got on the phone and called an officer at the train depot where William had been taken. He was told that it was too late—William was already on the train. The telephone conversation became a power struggle in which the SS officer threatened his counterpart. Braunwald later recalled, "My mother only overheard Pavlik's side of this conversation, in which he pulled rank on the officer at the depot, saying, 'I don't care if you are a full colonel in the German army—I am a captain in the SS, and I want this Jew returned!'" Pavlik then slammed down the phone and stomped out of the Braunwald home. A short while later a taxi arrived, and William staggered out, shaken but safe.

"It's incredible what life can hinge on," Eugene Braunwald said later when reflecting on this incident. "He had been gone for only eight hours, but it was a very close call. If my mother had not acted at that moment, none of our family would have survived."[3]

After that narrow escape, William knew that they had to leave Vienna and that time was short. He had begun preparations for an escape immediately after the occupation began, but after his brief arrest he accelerated his efforts. He had had several opportunities to leave Vienna alone, with contingency plans to bring the rest of the family along later, but he refused to allow the family to be separated. The family had to stay together, even though doing so made the plans much more complex.

~

On the morning of July 30, 1938, a Saturday, William and Claire told Eugene and his brother, Jack, that they were all going on a picnic. "That seemed quite strange to me," Eugene would recall in later years, "given what our life had become." At that point, the children had ceased attending school and were no longer allowed to play outdoors.

They set out for the "picnic" with only a few sandwiches and a thermos of tea. They took a trolley, then a taxi, and boarded a train. Braunwald believed that his father bribed a conductor or some official, so as to make crossing the border into Switzerland possible. Two days after they departed, with no possessions, they reached London.

"We arrived in England exhausted and frightened," Braunwald recalled. "I was the only English-speaking member of our family, because I had had a tutor in English. So I was the interpreter. It made me feel pretty good that I could help." Eugene was not yet nine years old.

The Jewish Relief Agency took the Braunwald family to a small apartment. Braunwald remembered the family's gratitude that they had escaped, but also their anxiety about what might happen next. The agency had provided a warm welcome, however. They had arranged English lessons for the family, as well as jobs for Braunwald's parents that began the following week: William and Claire would be wrapping packages in Selfridges Department Store, on London's Oxford Street. ("Every time I'm in London and pass by that store, I think of my parents working in the basement," Braunwald would later say.)

In the months that followed, other members of the family escaped and came to London. William's father and brother arrived (his mother had died long before). So did Eugene's maternal grandmother and other relatives from Claire's side of the family. They all stayed together in a large apartment in the Golders Green area of London. Eugene and Jack were immersed in family. Their grandfather often took them to a nearby park; he taught them how to make a kite and fly it.

William and Claire never stopped worrying about their sons' educations, and were delighted when the Jewish Relief Agency found a spot for Eugene at a boarding school about fifty miles away. It was in Hove, near Brighton, on the southern coast of England. The family thought it was a chance for him to get an excellent English education. But it was a difficult adjustment for a nine-year-old so recently displaced from his home. Eugene was desperately unhappy at being separated from his family, and refused to behave. In an era when corporal punishment was routine, he was frequently caned by the headmaster. When he returned home for vacation, his parents were shocked to see his bruises and the amount of weight he had lost.

By the end of the school year, though, he had adjusted to his new setting. He had made friends, regained the lost weight, and was earning excellent grades: "I was one of the boys." He rejoined his parents for the summer, but was looking forward to returning to school in the fall.

That was not to be. On September 1, 1939, the Nazis invaded Poland, and Great Britain declared war on Germany two days later. British authorities immediately launched Operation Pied Piper, aimed at evacuating young children from London to the countryside. More than half a million schoolchildren were moved to rural areas within a few days.[4]

Jack was only five years old, and his parents felt that he could not go to the countryside alone. So instead of returning to Hove, ten-year-old Eugene was sent on Operation Pied Piper with his brother. Both were issued gas masks and put on a train out of London. No one knew where they were actually going, not even the adults supervising and accompanying the dozens of London children. William and Claire gave Eugene a postcard addressed to them, with instructions to mail it with information on their new home once the two boys were settled somewhere.

The Braunwald brothers and forty to fifty other children boarded a train for Northampton, located about seventy miles north of London in what was then a rural part of England. There, the children were divided into smaller groups and were taken by bus to small villages in the countryside. The group that included Eugene and Jack were deposited at a local church, and then waited until they were picked up by the families that had volunteered to take them in.

Somehow, all of the children were matched with families—except Eugene and Jack. "Nobody picked us up," he later recalled. "I don't know if we looked strange or talked strange. Anyway, this was all voluntary." All of the adults had departed, and for about an hour the two boys were alone. Young Eugene was panic-stricken. "I had been charged by my parents [to look after Jack]. 'He's your responsibility. That's why you are going with him—that's why you're not going back to Hove,' they had said. I was very scared. I looked around, wondering, 'What am I going to do? Are we going to sleep in the church?' There wasn't any food."

Finally, an English family, the Whites, appeared, and took Eugene and Jack home to their farm. There were three White brothers, all of whom were in their teens. "They were wonderful to us," Braunwald recalled with gratitude.

Thus, in the fall of 1939, William and Claire were working in London and their two children were safely in the countryside about seventy miles away. But German bombs were just one of the threats the elder Braunwalds faced. The clock was ticking. Like other European refugees, they were welcomed in Britain but were given only eighteen months to find another country that would take them.

William had begun planning for this next step from the moment his family arrived in England. He knew that Australia was the only place his family could go without help—without someone to "sign" for them and guarantee that they would not become a burden to society. William and Claire began saving immediately, and eventually had enough funds to buy tickets for the family to sail to Melbourne. The other members of the extended family were making their own plans, and the clan seemed about to scatter.

But only a few weeks before the Braunwalds were due to leave for Australia, they heard from an aunt in New York on Claire's father's side of the family. The aunt had never met any of the family, and had very modest means herself. Nevertheless, she agreed to sponsor the Braunwalds as immigrants to the United States. Ultimately, she sponsored about twenty members of the extended family, most of whom settled within a few blocks of one another in Brooklyn.

In the English countryside, Eugene and Jack received a telegram from their parents. "It said, 'We're going to America,'" Braunwald remembered. "'Take the train' (and it gave us the train number) 'from Northampton, and then change to another train in Leeds, and that train arrives in London at this time. We will pick you up with joy!'"

Eugene and Jack made the journey and were reunited with their parents in London. Five days later, on November 15, 1939, they were aboard the steamship *President Harding*, leaving Southampton for America.

There was already a great deal of U-boat activity in the North

Atlantic in November 1939, and even though the United States was officially neutral, the Germans were well aware that the country was sending arms and other materials to England. Numerous ships with passengers had been attacked. Braunwald remembers a gigantic American flag ("Huge—about three stories high!") fluttering in the wind at the ship's stern, with lights shining on it at night. The crew wanted U-boat captains to know that this was an American ship.

The family was huddled in one cabin in the lowest passenger class—"the bottom of the barrel," as Braunwald described it. But "we were all so excited, because we never dreamt that after all the bad things that happened to us in Vienna, we might be able to get to America." On November 23, 1939, Thanksgiving Day, the crew served turkey to all of the passengers. Dessert was something Eugene and Jack had never experienced before: ice cream, served in small Dixie cups. The next day, the ship arrived in New York, sailing past the Statue of Liberty.

There was a tremendous commotion at the wharf, where Eugene and his family were met by his "good Uncle Joe and wonderful Aunt Rose." Rose had had to convince Uncle Joe to sign for the Braunwalds, since women were not allowed to sign for anything in those days. (Joe Richberg of 1325 Lincoln Place in Brooklyn was identified as the sponsoring relative for the Braunwalds, on the Manifest of Alien Passengers for the U.S. Immigrant Inspector.) The Richbergs rented a small house for the Braunwalds near their own modest home, on a long boulevard that cut through their city. The Braunwalds' new address was 892 Eastern Parkway, Brooklyn, New York.

~

The Braunwald family's escape and journey were extraordinary—but not unique. Take, for example, the parallel saga of Erik Kandel, who was born in Vienna three months after Braunwald, and who would later win the Nobel Prize for his research on learning and memory. Kandel's parents came from the same area of Ukraine that Claire did; they, too, had been driven out by pogroms, and they lived near their toy store just over a mile from the Braunwald home on Zelinkagasse. Halfway between lived Sigmund Freud and his family. All three families were forced to flee Vienna, and Kandel's and Braunwald's would settle only about three miles apart in Brooklyn.[5] Braunwald and Kandel would go to different high schools, but both would spend time at New York University, the NIH, and Harvard. Even though they were taking such similar journeys, they never really met until 2012. During their early years, they were too busy trying to get an education, like so many other war refugees who passed through Ukraine, Vienna, London—and, later, New York, Bethesda, and Boston.

: 2 :

An American Education

1939–1948

In the fall of 1939, Brooklyn was a destination that was obvious and ideal for families like the Braunwalds. Brooklyn comprised nearly 2.7 million people in 1940—more than double the number who had lived there in 1900 and more than fourfold the number of residents (600,000) in 1880. One reason for Brooklyn's rapid growth during this era was the opening of the Brooklyn Bridge in 1883, which allowed access to Manhattan without use of a boat. Shortly thereafter, Brooklyn joined the other four boroughs to form the modern New York City. Then, as now, Brooklyn had a good deal of open space and was relatively affordable. As described by Ilana Abramovitch and Sean Galvin in *Jews of Brooklyn*, it was "the flavorful, even pungent, working-class entity lying next to its slimmer, more cosmopolitan urban partner, Manhattan."[1]

Brooklyn became the destination for many immigrants—albeit not the final destination. Families like the Braunwalds passed through Brooklyn on their way to somewhere else. Sociologists estimate that "as many as a quarter of all Americans can trace their ancestry to people who once lived in its eighty-one square miles."[2] Abramovitch and Galvin wrote, "Brooklyn is the funnel through which much of the U.S. immigrant world has whirled."[3]

Like the Braunwalds, many of these immigrants were Jewish. During the late nineteenth century and early twentieth century, political turmoil and anti-Semitism forced hundreds of thousands of Jews out of the cities of Russia and other eastern European countries—and many made their way to Brooklyn. Brooklyn's Jewish population grew from 100,000 in 1905 to more than 800,000 in 1930. At this point, a third of Brooklyn's population was Jewish, and nearly half of all Jews in New York City lived in the borough.[4] Brooklyn became one of the great shipping and manufacturing centers of the world, with countless sweatshops filled with immigrants working at sewing machines.

Jewish immigrants settled in neighborhoods like Brownsville, Flatbush, Williamsburg, Borough Park, and Crown Heights.[5] The culture of the Jewish community in Brooklyn during this period became celebrated in literature. Chaim Potok, a rabbi who lived in Brooklyn, wrote the novel *The Chosen,* about two Jewish boys growing up in the Williamsburg section of Brooklyn. And William Styron set *Sophie's Choice* in Flatbush during the summer of 1947. Parents usually took any job they could find, while their children started down the academic paths that would make them leaders in business, law, the arts, medicine, and science.[6]

But to the Braunwalds, the early years of their life in New York did not seem like chapters from a novel—they had no time to waste, and no margin for error in the decisions they made. After arriving in Brooklyn in 1939, William set to work immediately, peddling neckties door to door. Eugene was promptly enrolled in a public school about a block from their new home on Eastern Parkway.

Once again, he was an outsider, the only refugee child in his class. He spoke English, but he had picked up a British accent during their year in England. An American friend of his mother said to him, "You must always keep talking like this. It's a pleasure to hear you speak with your English accent. It's terrific." Young Braunwald answered, "Well, I don't want to speak that way. I don't want to be different. I want to speak like everyone else as quickly as possible."

Braunwald did adapt rapidly, and graduated first in his eighth-

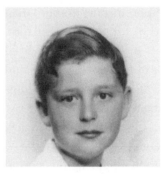

2. Eugene Braunwald, age ten. *Photo courtesy of Eugene Braunwald.*

grade class in 1943. He passed the demanding entrance examination required for admission to Brooklyn Technical High School, an elite public school specializing in engineering, mathematics, and science. Like Stuyvesant High School and Bronx High School of Science, Brooklyn Tech has been an entryway to academia, wealth, and fame for generations of brilliant New Yorkers, including many immigrants. Among its alumni are two Nobel Laureates: George Wald (Physiology or Medicine, 1967), the son of Jewish immigrants from Austria and Germany, and Arno A. Penzias (Physics, 1978), who, like Braunwald, was evacuated from London in 1939 and subsequently came to the United States with his parents. Braunwald entered "Tech" at age fourteen, at the height of World War II, when great cultural value was placed on electronics, mechanical engineering, and "hard" science. He assumed that he would become an engineer, and began studying electrical circuits, electronics, and hydraulics.

He was also to benefit from his status as the youngest of the "Four Eugenes." Claire Braunwald had reunited in Brooklyn with her siblings, three of whom had named their firstborn sons Eugene in tribute to their late father. Eugene Braunwald was constantly urged to follow the example set by his older cousins.

"I think there was a sense of competition among the siblings as to whose Eugene was the best," Braunwald commented. "I remember when the first Eugene got his Master's degree from Columbia, my mother said, 'We must go to the graduation.' The message was clear. They were setting an example for me."

The first Eugene, Eugene Reed, won some of the highest honors in electrical engineering for his work at Bell Labs, including election to the National Academy of Engineering (a division of the National Academy of Sciences) and Fellowship in the Institute of Electrical and Electronic Engineers. The second, Eugene Kleiner, was the founder of the legendary Silicon Valley venture capital firm Kleiner Perkins (now Kleiner, Perkins, Caulfield, and Byers), an early investor in hundreds of information technology and biotech firms, including Amazon, AOL, Genentech, Google, and Sun Microsystems.[7] The third, Eugene Wallach, enjoyed a successful career in real estate in New York.

The three elder Eugenes provided important role models and advice to their young cousin when Eugene Braunwald was growing up in the 1940s. "We were all living within a few blocks, and I was very much influenced by them," he later recalled. "They were like older brothers."

During Braunwald's second year at Brooklyn Tech, his mother and Eugene Kleiner helped him make two major decisions that would send him toward medicine and ensure that he would be the youngest person in his academic settings for years to come. Braunwald had always been an outstanding student, but he had difficulty with some of the drafting and shop courses that were considered essential to becoming an engineer. "I was no good in any manual activity. My mother was watching me struggle, and I was getting grades like B's. And she said, 'You are not a B. Maybe you should consider medicine.'"

He did not know much about medicine, and knew only one physician—a general practitioner with an office near the Braunwald home (Eugene occasionally did babysitting for the family). "But I did know that medicine was considered to be a noble pro-

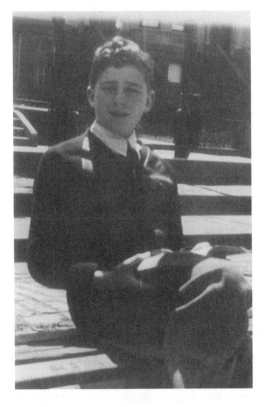

3. Eugene Braunwald, age fourteen. *Photo courtesy of Eugene Braunwald.*

fession, even though the emphasis was on engineering at that time. To be a physician was considered to be near the apex of the pyramid." Braunwald was attracted and intrigued by the prospect of becoming a doctor.

William had another idea. He was steadily rebuilding his career in textiles, and wanted his oldest son to join him in the family business. "We would be a dynamo," he told his son. Yet William understood when Eugene said he was more interested in medicine.

Still, Eugene was concerned about the length of time it would take to get a medical degree—four years of college and four years of medical school. And time seemed a luxury that the family could not afford. His cousin Eugene Kleiner offered a suggestion.

Kleiner had just returned to Brooklyn from duty in the U.S. Army. He had suffered an injury that was not major, but serious enough to lead to his discharge, and he was eager to get on with his life. He had not yet graduated from high school. "So he went to a private school that was basically a diploma mill," Braunwald recalled. "It was approved by the state, but it was in a factory building, and it really was a diploma factory."

Kleiner had gone to Boro Hall Academy in downtown Brooklyn, and had completed the coursework for two years of high school in one semester, passing the courses and exam necessary to receive a New York State Regents diploma. Using this approach, Kleiner short-tracked his way to a high-school diploma, and then began his undergraduate work at Polytechnic University of New York, in Brooklyn.

Kleiner took note of his young cousin's uncertainty and impatience. "Why don't you do this, too?" Kleiner said to Eugene. "You shouldn't waste any more time at Brooklyn Tech. Do what I did. Hold your breath, and jump in. You have more time than I had—you can do it in the summer and fall. That's a piece of cake, compared to what I did."

Following Kleiner's advice, Braunwald left elite Brooklyn Tech and enrolled at Boro Hall Academy in the summer of 1945, taking courses that made him eligible for a Regents diploma. He passed his exams that winter, and in February 1946 started college at New York University. He was sixteen years old.

The decision to go to NYU was simple for Braunwald. The family did not have the means to enable him to leave New York for college, and although Brooklyn College and City College of New York were financially accessible, it would be very difficult to get into medical school with a diploma from those institutions. NYU, in contrast, had an excellent medical school, and if admitted, he could save money by continuing to live at home. The financial challenge of college eased considerably after the first semester: he maintained a straight-A average and won a full-tuition scholarship.

Braunwald would have been young for a college student in any era—but in 1946, NYU and other U.S. schools were flooded with veterans like Eugene Kleiner who were returning from the service. These veterans were eager to acquire the training and credentials for the next phase of their lives. As focused as these mature veterans in their twenties were, the teenage Braunwald was just as determined to succeed.

He knew that the odds were stacked against him. He realized that medical schools had quotas that would make it more difficult for Jews to gain admission, and that preference would be given to veterans. He was attending a good college, but not a great one. He felt that he *had* to achieve a straight-A average. Any grade below an A would likely mean the end of his dreams of becoming a physician.

The high stakes made Braunwald's college years dismal much of the time. "I think I did all the things we wouldn't want to see in a college student we were interviewing for medical school today. I was at school or studying about a hundred hours per week, and the whole time I was thinking that I had to get straight-A's. I was thinking about which courses to take, which professors made it more likely that I'd get an A. I was living at home, taking the subway to and from school. My only escape from schoolwork was listening to music.

"So, basically, I didn't have a college experience—until I met Nina."

∼

Nina Starr was in Braunwald's organic chemistry class, a young woman who already had clear and unusual plans by the time they met. She had grown up in Flatbush, the daughter of a Brooklyn physician, and she was determined to be a surgeon. She had always had excellent manual dexterity, and she wanted to put that talent to good use.

As was true with William and Claire, music played a critical role in bringing Eugene and his future wife together. He had taken piano lessons all through high school, including the months when he was laboring under a heavy courseload at Boro Hall Academy, and during his first year or two as an undergraduate at NYU. But he finally gave up playing because he had his own talents in perspective. "I loved beautiful music, and tried so hard to make it, but it just wouldn't come out. I could understand it; I studied it; but I couldn't do it well. It was another manual activity that I was not good at."

Nevertheless—in New York, as in Vienna—a love of classical music and opera was central to the Braunwalds' lives. "I don't know how my father did it, but somehow he managed to get tickets to the Met year after year." Eugene managed to get even closer to the performances while a student at NYU. He would occasionally work as an extra—earning a dollar a night as a spear carrier in productions of *Aida,* for example. Being on the stage of the Metropolitan Opera during a grand production was an unforgettable experience for him, and he gave it up only when his schedule made such extracurricular activities impossible.

The other focal points for his New York cultural life were the concerts of Arturo Toscanini, who was widely recognized as the greatest conductor of his time. "There was nobody close to him," Braunwald believed. "He was such a superstar that NBC created an orchestra for him, and they played a concert each week in the famous NBC Studio 8H. Since it was a broadcast, they were not allowed by law to charge admission.

"To me, it was like opening a door to heaven. Through high

school, college, and maybe a year or two of medical school, I was there, getting in line a couple of hours early, bringing my books with me, sitting on the floor and doing my homework. I was oblivious to everything else. I didn't lose any time—just the subway ride, and I was working on the subway. And I'd sit in the first row for Toscanini concerts, and the orchestra was major league."

Braunwald estimated that he attended nearly a hundred Toscanini concerts over a six-year period. One of them was his first date with Nina Starr, which occurred at the end of 1946. "She was also interested in music. So I asked if she would like to come on Sunday afternoon to a Toscanini concert. She said, 'Oh, wow!' So I took her, and she had no idea that it was free. I said that we would just have to wait outside a little bit. It was open seating. The performance was Beethoven's Seventh Symphony. She thought I was a big spender, and it was much later before I told her that it was free. But she was so impressed—she was being taken on a date by a serious person!"

Eugene and Nina began dating. They were both determined and highly motivated students who did very well as undergraduates. Nina was accepted to NYU School of Medicine in March 1948, but Eugene initially did not receive any acceptances, despite achieving the straight-A's he had sought. The ensuing weeks were agony, but on May 1, 1948, he was accepted to NYU from the waiting list—the last student to be admitted to that entering class. "It felt like an incredible load had been taken off my back. Starting May 1, I could begin to learn, and I didn't care what my grades were."

That summer, he got a job as an attendant at Brooklyn State Hospital, a psychiatric hospital close to his home. He realized that he did not want to be a psychiatrist, but it was nevertheless an exhilarating time for him. A long, difficult phase had come to an end. During his first two years of high school, he had been plagued

by the thought that he was perhaps embarking on the wrong career. Then he had spent eight months at Boro Hall Academy,
which was hardly a true school environment. And then, having
chosen medicine, he had been unsure of whether he would be able
to get into medical school, despite a perfect academic record.
"Given the experiences we had in Vienna, it wasn't difficult for me
to accept that I had to work extremely hard. But when you put the
whole thing together, I didn't really have a childhood. There was
no chance to be carefree.

"On many Saturdays, while going to high school, college, and
medical school, I would not shave, not go out at all. I had an elec-
tric alarm clock. So after breakfast on Saturday morning, I would
turn that alarm clock to 12:00—and every time I would leave the
room, whether it was to eat lunch or dinner, I would stop that
clock. And I didn't stop studying until I had a cumulative thirteen
hours of work that day.

"My parents would be modestly upset with me. They would call
to me, 'Your aunt and uncle and your cousins are here!' And I
would say, 'Well, okay.' I certainly loved them and I wanted to see
them. I'd come downstairs, and be polite for about seven or eight
minutes. But then I would get back to work. Sunday afternoons
were for the Toscanini concerts."

Asked whether he had been confident in his abilities during
that period of high school and college, he said, "I was much more
confident in my abilities than I was in my future."

: 3 :

Medical Education and Training

1948–1952

Just as it was no accident that the family of Eugene Braunwald landed in Brooklyn in 1939, it was no accident that he enrolled at New York University School of Medicine nine years later. For a young Jewish immigrant in New York City who could not afford to leave the region, there were virtually no medical-school options besides NYU. And even that option was barely available to Eugene in 1948.

Jews had been accepted in increasing numbers to medical schools in New York and other American cities from 1880 to 1925, but a backlash against the rise in Jewish applicants developed in the 1920s. About two million Russian Jews had immigrated to the United States between 1880 and the beginning of the First World War, joining about 400,000 Jews already in this country.[1] That wave of immigration was followed by an increase in Jewish applicants to medical schools in the 1920s and 1930s. This surge occurred in the context of jingoistic, anti-Bolshevik, and ethnically biased reactions in the United States including the growth of the Ku Klux Klan and overt anti-Semitism.

New York City was the place where the backlash against Jewish applicants to medical school was most obvious and most intense. It had the greatest concentration of Jews in the country, and the greatest number of Jewish applicants to medical school. At Columbia's College of Physicians and Surgeons, enrollment of Jewish students dropped from 47 percent of the class in 1920 to 6 percent in 1940; at Cornell University College of Medicine, also in New

York City, it fell from 40 percent to 5 percent. By the 1940s, three out of four non-Jewish students were being accepted, compared with one out of thirteen Jewish students.[2]

Admissions officers generally denied that quotas were being used, but evidence of explicit and de facto quotas abounds. A 1949 survey of thirty-nine U.S. medical-school application forms showed that all asked for the applicant's religion, ten asked for the religion of the applicants' parents, and eleven asked if the family name had ever been changed.[3] The interview process was also used to identify applicants who might be masking their origins.

In 1951, Dr. Howard Wilson of the Carnegie Endowment was commissioned by the New York State Board of Regents to study anti-Jewish discrimination in medical admissions. His report provided statistical evidence of systematic discrimination against both Catholics and Jews, especially the children of recent Jewish immigrants. Wilson found that in 1950, 41 percent of applicants to New York medical schools were Jewish, 37 percent were Catholic, and 22 percent were Protestant. As shown in Table 1, the overall acceptance rates were 15 percent for Protestants, versus 8 percent for Catholics and 9 percent for Jews.

Wilson used some rudimentary statistics to adjust for differences in the applicant pool. He translated grade point averages into a scale with a mean of 500 and a standard deviation of 100, and found the following median academic achievement scores for the various religious groupings:

Catholic: 496
Jewish: 589
Protestant: 520

Nevertheless, only two institutions had higher rates of acceptance for Jews than for Protestants: NYU and the State University of New York at New York City. These two medical schools accounted

TABLE 1.

ACCEPTANCES TO NEW YORK MEDICAL SCHOOLS, 1950, BY RELIGION.

School	Total number of applications				Number of applications accepted				Percentage of applications accepted			
	All	Catholic	Jewish	Protestant	All	Catholic	Jewish	Protestant	All	Catholic	Jewish	Protestant
Albany	386	129	179	74	36	9	10	16	9.3	7.0	5.6	21.6
Buffalo	232	82	104	45	19	11	4	4	8.2	13.4	3.8	8.9
Columbia	407	123	199	78	25	5	10	9	6.2	4.1	5.0	11.5
Cornell	461	142	214	98	33	8	6	18	7.1	5.6	2.8	18.4
NY Med	607	227	293	82	43	20	11	12	7.1	8.8	3.8	14.6
NYU	516	154	283	71	65	11	45	7	12.6	7.1	15.9	9.9
Rochester	282	74	133	73	16	4	3	9	5.7	5.4	2.3	12.3
SUNY NYC	573	190	307	69	110	29	74	5	19.2	15.3	24.1	7.2
SUNY Syracuse	454	150	212	87	45	5	16	24	9.9	3.3	7.5	27.6
Totals	3918	1271	1924	677	392	102	179	104	10.0	8.1	9.3	15.4

Source: Howard E. Wilson et al., *A Study of Policies, Procedures, and Practices in Admissions to Medical Schools in New York State* (Albany: University of the State of New York, 1952), p. 25.

for two-thirds of the Jewish applicants accepted to medical schools in New York (119 out of 179, or 66 percent).

Wilson's conclusion: "The data show that at each level of academic achievement below the top level a larger proportion of Protestant applicants is accepted for admission than of Catholic or Jewish applicants, and that the Catholic applicants are accepted in greater proportion than Jewish applicants." He did note that one institution seemed to admit students without any suggestion of religious bias:

> The New York University Medical [School] record indicates close adherence to academic criteria, with virtually all top-level candidates accepted and almost no acceptances from the lowest academic categories. It tended to admit Catholics, Jews, and Protestants at each level of academic achievement in substantially the same proportions as they applied. . . . So far as these data indicate, only at New York University Medical were applicants selected in 1950 in such a way that, at each level of academic achievement, approximately the same proportion of applicants in each of the three religious groupings was selected for admission.[4]

If NYU was different from other medical schools, one reason was the influence of John Wyckoff, MD, a cardiologist who had been dean from 1932 to 1937. Wyckoff found that premedical students from the largely Jewish City College of New York (CCNY) tended to perform extremely well at NYU School of Medicine. In the 1930s, as Jewish quotas took effect, admission rates for CCNY students went down at most medical schools, including NYU, and administrators at CCNY discouraged students from applying to medical school.

But NYU did accept Jewish students from its own premedical program. Thus, for young Eugene Braunwald, pursuing an undergraduate *and* medical education at NYU was a pathway that was difficult but at least feasible. As was true so often in his career, he managed to be in the right place at the right time.

As Braunwald was preparing to apply to medical school, outrage about the quota system limiting Jewish enrollment was just beginning to generate a political response. In 1946, the New York City Council created a committee to investigate the difficulty that graduates of the city's public high schools and colleges experienced in getting graduate and professional educations. The committee recommended that the city take legal steps to ban discrimination by medical schools. In 1948, the state legislature in Albany passed the Fair Education Practices Act (also known as the Quinn-Olliffe Law), which asserted: "It is hereby declared to be the policy of the State that the American ideal of equality of opportunity requires that students, otherwise qualified, be admitted to educational institutions without regard to race, color, religion, creed, or national origin."[5]

Albert Einstein College of Medicine was created as an affiliate of Yeshiva University, a Jewish secular institution, in 1951, and planning for a medical school at Mount Sinai Hospital began in 1958. Both served as alternatives for Jewish applicants who faced obstacles at other schools. But if Eugene had not been admitted to the NYU School of Medicine in 1948, these alternatives would likely have come along too late for him to pursue a career in medicine.

Braunwald had in fact almost given up on the idea of a career in medicine when he learned that he had been accepted to NYU's medical school. He was only in his third year of college, so he could have continued as an undergraduate, but he was eager to move on with his life, and he would have gone to graduate school in biology or another science if he had not been admitted to NYU's medical school. He began his medical studies in September 1948, still commuting by subway from home, at a time when medicine was on the cusp of a new era.

~

A quarter-century earlier, the American writer Sinclair Lewis had written a novel about a bright young man who becomes a physician and researcher, and makes discoveries that help to curb an epidemic. *Arrowsmith* won a Pulitzer Prize in 1926, and is often described as the earliest major novel to portray the cultures of medicine and science. It described the rigors of medical training and the discipline of scientific research, and it romanticized the selflessness of the people who pursued this work. During the mid-twentieth century, it was eagerly read and provided inspiration for generations of young physicians and researchers, among them Eugene Braunwald and others who would eventually collaborate with him.

Arrowsmith reflected an optimism that was beginning to pervade medicine in the early twentieth century as the tools available to physicians evolved. To make diagnoses, doctors still relied predominantly on their eyes, ears, experience, and intuition. Even when they correctly diagnosed diseases, physicians had only a handful of drugs that could extend patients' lives, and surgery was fraught with hazard from bleeding and infection. In this context, medicine's culture had been characterized by stoicism and fatalism. Experienced physicians might have been able to predict what would happen to a patient, but there were few data on whether the potential benefits of a treatment actually exceeded the risks. The major progress in the nineteenth century had been in the disciplines of anatomy and pathology, achieved through careful dissections of cadavers and use of the microscope. Scientists examined immobilized tissues, but, for the most part, they did not yet have the tools or insights to describe the body's systems in action. They could describe the physical structure of the healthy and diseased human body, but they knew much less about its function.

Physiology, the science of the functioning of living systems, was a young but rapidly expanding field. In the 1920s and beyond, Carl Wiggers and others of his generation made tremendous progress in measuring the dynamic forces that characterize human life, such as the pressures generated by a beating human heart. However, these types of data were not yet routinely measured, and the notion that physicians might use such knowledge to alter the course of disease was not widespread. Events like myocardial infarction were usually diagnosed *after* patients had died, thus reinforcing beliefs that the outcomes of such conditions were dismal and could not be altered.

Around the time of *Arrowsmith*, however, new treatments were starting to make dramatic inroads against some diseases previously considered untreatable. On January 11, 1922, a fourteen-year-old boy named Leonard Thompson, who was dying from diabetes at Toronto General Hospital, was saved by the first injection of insulin into a human. On September 28, 1928, Alexander Fleming observed that bacteria on a culture plate had been killed by a contaminating mold—an observation that led to the discovery of penicillin.

Progress and cultural change were particularly conspicuous in cardiology. In 1924, Willem Einthoven won the Nobel Prize in Medicine for development of the electrocardiograph (ECG or EKG), the recording of the heart's electrical activity. Readings were obtained at first via immersion of the patient's limbs in buckets of salt water, and later via leads attached to the body. This technology allowed physicians to diagnose events and conditions such as heart attacks and abnormal heart rhythms. The EKG also helped to create the specialty of cardiology, by providing a test that doctors could administer and interpret only after receiving special training. Early in the twentieth century, general practitioners would call in a cardiologist to perform and interpret the EKG.

Another widely held belief—that the heart was too delicate to touch—was also beginning to erode. The conventional wisdom of the nineteenth century was summarized most famously in a quote widely attributed to the eminent German-Austrian surgeon Theodor Billroth (1829–1894): "A surgeon who tries to suture a heart wound deserves to lose the esteem of his colleagues." Whether and when Billroth actually made this comment is not clear, but other leading surgeons expressed similar sentiments in the late 1800s.[6]

Nevertheless, occasional reports of successful attempts to save patients who had been stabbed in the heart emerged, and in 1923 Elliot Cutler, a surgeon at Harvard Medical School and Peter Bent Brigham Hospital, operated successfully on a twelve-year-old girl with stenosis (narrowing) of the mitral valve—the opening through which blood enters the left ventricle, the heart's main pumping chamber. Cutler opened the child's chest, thrust a scalpel through the left ventricle's wall, and twisted it in the region where he guessed the narrowed valve would be, in order to widen the passageway through which blood could flow. Cutler guessed right, and the patient improved almost immediately.[7] Unfortunately, Cutler's next seven cases did not go as well; only one patient survived.[8] Heart valve surgery was rarely attempted again until the 1940s—just before Braunwald and Nina were about to enter medical school.

One of the most audacious medical acts of the *Arrowsmith* era had been performed in 1929, just two months before Braunwald was born. About four hundred miles to the north of Vienna, in a small hospital in Eberswalde, Germany, a urology resident named Werner Forssmann defied the direct orders of his supervisor when he inserted a thin tube (catheter) into his own heart, and took an x-ray to document what he had done—the first cardiac catheterization.[9] Until that moment (and for several years after), the conventional wisdom was that insertion of a catheter into the beating human heart would have disastrous consequences, such as perforation of the heart or fatal rhythm disturbances.

These and other advances in the early twentieth century set the stage for progress in subsequent decades by Braunwald and his contemporaries. A static view of the human body and of disease was giving way to a dynamic one, opening up the possibility that physicians might help patients through more precise diagnosis and more aggressive intervention. These changes did not come overnight, however; indeed, they were just gaining momentum at midcentury, when Braunwald entered medical school.

~

Anatomy was a core course that lasted throughout Eugene Braunwald's first year of medical school, during which Braunwald teamed with three other students in the dissection of a human cadaver. His most immediate partner in the anatomy sessions was Milford ("Mel") Parker, one of only two African Americans in that entire first-year NYU class. Braunwald got on well with Parker, but other students would occasionally ask Braunwald what it was like to work so closely with an African American. In that era, nonwhite medical students were a rarity in New York. The Wilson Report showed that there were only sixteen nonwhite applicants to medical schools in all of New York State in 1950—so few that statistics on their rates of acceptance were meaningless.[10]

"In that era, NYU's medical school seemed to have a policy of admitting at least one African American student per year, but never more than two," Parker recalled in a 2013 interview. "But we never felt unwelcome, and I had a wonderful relationship with my classmates, particularly Gene Braunwald." Parker, who would later become a psychiatrist based at the University of Medicine and Dentistry of New Jersey, remembered Braunwald as pleasant yet intense. "He had a good sense of humor, and he could be very light-hearted. But he was very focused and goal-oriented."

Braunwald, though he applied himself diligently, was not in love with that anatomy class. He viewed anatomy as a necessary rite of passage, yet he wasn't sure that the information was going to be relevant to him in the long term. "I knew that doctors all seemed to have human skeletons displayed in their offices," he said. "But I suspected that I was not going to be an orthopedic surgeon, so learning the names of all those bones in the wrist and ankle seemed a bit silly."

In contrast, Braunwald liked biochemistry, another core course, and he excelled at it almost immediately. He did so well that his professors asked him to take one year off and pursue a Master's degree. That was an unusual request at the time, because virtually all medical students proceeded in lockstep through the four-year curriculum. Braunwald was flattered, but passed up the opportunity because he did not want to interrupt his medical education.

It was the third course, physiology, that thrilled Braunwald. The course was run by Chester Hampel, a physiologist who was also an extraordinary teacher. Braunwald began doing experiments using cats and other animals to learn about cardiovascular physiology. "The laboratory classes were *real*," he recalled. "They were not dry. There was blood and guts.

"Anatomy was drudgery but was a badge of honor—like pulling an all-nighter as an intern, and coming through it having learned something, but you just don't quite know if it's ever going to happen again. Biochemistry was an important core course. But physiology is what really got me interested. It was qualitatively different from the other courses, because you began to see how disease could interrupt something."

The chairman of the Department of Physiology at NYU at that time was Homer Smith, who was famous both for his kidney research and for his philosophical musings. Smith was jokingly described by the medical students as "the person who discovered the kidney." Each year, he gave NYU students of that era a legendary series of ten lectures on the kidney—lectures that Braunwald remembered as "truly magnificent."

Smith surrounded himself with extraordinary scientific and teaching talent, and Braunwald developed close relationships with several of his instructors, including Lawrence G. Raisz, MD, who later became a well-known expert on bone disease, and George E. Schreiner, MD. Schreiner was a thirty-six-year-old kidney specialist who had come to NYU to perform kidney research in Smith's laboratory, and was pressed into service as a physiology instructor during Braunwald's first year of medical school. In a 1997 interview, Schreiner recalled his surprise when he'd been told to teach in the physiology course: "I began to sweat bullets and realize that I had to stay up all night in order to stay a few hours ahead of the class in my reading because I really hadn't had that much background."[11]

Schreiner had vivid memories of his initial encounter with Eugene Braunwald on the first day of class. "The students sat in alphabetical order, so Braunwald was right up front. I thought it was important to show the students who was in charge, so I picked on the first student handy and started asking him questions to demonstrate how much they needed to learn. Unfortunately, that first student was Braunwald. He answered all my questions in a way that made it very clear he understood everything—and better than me! I thought to myself, 'I am in deep [trouble].' Fortunately, it turned out that Braunwald was extremely unusual."[12]

To use a biological metaphor, that first physiology course was, for Braunwald, like a hormone fitting into a receptor: a perfect combination that sets larger processes in motion. But it was also clear to Braunwald that he did not just want to study physiology and describe how the body's processes worked. He wanted to study *pathophysiology*—that is, how diseases affected these processes—so that he might learn how to mitigate the diseases' effects. He was more focused on the clinical implications of physiology than were the physiologists who were his teachers.

⁓

During the summer of 1949, Eugene Braunwald and Nina Starr became engaged. They did not plan to marry until they had completed medical school, because they did not feel that they should be married until they could support themselves. Braunwald's father was becoming successful once again, and the family moved to Queens. Braunwald continued to live at home even after the move, commuting to school and studying on the subway. Nina Starr worked in the physiology department at NYU in the summer of 1949, performing kidney research. Eugene Braunwald spent the summer working as a technician in the chemistry laboratory at Mount Sinai Hospital, on the Upper East Side of Manhattan.

The laboratory was run by Harry H. Sobotka, who was, like Braunwald, a refugee from Vienna. In that lab, Sobotka and his colleagues performed the routine laboratory tests for Mount Sinai Hospital, as well as some research. Braunwald learned how to conduct routine tests and became familiar with cutting-edge techniques such as serum electrophoresis, for which Sobotka was a leading researcher. "I learned my way around a laboratory," Braunwald later recalled. "I felt that I was going to be involved in laboratory work in the future, although I didn't know how."

But the highlights of the summer for Braunwald began in the afternoons, when his work in the lab was completed. He would go to the floors of the hospital, and stand in the back while the senior physicians performed their rounds on patients each day between

2:00 and 4:00 P.M. "I cleaned myself up and put on a white coat. This was actually my first exposure to sick people, and it was very exciting."

The chief of one of the medical services was Isidore Snapper, a native of Holland. Snapper was respected as a researcher, but he was most famous as a master clinician who was often described as the "champion of bedside medicine."[13] At that time, the patients who were most ill and had the most complex conditions sought care from excellent internists, not specialists. Physicians like Snapper were the peak of the profession.

"He was old-fashioned," Braunwald said. "When Dr. Snapper was going to make rounds, it was announced, the place was cleaned, and there was not a speck of dust. Nurses put on clean uniforms, and the interns stood at attention. Of course, as a summer technician, I was way in the back of the crowd, observing this ritual. Snapper was a large and heroic man, and he was appropriately distant to all of his underlings. But he was something to aspire to."

Charles K. Friedberg, another internist, whose subspecialty was cardiology, also took part in these summer rounds. "He had an encyclopedic mind, and his analysis of cases was brilliant," Braunwald said. During the summer of 1949, he watched Friedberg on rounds, again from the back of a crowd, never speaking, but thinking, "This is what I want to be. I want to be an internist in the grand way."

When the fall arrived, Braunwald returned to NYU and discovered another course that he loved: pharmacology. It was a continuation of physiology, both intellectually and physically; the same laboratories were used by students in both courses. The chairman of the department was another immigrant, Severo Ochoa, who would win the 1959 Nobel Prize in Physiology or Medicine. And

Braunwald's laboratory instructor was another refugee from Austria, Otto Loewi, who had already won a Nobel Prize in 1936 for the discovery of acetylcholine, a chemical essential to actions of the body's nervous system.

Loewi had been a professor of pharmacology at Graz University for twenty-nine years, until he was arrested by the Nazis on March 11, 1938, the night of the German invasion of Austria. That day, he was conducting experiments on how sensory nerves carry signals to the brain. After he was arrested, he was certain that he was going to be executed, and persuaded a prison guard to send a postcard with his findings to the journal *Die Naturwissenschaft,* so that his data would not be lost.[14]

After two months in prison, Loewi was released, in part because British and American members of the Physiology Congress threatened to end all contact with German researchers as long as he was imprisoned. Loewi first went to London, then to New York. He was in his seventies, and did not speak English particularly well. (The physician who evaluated him as part of the immigration process wrote on the medical certificate: "Senile, not able to earn his living.") Loewi felt fortunate to find a teaching position at NYU, and he became part of a vibrant Jewish expatriate scientist community that summered each year in Woods Hole, Massachusetts, where he was interred after his death in 1961.

For Braunwald, working with such outstanding faculty was exhilarating. He remembered Loewi as a brilliant teacher, albeit with a heavy accent, who "saw the grand picture of biological science." Braunwald took microbiology that year from Colin MacLeod, who had come to NYU from the Rockefeller Institute (now Rockefeller University), where he had become famous for his research on the role of nucleic acids in heredity. MacLeod taught Braunwald and the other students about how genetic material determines which antigens are present on the surface of the bacteria that cause pneumococcal pneumonia. (Antigens are substances foreign to the body that evoke an immune response.) For Braunwald, it was a fascinating first look at the potential importance of genetics.

The other transformational influence on Braunwald during his second year came after hours. The cardiologists at Bellevue Hospital had set up a program called the Thursday Night Cardiac Clinic (TNCC). Second-year students like Braunwald were allowed to volunteer to help, and in return could see patients with the faculty. The patients were working people who could not afford to take time off from their day jobs. Patients with heart failure would come in on Thursday nights and receive their weekly injections of mercuhydrin, a medication that helped them to get rid of excess fluid. The injections went deep into muscle and were exquisitely painful; patients needed the weekends to recover. The clinics were held on Thursday nights instead of Fridays, though, because no one would volunteer to staff a clinic on Friday night.

"I remember the thrill I got from sitting across the desk of the first patient I ever saw," Braunwald said. "Of course, it was done under good supervision. But he was *my* patient. I thought, 'This is why I am here—this is what I was born for.'"

At TNCC, patients with heart murmurs were asked to stay late, and sometime around 9:30 the junior instructors would help students like Braunwald listen to their patients' hearts and learn the characteristic manifestations of various forms of heart disease. This early experience cemented Braunwald's growing interest in cardiology—though, as he later said, "I was so anxious to have patient contact, that if it had been a clinic in orthopedic surgery, I would have volunteered for that."

But there was no orthopedic clinic, and Braunwald experienced his first real patient contact with people afflicted with cardiac conditions. The effect was powerful. "I will never forget how he star-

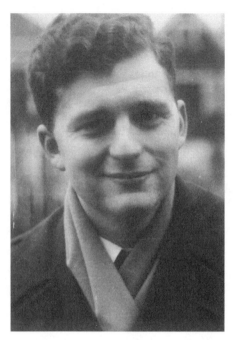

4. Eugene Braunwald in
1952, at age twenty-two.
*Photo courtesy of Eugene
Braunwald.*

tled us by saying that his goal was the heart," Mel Parker said.
"Most of the rest of us still had no idea of what we wanted to do."

Nevertheless, Braunwald did not consider himself as focused
on being a cardiologist or a researcher. His goal was to become a
doctor who could take care of any and all sick patients. He admired the researchers he was meeting at NYU, such as Loewi and
MacLeod, but he still saw the master internists Isidore Snapper
and Charles Friedberg at Mount Sinai as his role models.

Braunwald became even more deeply immersed in patient care
during his third and fourth years of medical school, when he took
"clerkships." These were several-week rotations in which medical
students worked on various services within Bellevue Hospital. His

first clerkship was a two-month block on surgery, followed by two months of pediatrics. At that time, Bellevue Hospital had an entire floor for children with rheumatic fever, a disease that is rarely seen in the United States today. Braunwald also spent two weeks learning about the care of children with tuberculosis—which today is not as rare as rheumatic fever, but still far less common than in 1950.

Braunwald served his internal-medicine clerkship in the winter of 1950–1951, working on the great open wards of Bellevue Hospital. They were full of patients with pneumonia, many of whom were poor and homeless. Penicillin was just becoming widely available, but often people were not hospitalized until their disease was quite advanced. In some cases, infection had caused "adhesions" to build up between the chest walls and the lung. The chairman of medicine at NYU, William Tillett, was interested in using a bacterial product called streptokinase to break up those adhesions.

A vivid memory for Braunwald from that time was his experience of crossing First Avenue from Bellevue Hospital to NYU School of Medicine, and seeing homeless people lying on the sidewalk. Some were inebriated, but others were simply sick. Braunwald saw hospital residents in their starched white uniforms and faculty members in their white laboratory coats walk right by, and was appalled. These observations made him realize that society needed more from the medical profession than individual doctors doing the best they could for the individual patients under their care. But for the time being, his job was learning medicine.

~

Braunwald did well on his third-year rotations, and seemed well on his way to his goal of becoming a master internist—ideally, a consultant with an office on Park Avenue in Manhattan. Then he ran into William Hubbard, who was the assistant dean at NYU responsible for helping fourth-year students plan their final medical-school experiences. Hubbard had different ideas about what was right for Braunwald.

Hubbard had developed the concept of electives—three months in the senior year of medical school during which students could choose what they wanted to do. When Hubbard interviewed Braunwald, Braunwald said he wanted to take a month of dermatology, a month of otorhinolaryngology (ear, nose, and throat medicine, or ENT), and a month of ophthalmology. Braunwald's reasoning was that these areas were covered lightly in the curriculum, and he wanted to deepen his expertise in preparation for the time when he would be a master clinician like Isidore Snapper or Charles Friedberg, dealing brilliantly with any and all cases presented to him. "To be the Grand Snapper, you had to understand the cutaneous manifestations of internal disease," he believed. "To be the next Charles Friedberg, you had to be able to examine the eye and ear, nose and throat."

For reasons that Braunwald never understood, Hubbard did not agree to this plan. "No—I'm not going to do that for you," Hubbard told Braunwald. "I want you to do research. You are the kind of person who should do research and work in a laboratory."

Braunwald was unhappy with the "recommendation," and Hubbard told him to go home and reflect on his advice. One week later, Braunwald returned, and said he still wanted to do dermatology, ENT, and ophthalmology: "Look, if it's an elective, it seems to me that means that I do the electing." But Hubbard was adamant.

"What flashed across my mind is that he's going to be writing the internship letters," Braunwald said. "He's got 110 students, and I didn't want him to think of me as just this kid who was the youngest in the class and who wouldn't follow his advice. So during that second interview, I decided I would just do what he said. I became totally submissive."

Hubbard picked up the phone and called Ludwig Eichna, a clinical cardiovascular physiologist—a "new breed"—whom Braunwald knew from volunteering in the TNCC. Eichna was running NYU's research cardiac catheterization laboratory, one of the few such facilities in the country at the time, and was studying heart failure and other medical conditions that caused accumulation of fluid in the lungs and elsewhere. As Braunwald sat there, Hubbard told Eichna: "I have a young man here who is excited about working in the catheterization laboratory in our new elective program."

Braunwald did not roll his eyes. "I was smart enough to know when not to fight. But, my God, he was right. Three months later, I got to work with Eichna. It was a magnificent experience. I saw patients with heart failure. I would go over the tracings, and then learn the various wave forms of the pressures. I liked it so much that I extended the period. It lit the same flame that had been lit two years earlier, in the Thursday Night Cardiac Clinic."

Hubbard himself went on to become dean of the medical school at the University of Michigan and later the CEO of Upjohn, the pharmaceutical company. He would become and remain Braunwald's friend for years to come. Amid many hours of conversation on other topics, however, they never discussed why Hubbard had refused to let Braunwald spend his last months of medical school learning dermatology and other clinical topics, but instead had sent him toward research.

～

As much as Braunwald enjoyed his experience with Eichna, he was still focused on becoming a master Park Avenue clinician. "At that point, I was thinking Charles Friedberg. In other words, I wanted to be a great internist and *also* a clinical heart specialist. I had so enjoyed the rounds I did after my first year that whenever I could, I would take the subway up to 101st Street and go on rounds at Mount Sinai, and try to be there for Friedberg or for Snapper."

That impulse—to be a clinician—was reinforced during a "substitute internship" rotation during his fourth and final year of medical school. Braunwald applied and was appointed to serve for three months as an intern on one of the medical services at Bellevue. He was on call every other night, functioning in the role usually occupied by physicians who had just graduated from medical school. He and one regular intern were responsible for sixty patients, with little supervision.

From his experience on other rotations, Braunwald knew his way around the 1,200-bed medical pavilion. During the nights, there was only one registered nurse, so Braunwald and the other interns had to mix drugs, give injections, and essentially do anything and everything required to keep their patients alive. The culture was one in which interns only rarely called for help.

Braunwald was not overwhelmed. "I was thrilled, just like I'd been with that first patient in the Thursday Night Cardiology Clinic two years earlier. Of course, I didn't know anything, but there wasn't that much to know. I was excited just having my own floor, my *two* floors, at night. It didn't matter whether you worked four hours or forty-four hours. You didn't complain."

Soon, it came time for Braunwald to look for an internship, a place to train after he graduated from medical school. "The two prestigious hospitals were New York Hospital and Columbia Presbyterian. Nobody thought of a Jewish kid going to Boston. The assumption was that you grow up and train in New York City, and then have a practice, and the apex of the practice would be to become a consultant internist with an office on Park Avenue. I think, if I went back and looked at my class in medical school, the farthest that anybody went for an internship was Philadelphia."

Braunwald did not apply to New York Hospital or Presbyterian Hospital, because he believed that Jews were even less likely to be admitted to those training programs than to their affiliated medical schools. He knew he was a good medical student, but he concluded that "it wasn't worth the three-cent stamp" needed to mail in his application.

That left Mount Sinai and Bellevue. Braunwald had been immersed in the Bellevue experience as a medical student, but he decided he was more comfortable at Mount Sinai. That was where his role models, Snapper and Friedberg, worked. And it had a "rotating" internship in which he would gain experience in anesthesia, surgery, gynecology, and other disciplines—experience that would help him to become the multidimensional master physician. He picked Mount Sinai.

When his courses ended, he and Nina Starr married, and then left for a four-week honeymoon in Bermuda. "We stayed at a place that cost two dollars a day. We bought second-hand bikes for about a dollar, and then we sold them for about two dollars a month later." It was the longest period he would spend away from work throughout his career.

Because he and Nina were on their honeymoon, he did not attend his graduation. Only after his return did he learn that he had graduated first in his class. His father had gone to the graduation ceremony to pick up Eugene's diploma, and was there to hear the announcement that his son had graduated number one. Eugene had earned the highest grades in his class, and received the research prize. William Braunwald declared it was the proudest day of his life.

⌢

As Braunwald finished his medical-school training and started his internship at Mount Sinai, he was deeply affected by a new textbook of medicine—one that was arguably as important culturally to Braunwald's generation of physicians as the novel *Arrowsmith* had been. The first edition of *Principles of Internal Medicine* was

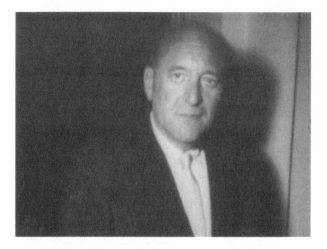

5. William Braunwald, circa 1952. *Photo courtesy of Eugene Braunwald.*

published in 1950. The book's main editor was Tinsley R. Harrison, MD, who at that time was chairman of medicine at the University of Texas Southwestern, in Dallas. The textbook eventually became known simply as *Harrison's*.[15]

This was not just another textbook; it was visionary in its ambitions. The editors of *Harrison's* understood that medicine was changing, and that new generations of physicians had to do more than imitate the methods and manners of their predecessors. Medicine was no longer a craft. *Harrison's* asserted that the time had come to integrate the science and the practice of medicine. The philosophy was summarized in the second paragraph of the preface:

> The modern view of clinical teaching holds that the classic approach, with primary emphasis on specific diseases, is inadequate, and that the student or practitioner cannot be expected to recognize disease in its various manifestations and to manage it intel-

ligently unless he also understands the basic mechanisms of its cardinal manifestations. The basic mechanisms of disease are no longer solely of academic interest to the investigator and to the teacher, but have now become of immediate practical importance in the care of patients.

Harrison's thus declared that medicine was progressing rapidly enough that there actually *was* a "modern view." This modern view was a break from the past, since it required that physicians understand the physiological basis of disease and integrate those insights into their work if they were to provide state-of-the-art care. Previously, there had been too little relevant scientific knowledge for science to play much of a role in clinical care. The editors of *Harrison's* knew that young physicians like Eugene Braunwald would be practicing their craft in a different world.

That bold and optimistic statement in the book's preface revealed more about how visionaries saw the future than about the state of medicine in 1950. In the main part of its text, the first edition reflected the tools that were available to physicians at the time, and those tools were severely limited when it came to diagnostic testing and treatment. There were lengthy descriptions of what might be detected through thorough physical examinations, but precious little information on the long-term outcomes that might be expected with one treatment strategy or another.

"Everything was based on experience," Braunwald would later comment. Whole pages of text included no numbers at all—just prose descriptions of what physicians might observe when seeing patients with a specific disease. For many conditions, of course, no treatment options could be described at all.

A sense of the state of the medical field that Eugene Braunwald was entering can be gleaned from a review of the chapters on cardiovascular disease in the first edition of *Harrison's*. In this section, the authors devote many pages to the physical examination, with detailed prose descriptions of the sounds that might be appreciated by a careful examiner. For example, nearly one full line of text with varying font sizes is used to describe the murmur produced by narrowing of the mitral valve: "R-R-R-UP-DUP-R-R-R-R-R-R-R-UP-DUP."[16] The care with which these descriptions were rendered reflects physicians' reliance on the physical examination, in the era before ultrasound and other technologies would illuminate the structure and function of the heart. In the absence of such technologies, *Harrison's* dispensed clinical pearls of wisdom that relied on low-technology methods to identify those relatively rare conditions for which effective treatments existed. For example, the textbook advised:

> In all cases of congestive heart failure one should feel the hands carefully. If, in the absence of fever, they are warm, the pulse pressure is large, and the heart sounds are loud, one should think of high output failure which is often curable and most commonly due to thyrotoxicosis.
>
> In every case of hypertension one should palpate the femoral arteries. Feeble or absent pulsations point toward coarctation of the aorta, a curable condition . . .
>
> In every case of auricular fibrillation, one should think of mitral stenosis, senile heart disease, and thyrotoxicosis, but first of all thyrotoxicosis, because it is curable.[17]

Physicians might go decades without seeing a case of hypertension due to coarctation (narrowing) of the aorta, or heart failure due to thyrotoxicosis (high levels of thyroid hormone). But these were among the few conditions for which treatments existed in 1950, so overlooking them would be particularly tragic.

The treatments described in the first edition of *Harrison's* were often based on mechanical maneuvers, rather than on medications. For example, a common form of rapid heart rate (paroxysmal atrial tachycardia) today can usually be restored to normal within a few minutes via medications (such as verapamil or adenosine) given through an intravenous line, or instantly with a small burst of electricity. But here are the recommendations from the 1950 edition of *Harrison's*:

> Have the individual take a deep breath and attempt to expire against a closed glottis (the Valsalva experiment).
>
> Massage the back of the pharynx with the finger or any convenient instrument, to induce vomiting.
>
> Massage the carotid sinus region (first one side, then the other) while listening to the heart, discontinuing the massage if the rate slows abruptly.
>
> Press on the eyeballs firmly enough to produce mild but easily tolerable discomfort.
>
> With the aid of bystanders, carry out procedures 1, 3, and 4 simultaneously.
>
> Induce vomiting either by administering ipecac or by the administration of hot water, followed by the massaging of the pharynx. While the patient is retching, repeat procedures 1, 3, and 4, singly or simultaneously.
>
> If the attack persists despite these measures, administer morphine and digitoxin . . . and repeat the above procedures four to six hours later.[18]

In the section entitled "More Common Underlying Causes of Heart Disease," the first condition described was rheumatic heart disease. The different types of damage to heart valves often seen in patients with rheumatic heart disease were well described, but the section on treatment was quite short. Cardiac surgery for rheumatic valvular disease had fallen by the wayside since Elliot Cutler's bold experiments in 1923, and new attempts to repair damaged heart valves were still a few years in the future.

After a discussion of rheumatic heart disease, *Harrison's* turned to "arteriosclerotic heart disease"—that is, cardiac disease due to atherosclerosis. This passage did not use the phrase "risk factors." Instead, *Harrison's* provided qualitative descriptions (that is, no numbers were involved) of characteristics that seemed more common among patients with heart disease. The textbook noted a growing body of evidence that cholesterol had something to do with the development of atherosclerosis. It also observed, "Many believe that this disorder is more frequent in individuals who carry on sedentary occupations, associated with relatively great emotional tension. Thus there is some evidence that the disease is more common in business executives, physicians, and the like, as compared with laborers."

The section on treatment of heart attacks and angina began with the sentence, "The treatment of the underlying disease rarely is completely successful." The emphasis was on rest, losing weight, and treating conditions that might increase the heart's workload, such as anemia and hyperthyroidism. For patients having heart attacks, the goal was to decrease the heart's work as much as possible. The text said, "As a rule, the patient should be kept in bed, except for bowel movements, for a period of two to three weeks after pain and shock have subsided, and then allowed a little more activity each day, with gradually increasing walking about the room." In 1950, exercise tests were occasionally performed, but never on patients who had just had a heart attack.

The list of medications available to physicians for treatment of cardiovascular disease was short. Heart failure could be treated with digitalis, an old drug that makes the heart contract more strongly. But digitalis can sometimes cause heart rhythm abnormalities, and therefore is used only rarely today. Diuretics—medications that cause the kidneys to increase urine output—were considered of great value then, as they are today. But the diuretics available in 1950 were based on the metal mercury, and fell by the wayside when less toxic options became available soon thereafter.

Harrison's also listed venesection (removing blood by withdrawing it from veins) and venostasis (applying tourniquets to the legs) as other acceptable ways of treating congestion in the lungs.

The final passage of the chapter on arteriosclerosis suggested that fatalism in medicine had not died quite yet. It argued that early death from cardiovascular disease might well serve the purpose of reducing burdens on younger generations. It reflected a philosophical acceptance of death from heart conditions and many other diseases that was convenient, since the ability of physicians to change the diseases' natural histories was so limited.

> Arteriosclerosis, removing people from active life when the period of maximum fertility has passed, is of benefit to the young if it relieves them of the care of parents, or brings them an inheritance as they enter adult life. . . . Any attempts to eradicate such a disease from the urban population will be frustrated by natural selection and the survival of more grandchildren in families with few grandparents. Those best fitted to survive in a world growing more urban are those who cease to require support as soon as their roles as parents have been completed. Atherosclerosis and hypertension are now the chief factors in determining that we do not overstay our allotted span of life too long.[19]

Much of Eugene Braunwald's career would be devoted to changing that fatalism about myocardial infarction—to finding medications and other treatment strategies that can extend life for patients with atherosclerosis. But as he prepared to start his internship, Braunwald was concerned more about learning medicine than about changing it. And he had several shorter-term issues on his mind.

: 4 :

Internship and Research at Mount Sinai and Bellevue

1952–1955

Life was changing in almost every way imaginable for Eugene Braunwald in the summer of 1952. He had always been a student and had never lived outside his parents' home. But now, not quite twenty-three years old, he was a doctor, and he was married. He and Nina moved into a small apartment at 235 East 70th Street—midway between the two hospitals where they were doing their internships.

Eugene Braunwald was at Mount Sinai Hospital, on the Upper East Side, while Nina remained downtown at Bellevue. Both of them had every-other-night call schedules—meaning that on alternate nights and weekends, they would remain in their hospitals to take care of patients. They often pulled all-nighters, when they would never get to sleep. On the other nights, they might be exhausted and go directly to sleep, but at least they could do so in their home.

The problem that obsessed Eugene Braunwald before their internships began was: What if their call schedules were out of sync? What if he had to sleep in the hospital on the days that Nina was allowed to go home, and vice versa? It was a coin flip situation, and if Braunwald lost, he would hardly see his new wife for a year. The uncertainty was maddening.

Fortunately, Braunwald was paired at Mount Sinai with another intern, Jonathan Uhr, who had been a close friend of his in medical school at NYU. He and Uhr were assigned to one small "on-

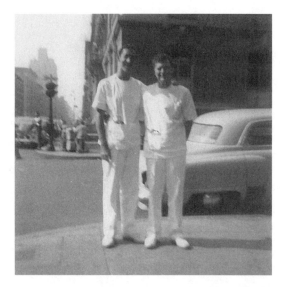

6. Braunwald (right) and Jonathan Uhr during their internship. *Photo courtesy of Eugene Braunwald.*

call" room at the hospital. They would be on call on alternate nights—thus, only one of them would sleep there on any given night. In a sense, they were roommates, but they were roommates who would never actually sleep in the room simultaneously.

Once Uhr understood Braunwald's situation, he told him not to worry—he would switch schedules with him if necessary, so that the new husband and wife could see each other. Braunwald was relieved and grateful to Uhr for his flexibility. As it turned out, Eugene and Nina Braunwald were both assigned to be on call on the same days.

According to Uhr, the Eugene Braunwald of those years was "extremely humorous, given to practical jokes." "He got me in trouble," Uhr recalled during an interview in 2010.[1] "Once, the interns were unhappy about something, and I was selected to represent them. Dr. Horace Hodes was the head of pediatrics, and was the representative of the faculty. So Hodes called our room one day, and asked to speak to Dr. Uhr."

Braunwald happened to be in the room, and answered the phone: "I'm Dr. Uhr. What can I do for you?"

Hodes said, "I'd like you to come over and have coffee with me, and we can discuss the problem."

Braunwald said, "Well, I don't drink coffee."

Hodes then exploded in anger: "You'd better get your ass over here right away if you know what's good for you!"

Practical jokes aside, Braunwald was focused that year on becoming an excellent clinician—a great diagnostician in the tradition of his role models. Uhr recalled that Braunwald would spare no effort to try to come up with the right diagnosis. "Once we admitted an elderly man who was thought to possibly have a tumor in his abdomen, but his abdominal wall was really rigid, so we couldn't feel anything well. I remember, in the middle of the night, Gene lowering him gently into a big, hot bathtub, to see if he couldn't feel something if the patient's abdomen was more relaxed."

Snapper had taught them that in patients with tumors of the kidney (hypernephroma), a soft noise ("bruit") could sometimes be heard if one listened with a stethoscope over the kidneys. But the wards were noisy, and such soft sounds were hard to hear, especially during the day, when the hospital was buzzing with activity and traffic noises filtered in from the streets outside. Uhr remembered that Braunwald "would take people into the back rooms at night, and listen very carefully if [hypernephroma] was suspected."

Braunwald quickly emerged as one of the top interns. In his few off hours, he went to the library and read journal articles relevant to his cases. "I read when other people were too tired to read," he recalled. Sometimes, late at night in that library, he would see Charles Friedberg working on his famous textbook, *Diseases of the Heart,* from which Braunwald would learn cardiology. Inspired by Friedberg, Braunwald began to write as well. One of his first papers, written with Jonathan Uhr, was a study of a syndrome in which the chest cavity becomes filled with fluid from the lymphatic system. It was published in a Mount Sinai journal in 1954.[2]

Late in the summer of 1952, just months into his internship, Braunwald went back to Bellevue Hospital to visit Charles Kossman, an expert on electrocardiograms, who had been the director of the Thursday Night Cardiac Clinic where Braunwald had seen his first patients. Kossman was fond of Braunwald, and suggested that he think about coming back to Bellevue to pursue cardiology at some point. Braunwald received similar advice from Ludwig Eichna, who had been impressed with Braunwald's work during his research elective the prior year.

Although Braunwald was attracted to the notion of becoming a cardiologist like his Bellevue mentors, his plan was to stay at Mount Sinai to do his junior residency. He hoped that he would then be picked to be one of the two "chief residents," an honor that would position him well to become one of the internists who admitted patients to Mount Sinai Hospital.

∼

But once again, turmoil in world politics played havoc with Braunwald's plans. In 1953, the Korean War was grinding toward a stalemate, and the Communists in the Soviet Union and China seemed an ominous threat. In response, the United States was building up its military forces—including its physician corps—through what became known as the "Doctor Draft." Young physicians of Braunwald's age were at high risk of being inducted into the armed services at any time, an event that would interrupt their training and alter the course of their lives.

At Mount Sinai, when young physician residents were drafted, they would leave a gap in the hospital's on-call schedule that needed to be filled for the rest of the year. To avert that situation, Alexander Gutman, chief of the medical service at the hospital, decided that he would not accept any residents who had not yet completed their military service. Gutman told Braunwald that he would be welcome back at Mount Sinai at any time, but only *after* he had completed his military duty. Braunwald briefly considered enlisting and getting his military obligations out of the way, but Nina quickly vetoed that notion. She did not want to interrupt her own training as a surgeon. "I'm not going to some base in Germany or Korea, and sit around and knit," she told Eugene.

With only a few months left in his internship, Braunwald suddenly found that he did not have a job lined up for the next year. He could try to get a residency in another program, but it would have to be at one of the less prestigious institutions—a hospital that would be willing to risk having its residents drafted at any moment.

Braunwald had one other professional option, which was to obtain a fellowship—a year-long appointment as a researcher. But fellowships were usually given to physicians who had completed their residencies and wanted to further their careers in research. Even though he was younger—chronologically and professionally —than other fellows, Braunwald was able to get an appointment doing cardiology research at Mount Sinai. Nina could continue her training at Bellevue, and, if he got drafted, this would not have a profound impact on anyone other than Braunwald and his wife. So in 1953, driven less by love of physiology than the need to find a job in New York, Eugene Braunwald started his first extended research experience: a year as a cardiology fellow at Mount Sinai.

His salary for that year was $2,000—a nontrivial sum in an era when subway fare was a nickel, but not quite enough to enable the couple to get by. He and Nina refused offers of financial support from their families, now that they were "grownups"—physicians who were finally married after their three-year engagement—but their household budget was tight. During the previous year, when Eugene had been an intern at Mount Sinai, the hospital had provided him with free food. In 1953 Nina could still eat at Bellevue Hospital, because she was a surgical resident; but as a research fellow, Eugene had to feed himself, and there was also the $50 monthly rent on their studio apartment at 235 East 70th Street. So when Nina was on call at the hospital, and when Eugene was not analyzing pressure tracings and writing papers, he worked night and weekend shifts in the Mount Sinai emergency department, and read electrocardiograms for $2 per tracing at a small private hospital in the Bronx. He earned another $2,000 through these "moonlighting" activities that year, and life was good.

The funds that provided Braunwald's modest salary as a researcher came from Mount Sinai's cardiology group, which had received enough philanthropic donations to support one research fellow per year. Organizing a respectable research program cost fairly little in those days, because help like Braunwald was relatively cheap and the other costs of clinical research were blurred with those of the clinical care of patients; no one tracked the additional costs and time that went beyond routine patient care.

During that first year as a fellow, Braunwald initially worked on what was a hot topic in the early 1950s: sophisticated analyses of electrocardiograms, a technique called vectorcardiography. That work led to several papers in respected journals, but vectorcardiography never proved a useful tool for physicians caring for patients, and Braunwald was soon attracted to a subject that had greater durability: diseases of the heart's valves.

In those very early days of cardiac surgery, Braunwald started to work with Mark Ravitch, who had just come from Johns Hopkins to be the first full-time chief of surgery at Mount Sinai. Rheumatic fever was still common, and one of its most frequent long-term complications was narrowing of the mitral valve, a condition known as mitral stenosis. During operations to dilate those narrowed valves (mitral valvuloplasty), Ravitch would insert catheters directly through the walls of the heart into the left ventricle and the left atrium, allowing Braunwald and his colleagues to measure pressures inside those chambers. By comparing the pressures, the researchers could assess the impact of the valve narrowing (stenosis). The more severe the narrowing, the greater the buildup in pressure in the left atrium compared to the left ventricle—that is, the greater the pressure gradient across the mitral valve. Then they could document the drop in that pressure gradient after the valve-opening surgery had been performed.

Braunwald had plenty of time to plunge into this work, as Nina was rarely off duty from her surgical residency. His research produced a series of papers, including one in the prestigious journal *Circulation,* as well as studies of the hemodynamic changes that accompany pregnancy, and research on the relationship between the heart's electrical and mechanical activities.[3] One curious observation from Eugene Braunwald's research during his Mount Sinai fellowship appeared in a paper published in 1956. He and his colleagues had measured levels of C-reactive protein (CRP) in patients with heart failure. Somewhat to their surprise, they found elevated levels of CRP—a blood marker generally used to detect inflammation due to rheumatic disease—in patients with heart failure caused by chronic hypertension or coronary artery disease, but without any evidence of rheumatic disease.

In retrospect, it seems likely that Braunwald and his colleagues were uncovering early evidence of the role of inflammation in the development of atherosclerosis. Worse atherosclerosis led to higher CRP levels, due to the chronic process of injury and repair inside scarred arteries. Yet Braunwald, after that single paper, did not pursue research on inflammation and heart failure. Half a century later, one of his protégés, Paul Ridker, would pick up the scent and demonstrate the important role of CRP in heart disease, and large studies of the impact of inflammation-reducing medications on patients at risk for heart disease have now been launched. But in the early 1950s, Braunwald's interests lay elsewhere.

Braunwald was instead focused on hemodynamics, an area where he was beginning to demonstrate the type of thinking that would characterize his research career. He thrived at the interfaces of different disciplines. Working with surgeons, he was able to connect physiology to anatomy and pathology—and then to clinical medicine. Describing the hemodynamics in the hearts of patients with valvular heart disease was like going from photography to cinema. The differences in pressures that he measured between one chamber of the heart and the next gave him a visceral sense of what was happening inside the bodies of patients with conditions such as narrowed or leaking valves. These types of data also enabled him to gauge the success of operations; and despite assertions by surgeons to the contrary, he could see that good results were being achieved in fewer than half of cases.

Braunwald's work led to several publications—the standard measure of success for a research fellow. Nevertheless, as the year progressed, Braunwald's future remained uncertain, and he was well aware that he had no plan. He enjoyed the research, but he still had his heart set on becoming a great clinician. Although he could not return to Mount Sinai to complete his clinical training, he spent many evenings working in the Mount Sinai emergency department to earn extra income and to maintain his clinical skills. He was still in danger of being drafted at any time, but he could not enlist to get his military obligations out of the way, because Nina was committed to her training program and he did not want to be separated from her.

There was only one answer, even though it was just a short-term solution: he needed to find another research fellowship. So he returned to talk to his old teachers at NYU. As a result, in the summer of 1954, Braunwald started working in the laboratory of André Cournand on the Columbia University service at Bellevue Hospital.

~

Cournand represented a rare species in the academic world: a full-time clinical researcher whose salary was covered by money from a foundation. In addition to Cournand, the laboratory included one full-time and three part-time faculty researchers (who also had private practices), as well as Braunwald and another research fellow. Cournand had funding for Braunwald—he had secured one of the NIH's first research fellowships. Suddenly, Braunwald's income from research leapt from $2,000 to $4,000 per year. This increase enabled him to give up his moonlighting activities and devote all of his time to the laboratory. With Nina's life consumed by her surgical training, Braunwald spent nearly a hundred hours per week on his work with Cournand. He also enrolled in night courses in advanced mathematics at Hunter College, to enhance his understanding of the pumping function of the heart.

The members of Cournand's lab met virtually every day. It was a "Mom and Pop" enterprise, offering all the intellectual and interpersonal rewards that accompanied daily collaboration with a brilliant researcher on the cutting edge of his field. Cournand was to share the Nobel Prize the following year. He did not need to travel to raise funds or burnish his reputation, so he was a constant presence for Braunwald and the others in the laboratory.

André Cournand was already famous and enormously respected when Braunwald joined his lab. He was yet another representative of the wave of American immigrants who had been buffeted by history—someone who had very nearly died during the First World War, and whose career was greatly advanced by the Second.

Born in Paris, Cournand had begun his studies in the Faculty of

Sciences at the Sorbonne in 1914, but with the outbreak of World War I most of the professors left to serve in the army. After a few months, Cournand decided to volunteer. He enlisted in an infantry regiment, and was assigned to an advanced ambulance service and later became an auxiliary battalion surgeon—a rank created for medical students, because there were so many casualties among army physicians that students had to be pressed into service.

Cournand worked on the Chemin des Dames front, in the *département* of Aisne in northeastern France, the site of a series of trench warfare battles in which hundreds of thousands died. Cournand's duties included searching for wounded soldiers in no-man's-land, giving first aid on the spot, and then helping to evacuate them. He was ultimately awarded the Croix de Guerre with three bronze stars.

On August 8, 1918, Cournand was wounded and gassed. He spent the entire fall and winter recuperating in Paris, before he renewed his medical studies in the spring of 1919. It was an exciting time to live in Paris, and, feeling fortunate to be alive, Cournand took full advantage of the city's cultural life. He befriended French artists such as Yves Tanguy, Jacques Villon, Jacques Lipchitz, Max Ernst, Robert Delaunay, and Max Jacob; and composers including Darius Milhaud, Igor Stravinsky, and Edgard Varèse.[4] Perhaps as a result, his training process was long: he finished his thesis ("Acute Disseminated Sclerosis") and obtained his medical degree only in 1930. He was ready to start work as an assistant in medicine at a hospital in Paris, but thought he would like to spend a year in the United States first. The chief of the chest disease service at his Paris hospital had a friend in New York, Dr. James Alexander Miller, who was director of the Columbia Chest Service at Bellevue Hospital. A visit was thus arranged.

Cournand spent three months caring for patients with tuberculosis at the Trudeau Sanatorium in Upstate New York, to improve his English, and then moved to New York City to begin working with Miller. Miller was sufficiently impressed to suggest that Cournand might stay longer and do research with Dickinson Richards, who was studying pulmonary physiology at Columbia-Presbyterian Hospital, uptown in Washington Heights. Cournand and Richards began working together in 1932, when both were thirty-seven years old.

The question that Miller asked them to address was why some patients who underwent chest surgery for tuberculosis died, but others did not. The two researchers realized that they had to study not just the lungs, but the entire thorax and circulatory system. Over the next few years, they methodically studied all the structures involved in circulatory and pulmonary function: the chest wall, the muscles, the lung, the heart, the blood, the arteries, the veins.

By the mid-1930s, Cournand and Richards knew that they had to go beyond currently available research techniques. To measure the heart's output (and thus the amount of blood flowing through the lungs), they needed to obtain blood from the right side of the heart. The formula for measuring the heart's output was known as the Fick principle:

$$\text{Blood flow per minute} = \frac{\text{Oxygen consumption per minute}}{\text{Difference in oxygen content between arterial and venous blood}}$$

Cournand and Richards could measure the numerator of the equation (oxygen consumption) by having a patient breathe into a collecting bag, and then analyzing the gas contents. And they could measure the first part of the denominator (oxygen content of arterial blood) by sampling blood from an artery in the arm or groin. The problem was getting a valid measure of the oxygen content of the venous blood. They couldn't rely on blood drawn from a vein in the arms or legs, because the veins draining the various parts of the body all contained different amounts of oxygen, depending on the oxygen consumption of the organs in that part of the circulatory system. The researchers needed "mixed venous" blood, which they could obtain only by analyzing blood from the right side of the heart or from the pulmonary arteries.

Cournand and Richards were aware of the experiments by Werner Forssmann, who had inserted a catheter into his own heart, and they also knew that some pioneering European radiologists had repeated those experiments. So in 1936 Cournand visited Paris and brought back some catheters, as well as large needles through which the catheters could be inserted into the bloodstream.

From 1936 to 1940, Cournand and Richards studied dogs, and improved their expertise in manipulating the catheters; they were also able to study a chimpanzee. One of their trainees inserted catheters into the right atrium of human cadavers, in order to calculate the necessary catheter lengths for human cardiac procedures.

In 1940, Dr. Walter Palmer, the chairman of the Department of Medicine at Columbia, gave them permission to do a right heart catheterization, but he insisted that the patient be very ill, so that any tragedy resulting from complications would not be considered too great. The patient who was chosen had extensive metastases from cancer, including large lymph nodes in his axilla (armpit). The researchers were unable to get the catheter past those bulky lymph nodes and into the patient's chest.

Their next chance came at Bellevue, where researchers under the leadership of Homer Smith (chairman of physiology at the NYU School of Medicine) were studying blood flow to the kidney in patients with hypertension. Cournand sat with Smith in the dining room in the Bellevue nurses' dormitory, and they talked about measuring cardiac output. Cournand said the best method for obtaining an accurate cardiac output would be to pass a catheter into the right atrium, as Forssmann and others had done. Smith was intrigued, and lobbied for permission for Cournand to try this approach at Bellevue. Smith's support led, in 1941, to the first reports of cardiac output measurement in humans.

Cournand and Richards's research took major leaps forward with the onset of World War II. On December 7, 1941, the Japanese attacked Pearl Harbor. Almost immediately thereafter, the American Thoracic Surgical Society held a conference in New Orleans. There, Cournand met with the Johns Hopkins surgeon Alfred Blalock, who was chairing the so-called Shock Committee commissioned by the federal government to find ways of reducing mortality among severely wounded soldiers.

Cournand showed Blalock their new approach to measuring cardiac output. At the time, Cournand was having difficulty getting grant funding for work in cardiac catheterization, but he knew Blalock had the influence to eliminate that problem. Blalock himself had studied shock in dogs, but he knew that physiology in man might well be different. Cournand argued that this new approach might be useful for treatment of the wounded. "You have your grant," Blalock assured him.[5]

In the war years that followed, Cournand and Richards studied all kinds of shock: traumatic shock, hemorrhagic shock, burns, and shock due to perforated bowels. They also studied all sorts of potential treatments: plasma, blood, drugs. They arranged to have most of the severe traffic injuries in New York City brought to Bellevue, so they could participate in the care of these patients.

"We had a very good team, with a surgical resident on call twenty-four hours a day," Cournand later recalled. "I had my technicians in contact with me by phone, and as soon as a surgical resident had a case, he would call me and I would go to the hospital to see the patient with him. I could then call in my technicians at any time, the middle of the day or night, to study these patients and evaluate their treatment."[6]

During the war, automobile traffic decreased as gasoline was rationed, and the number of trauma cases fell accordingly. Cournand and Richards then turned to study of the cardiovascular system in burn cases. From 1941 to 1945, Cournand and Richards improved their equipment and their techniques, and, with time, right heart catheterization became an accepted procedure. Cournand and Richards used cardiac catheterization to study a whole range of cardiac diseases, including congenital heart disease, heart failure, and rheumatic heart disease. This was the research that Cournand was pursuing at the time Eugene Braunwald joined his laboratory, in the summer of 1954.

When Braunwald became a member of Cournand's laboratory group, they were systematically studying patients with valvular heart disease. Braunwald performed some cardiac catheterizations and spent many hours measuring the pressure tracings that they obtained. Cournand was a constant presence, and Braunwald was able to work closely with him virtually every day.[7]

Braunwald focused on distinguishing mitral stenosis from mitral regurgitation—an important issue, since cardiac surgery was being performed with increasing frequency on patients with mitral stenosis. The operation was one in which the narrowed valve was widened with a finger or a mechanical device. Patients whose major problem was mitral stenosis benefited considerably from this operation, but it could actually worsen problems for patients who also had leaking (regurgitation) of the mitral valve. So it was important to be able to determine, before surgery, whether patients had mitral regurgitation along with their mitral stenosis.

As Braunwald and his colleagues performed these catheterizations and collected these data, another year was ticking by, and
Braunwald was all too aware that his career remained in a holding
pattern. He had to do more training to become a clinician, but he
had still not fulfilled his military obligation, and the risk of being
drafted remained high.

Then he learned about a new potential option: he heard about
the NIH's extraordinary "Building 10," a clinical center where researchers could also help care for patients. The idea of doing research and patient care simultaneously was enormously appeal-
ing. Braunwald knew that an appointment at the NIH meant being
a member of the Public Health Service—which was equivalent to
serving in the military. (The clinical associates at the NIH were
later called "Yellow Berets," because so many were there in part
because of the military exemptions.) But of increasing importance
to Braunwald were the opportunities the NIH afforded to conduct
research—opportunities that were unmatched at the time.

Had there been no Doctor Draft, Eugene and Nina would
doubtless have stayed in New York. He would have completed his
clinical residency at Mount Sinai, and would perhaps have become
a private-practice internist on Park Avenue. Instead, in the winter of 1954, the Braunwalds considered moving to the Washington, D.C., area. It would be the first time in their adult lives that
they had lived outside New York. Eugene Braunwald would seek
an appointment at the NIH, and Nina would transfer her residency training to Georgetown University Hospital.

To contemplate leaving Bellevue was painful for Nina, but
Georgetown assured her that, if she performed well as a resident,
she would become chief resident—a position that, for a surgeon
in training, would provide tremendous opportunities to accumulate experience in the operating room. Georgetown also required
that she spend a year as a research fellow, and Nina liked the idea
of working with an innovative surgeon at Georgetown named

Charles Hufnagel. Hufnagel had developed the first artificial valve used to treat a cardiac disease, a ball-and-cage apparatus that he sewed into the aortas of patients with leaking aortic valves. It prevented blood from the lower half of the body from leaking backward, and thus decreased the strain on the heart's main pumping chamber, the left ventricle.

Eugene Braunwald applied for an NIH clinical-associate position in the winter of 1954–1955; he was interviewed by Robert Berliner, MD, the NIH's research director. The interview went well, and Berliner asked Braunwald to wait outside the office. Berliner then telephoned André Cournand; after a brief conversation, he summoned Braunwald back in and offered him a position. It was the strength of Cournand's name and his recommendation that got Braunwald the job. There were only four such appointments out of more than two hundred applicants that year.

Braunwald finally had a plan—one that allowed him to avoid being drafted and being separated from his wife, and that would enable him to pursue *both* research and patient care. But it was at precisely this moment that the military finally decided it needed Eugene Braunwald. He received a letter summoning him to report for duty in Brooklyn in just a few days—not even as a physician, but as an ordinary seaman in the U.S. Navy.

Braunwald panicked, and called Berliner. Berliner made some phone calls over a weekend, and got Braunwald appointed to the Public Health Service, effective immediately, and stationed in the laboratory of André Cournand. So Braunwald completed the spring of 1955 in Cournand's laboratory, as a member of the U.S. Public Health Service. On July 1, 1955, he reported for duty at the NIH.

: 5 :

Clinical Associate at the NIH

1955–1957

In the summer of 1955, Eugene and Nina moved from 235 East 70th Street in Manhattan to a new apartment on the grounds of the National Institutes of Health (NIH) in Bethesda, Maryland. They were exhilarated. "Everything was brand new," he recalled. "The apartment house was brand new, and we were the first occupants of our little apartment. Everybody was moving in, and it was an extraordinary feeling. For the first time since leaving Vienna in 1938, I felt that I belonged to something.

"During the whole period from the age of nine, I had always felt like an outsider. I felt pretty good about things when I was in medical school, and certainly during my internship—until I learned that I couldn't continue the residency. I felt like a transient during the fellowship at Mount Sinai, even though it was enormously productive. And I certainly felt like a transient outsider during the Cournand-lab year, even though it was intellectually rewarding. But when I got to Bethesda, I got a different kind of feeling, a very good feeling."

Braunwald had found the place that would be his home for most of the next thirteen years.

There was a good reason that everything seemed new to the Braunwalds on their arrival at the NIH: everything actually *was* new. The Bethesda campus had arisen only recently, from fields that had been private property, a golf club, and a monastery for the Sisters of the Visitation. President Harry Truman had laid the cornerstone for the Clinical Center in 1951, and the first patient had been admitted in 1953. A dynamic and distinguished renal physiologist, James Shannon, was just assuming the leadership role of NIH director in 1955. The country was at peace and prospering. Funding for the NIH was expanding rapidly, and researchers were beginning to bang on the door in hopes of getting fellowships or more permanent positions. Visitors were coming from around the world to see what NIH researchers were doing. Those visitors added to the excitement, and sometimes, as we shall see, to the creativity.

⌒

The nation's commitment to medical research had begun much more humbly, in 1887, with a one-room laboratory created within the Marine Hospital Service (MHS). The MHS was a government agency established in 1798 to provide medical care for merchant seamen. During the early twentieth century, however, the MHS evolved into the U.S. Public Health Service (PHS) and that one-room laboratory developed into the National Institutes of Health.[1]

These changes were stimulated in no small part by the waves of immigrants coming to the United States in the late nineteenth century. The immediate concern in the 1880s was whether these immigrants were infected with contagious diseases. The MHS was charged by the U.S. Congress with examining arriving passengers for signs of infectious diseases, especially cholera and yellow fever, and was given the authority to quarantine them.

Scientists in Europe had only recently shown that microscopic organisms were the cause of several infectious diseases, and the MHS wanted to use this new knowledge to prevent epidemics on U.S. shores. In 1887, a young physician named Joseph Kinyoun, who had been trained in bacteriology, set up a small laboratory at the Marine Hospital on Staten Island, New York. In the German tradition, it was called a "laboratory of hygiene," reflecting its public health purpose. Within a few months, Kinyoun had shown the MHS that he could detect the bacteria that caused cholera.

For more than a decade, Kinyoun labored in obscurity as the Hygienic Laboratory's sole full-time employee. In 1891 his laboratory was moved to Washington, D.C. Its existence was officially acknowledged by the U.S. government in 1901, when Congress authorized $35,000 for construction of a new building for investigations of "infectious and contagious diseases and matters pertaining to the public health."

A year later, the MHS was reorganized and renamed the Public Health and Marine Hospital Service (PH-MHS). Other legislation launched a genuine federal program of research by authorizing three new divisions, in addition to the existing Division of Pathology and Bacteriology at the Hygienic Laboratory. The new divisions focused on chemistry, pharmacology, and zoology.

In 1912, the PH-MHS became simply the Public Health Service. Infectious diseases remained the preoccupation of the PHS, a concern that reflected the needs of the times. The PHS reserve corps was established in 1918, to help generate the manpower needed to cope with the global influenza epidemic of that year.

With the prosperity of the 1920s, other medical issues gained public attention. In 1922, the PHS established a Special Cancer Investigations Laboratory. In January 1929, the PHS Narcotics Division was created, and two hospitals for drug addicts were authorized. This PHS Narcotics Division would eventually become the Division of Mental Hygiene.

The growing federal research enterprise needed a home, and it found at least the site for one in 1935. when Mr. and Mrs. Luke I. Wilson donated forty-five acres in Bethesda, for use by the National Institute of Health (at that time the name was singular, not plural). The Wilsons made a succession of additional gifts of land in the next few years, and the cornerstone for Building 1 was laid in June 1938. Franklin Roosevelt opened the building and grounds of the NIH on February 1, 1942.

Great wars often foster great advances in science, and the NIH grew rapidly in the years during and after World War II. Researchers in Bethesda and around the country worked on vaccines for soldiers and on treatments for shock among the wounded. André Cournand was just one of the medical investigators whose research was accelerated because of federal funding related to the war effort. NIH researchers studied an enormous range of problems related to military issues. For example, their work on high-altitude flying explored the height above which oxygen is needed to prevent pilots from blacking out.

In the postwar period, U.S. confidence and ambition spilled over into medical research. Dr. James Shannon, who would later become director of the NIH, wrote:

> The war had revealed the enormous economic capability of the Nation and the heights to which man's efforts can reach, particularly when aided by science and technology. A conviction that a significant portion of the resources of the Nation could be productively directed towards the conquest of disease and for the well-being of man underlies these events. . . . For the first time, areas within these fields [medical and biological sciences] were ripe for intensive exploitation. . . . This happened in an era when the required funds could not be produced by private activity alone. These forces underlay the postwar development of the Federal role in medical research.[2]

Advocacy groups began pushing Congress to create institutes devoted to other specific disease areas, including cancer and heart disease. In 1948, legislation was passed creating the National Heart Institute, and renaming the National Institute of Health—the umbrella organization—the National *Institutes* of Health (see Figure 7).

Congress also provided funding for the world's largest research hospital, to be built on the NIH campus in Bethesda. The Warren Magnuson Clinical Center, which opened in 1953, was designed to

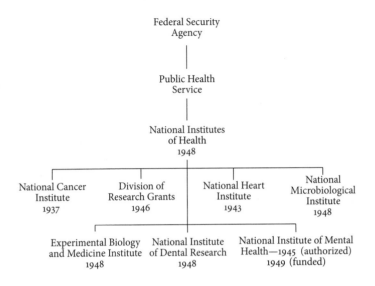

7. Structure of the NIH in 1949. *Courtesy of the NIH Office of History.*

allow researchers to work in close proximity to doctors taking care of patients. Leading researchers quickly adopted the Clinical Center's other name: Building 10. Casual references to Building 10 let listeners know that one had been to Bethesda, the Promised Land of medical research. The United States now had a place for scientists to congregate and do research, and thus, for the first time, a real vehicle for large-scale investment in research.

Figure 8 shows the annual amounts of federal funding for the NIH from 1950 to 2010. By later standards, of course, the funding for the NIH in the 1950s was modest. But excitement is generated by the rate of change of funding, and the scale of this long-term perspective masks the rate of the increases that were made in the first two decades. When funding is shown on a smaller scale just for 1950–1970 (Figure 9), the reason that so many promising researchers sought support from the NIH becomes apparent.

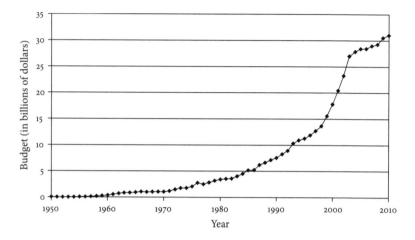

8. NIH Congressional Budget, 1950–2010. *Courtesy of the NIH Office of Budget.*

The inflection point in Figure 9 at which funding increases really began to accelerate was just around the time when Eugene Braunwald arrived at the NIH. A second inflection point is apparent in 1968, when growth of the NIH budget temporarily halted. The years between those two points, from 1955 to 1968, are often called the "Golden Years" at the NIH, and the expansion of funding was just one of the reasons. James Shannon's leadership of the NIH was visionary and would have tremendous impact on the nation's research landscape, far beyond Bethesda.

Shannon's wife had serious cardiac problems, including abnormalities of her mitral valve—a disorder that would ultimately prove fatal to her. But for several years during this period, she received her care from a young cardiologist with whom Shannon would become quite close: Eugene Braunwald.

The availability of research funding and the chance to work with stimulating colleagues were not the only reasons that promis-

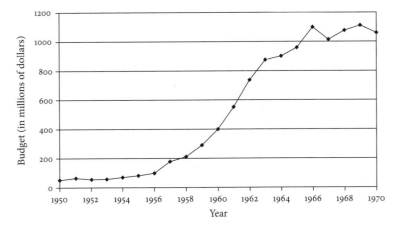

9. NIH Congressional Budget, 1950–1970. *Courtesy of the NIH Office of Budget.*

ing researchers sought appointments at the NIH. The doctor draft, which was created when the Korean War began in 1950, loomed large in the lives of all male physicians, and for the next twenty years the NIH essentially had its pick of the best and brightest young physician-researchers. The clinical-associate track was created to fulfill this aspiration. Physicians like Braunwald who were appointed as clinical associates cared for patients while pursuing research under the supervision of permanent intramural scientists. At the time, medical schools could not match the NIH's ability to provide good clinical and research training, along with an exemption from the draft. Bethesda was the place to be if you were a serious, ambitious physician-scientist.

Braunwald was appointed to work in the laboratory of Stanley Sarnoff, a noted cardiovascular physiologist who had taught at Harvard. Braunwald immediately realized that he could walk back and forth between his patients and his research in just a few min-

utes—a situation that was ideal from his perspective, and that influenced his thinking about the training of young physician-
researchers in later years.

"I realized that when you are young, bright, motivated, willing
to work upwards of a hundred hours a week, and you get the right
conditions, you can grow simultaneously as a researcher and as a
clinician," he would comment later. "You can multitask. It's one
plus one equals three—or at least 2.5."

Sarnoff posed a research question for his laboratory that started
Braunwald on one of the major themes of his career: What controls myocardial oxygen consumption? In other words, what factors influence how much oxygen is used by the beating heart? "It
was more of a question than a hypothesis," Braunwald said. "We
all put our heads together about how to design the experiment. It
was 'pure' science, a fascinating question that at first had no clinical connection. As we delved into it, it turned out to have enormous clinical implications."

In Sarnoff's laboratory, Braunwald and his colleagues performed studies in which they inserted small catheters into the coronary arteries of dogs to measure coronary blood flow. After two
years, they realized that myocardial oxygen consumption was important not just for intellectual reasons. They came to understand
that oxygen consumption was half of the dynamic that caused the
heart to develop ischemia—the condition in which the heart's demand for oxygen exceeds its supply. Myocardial oxygen consumption was the demand side of the equation.

Sarnoff was a laboratory physiologist, and was not particularly
focused on the implications of myocardial oxygen consumption
for patient care. But Braunwald was a member of the new generation of physicians who were adopting the perspective described in
the preface to Harrison's *Principles of Internal Medicine*—the perspective of clinician-researchers who integrated science and clini-

cal medicine. Until that point, Braunwald had not done any work related to coronary artery disease, but he would become famous in the next half-century for studies that flowed from this research in 1955.

It was while working in Sarnoff's laboratory that Braunwald first met Carl Wiggers. Wiggers was a legend—unquestionably the most accomplished cardiovascular physiologist in the world, and the founding editor of *Circulation Research,* the most prestigious journal for cardiovascular investigators—and he came to Washington to give a lecture. Sarnoff heard about the visit and brought Wiggers to the laboratory at the NIH.

"We were all prepared," Braunwald recalled. "There were five research fellows who had worked on the oxygen consumption study over a period of two years, and we had a chance to show the great man what a new physiology laboratory in a new facility, working for the government with extremely able fellows, could do. And we wanted to pave the way for the work's acceptance into *Circulation Research.*"

Wiggers was a gruff man who was not given to compliments, but he acknowledged that the research was very interesting. Sarnoff indicated that they wanted to submit the three papers on this work to *Circulation Research,* and Wiggers's response was positive.

There was one problem. Wiggers had a firm rule that there could be no more than three authors on any paper. He felt that research groups were getting bloated, to the point where it was increasingly difficult to know who had contributed what to experiments. Yet Sarnoff's lab had more than three collaborators on *every* project. This higher number was an early sign of an important trend: the challenges of modern science were going to require larger groups of investigators.

Sarnoff told Wiggers that the research had been a group effort, and that the complexity of the experiments required more than three investigators. He asked Wiggers to make an exception to his well-known rule.

Wiggers refused. He said that if he made an exception for Sarnoff, his position on authorship would no longer be defensible. Wiggers had a suggestion, however: "You are already well recognized, so why don't you take yourself off. And if we get one person of the other four to relinquish his role on each of the three papers, that would get us to three instead of four."

Sarnoff replied that this approach would not work—that it would be misleading to submit the papers without his name on them: "Authorship on a paper is not only a reward, but it's also a responsibility." This perspective would later become an accepted standard. Today it is inappropriate and potentially misleading *not* to include someone who has contributed to the intellectual groundwork, the conducting of the experiments, or the writing of a paper.

Wiggers would not bend. Thus, the three papers were not published in *Circulation Research,* and instead were submitted to the *American Journal of Physiology,* which published them in 1958, with five to six authors on each. They became among the most widely cited studies that Sarnoff ever published, and the same was true for Braunwald.[3]

～

Researchers' frustration with the limitations of the techniques available to them can sometimes spur important progress. Just as Cournand and Richards realized that they could not answer their research questions unless they were able to get catheters into the pulmonary arteries of patients, Braunwald understood that he had to go beyond existing research techniques in order to make a real contribution to medical knowledge. "I was practicing the medicine of the day, but I knew that wasn't moving medicine along.

The two places where there seemed to be movement were in cardiac catheterization and in mitral-valve surgery."

Thus, soon after he arrived at the NIH and entered Sarnoff's laboratory, Braunwald also started working with Andrew Glenn Morrow, a Hopkins-trained cardiac surgeon who would become one of Braunwald's most important influences and friends. A native of Indianapolis, Glenn Morrow had gone to Wabash College in Crawfordsville, Indiana, and then had enrolled at Johns Hopkins for medical school. He graduated with his MD in 1946, and remained at Hopkins for his surgical internship and residency under Alfred Blalock. Along the way, he joined the Public Health Service, presumably to help pay off the debt related to his education. Working at the NIH was a convenient way to fulfill his PHS obligations and start his career. In 1952, when Morrow was only 30 years old, he was asked to become the first chief of the Clinic of Surgery at the NIH.

The NIH was not quite ready to start its surgery program, so Morrow went to Oxford to study thoracic surgery. The Clinical Center of the NIH opened in 1953, and Morrow returned shortly thereafter. A year later, Braunwald arrived, and their collaboration began.

From Morrow's perspective, Braunwald was valuable because he had had two years of experience doing hemodynamic research and cardiac catheterization at Mount Sinai and then at Bellevue with Cournand. Braunwald knew how to analyze pressure tracings obtained from patients. From Braunwald's perspective, Morrow was a bold cardiac surgeon who could help him gather data from places where no physiologist or cardiologist was able to go.

The most important of these places was the left side of the heart. Braunwald had inserted many catheters into the right side of the heart and into the arteries supplying the lungs (pulmonary arteries). But the standard approach to obtaining blood and pressure tracings from the left atrium or ventricle required having surgeons puncture the left heart during surgery, as Mark Ravitch had done during Braunwald's research fellowship at Mount Sinai. That approach might suffice for the writing of research papers, but not for patient care. When considering whether to operate on a patient's heart, physicians needed to know what was going on in the left side of the heart before sending a patient to surgery, not during the procedure.

Morrow had developed an approach to reaching the left atrium that did not require opening the patient's chest—but it was brutally direct in its own way. He would insert a rigid tube through the patient's mouth with the patient's neck fully extended backward. (The patient was heavily sedated and the throat well anesthetized; Braunwald was assigned those tasks.) The tube (called a bronchoscope) was then inserted down the trachea into the lungs to the carina, the point at which the trachea divides into branches to the left and right lungs. The left atrium of the heart lies just beneath the carina. Morrow would insert a needle and a catheter through the bronchoscope into the carina—and into the heart. Then, Morrow and Braunwald could obtain blood and pressure tracings from the left atrium or left ventricle.

"It was a difficult procedure for patients," Braunwald remembered, but it provided critically important information for the evaluation of patients who were candidates for mitral-valve surgery. Moreover, it allowed Braunwald and Morrow to collect data that were important for their research. Morrow performed five to ten of these catheterizations every Friday morning, and Braunwald would analyze the tracings on the weekends.

Morrow's relationship with Braunwald deepened during those first two years at the NIH. In 1957, Morrow sent Braunwald to the University of Minnesota to observe the medical management of patients undergoing open-heart surgery, in which the heart would actually be stopped and opened up. Only a few such cases had ever been performed, and on that trip to the University of Minnesota, Braunwald saw open-heart surgery for the first time. He was in awe of what he observed. During that visit, Braunwald learned about techniques for putting patients on cardiopulmonary bypass and weaning patients from ventilators.

Morrow also taught Braunwald how to write papers. Braunwald was not a native speaker of English, but he was a clear thinker—an essential first ingredient for writing clear papers. The two would compose papers sitting side by side, with Morrow writing on a yellow pad. "We would talk about every sentence," Braunwald later recalled. "He was very concerned about split infinitives; he would *not* split infinitives. And he was extremely concerned about noun modifiers. Today, noun modifiers are used all the time." Over the next several years, they would write 115 papers together.

~

During this period, a major pattern in Braunwald's professional life began to emerge: the ability to integrate insights from various streams of research, leading to the creation of something new. Braunwald's clinical work with Morrow, combined with his research on animals in Sarnoff's laboratory, set the stage for him to devise ingenious models in dogs for studying valvular heart disease.

Braunwald began to study the sudden development of aortic or mitral-valve regurgitation (leaking)—often the result of damage to heart valves from infection, inflammation, heart attacks, or other diseases. When either the aortic or the mitral valve leaks, some blood travels in the wrong direction with every heartbeat. The amount of blood that the heart must pump increases abruptly. In both conditions the result is often severe shortness of breath, as the lungs become congested with fluid. Blood pressure falls, and other organs in the body suffer as the heart's ability to pump blood to them is severely diminished. This constellation of problems constitutes the syndrome known as "shock."

Although acute mitral regurgitation and acute aortic regurgitation are both potentially life-threatening problems that require the left ventricle to do much more work than usual, Braunwald could see that the two conditions are actually quite different from the perspective of the heart. In mitral regurgitation, the heart pumps blood in the *wrong* direction, into the low-pressure bed of the lungs. In aortic regurgitation, the heart pumps *all* of the blood into the high-pressure bed of the aorta and into the body's arteries. In both cases, the heart is doing "rework"—that is, pumping blood more than once. In the case of mitral regurgitation, that extra work is eased by the lower pressure in the left atrium, at least in the short term—but the lower pressure in the left atrium makes it easier for a great deal of the blood to flow in the wrong direction.

During that first two-year stint at the NIH, Braunwald developed sophisticated models for such damage in dogs. Braunwald knew that it would not be particularly helpful just to damage the heart valves and observe what happened to the dogs. He wanted to measure and control the increases in blood that the left ventricle had to pump. He wanted to quantify what had heretofore been only a qualitative concept: leakage through a damaged valve.

To do so, he created external shunts between the aorta and the heart. To mimic the impact of aortic regurgitation, he inserted a shunt with a flow meter from the aorta to the left ventricle. Braunwald could now control the amount of blood flowing back into the left ventricle with a clamp on the shunt and a thumbscrew, and could measure the simulated "leakage" using the flow meter.[4] He also controlled and measured the flow of blood through the aorta, so he could adjust upward and downward the amount of blood flowing out of the heart to the rest of the body, along with

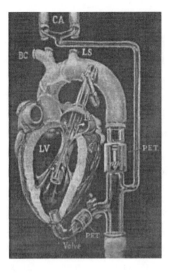

10. Schematic diagram showing preparation for producing and recording ventriculoatrial regurgitation while simultaneously recording effective cardiac output. PET = Potter turbine flow meter; LS = left subclavian artery; CA = carotid arteries; A = aorta; LA = left atrium; LV = left ventricle. *Courtesy of Eugene Braunwald.*

the amount of blood flowing back into the heart that had to be pumped once again. To mimic mitral regurgitation, he plugged the shunt into the left atrium instead of the left ventricle (Figure 10).[5]

Braunwald's model allowed him to control the major variables affecting the left ventricle when heart valves became defective. These variables were the amount of blood flowing in the wrong direction, and the resistance against which the left ventricle must work as it struggled to send blood to the rest of the body. He could now demonstrate what expert clinicians already sensed: that mitral regurgitation and aortic regurgitation were two quite different problems, with different likely courses.

At age twenty-six, Braunwald had begun to expand what was understood about hemodynamics and cardiovascular physiology, by measuring what had previously been unmeasured and by doing experiments in which he tightly controlled what had previously seemed uncontrollable. He was drawing on skills and experiences only recently acquired. He knew how to perform cardiac catheterizations, and was comfortable doing invasive procedures. He was learning about the new specialty of cardiac surgery and what it could potentially offer the patient. He could go from animal experiments to studies involving human subjects by just walking down from the seventh to the fifth floor of Building 10. He was constantly stimulated with new ideas in all of these settings. Through exposure to the cutting edge of several disciplines and through regular experience with patients, Braunwald was beginning to epitomize the "bench-to-bedside" physician-researcher.

This fortuitous situation required generosity on the part of Sarnoff, Braunwald's formal sponsor and boss, but also necessitated hard work by Braunwald himself. He was officially working for Sarnoff and carrying out catheterizations with Morrow; in addition, he was responsible for patients. When asked in later years how he managed to satisfy two demanding bosses, he recalled: "They had totally different work schedules. Like other surgeons, Glenn worked from 7:00 A.M. to 4:00 P.M. On the other hand, Stan was a 'night owl.' He came to work at 4:00 P.M. and worked until midnight."

Braunwald was able to work both "shifts" in part because Nina was a surgical resident in a hospital ten miles away and on call virtually all the time. When she had time off, Braunwald was able to adjust his schedule so he could be with her. Otherwise, he worked almost constantly.

That pattern had been established during July and August 1955, the first two months that Braunwald was at the NIH. Because there was a transit strike, Nina had needed the car in Washington; and without a car, Braunwald had been unable to leave the NIH campus, which was still very rural, with cow pastures and an active religious cloister.

"I was basically a prisoner," he recalled. Braunwald, of course, did not really mind being stuck at the NIH. He knew he was on an extraordinary run, in a time and place where creativity and hard work were going to change medical care. "Glenn and I felt like Lewis and Clark discovering the West."

~

One of those Lewis and Clark moments occurred during his second year at the NIH, when he began to spend some of his Nina-less evenings with a young surgeon who had moved into an apartment at the other end of the hallway. The surgeon, John Ross, rotated through the cardiac catheterization laboratory, where Braunwald was spending one day a week. Braunwald was more experienced in the catheterization laboratory than Ross, but Ross had the greater mechanical dexterity of a surgical trainee.

Ross also had another important way in which he used his head and his hands: he could cook. Every week or so, Ross would invite Braunwald to dinner, and Braunwald was virtually always available. It was during one of Braunwald's dinners with Ross that the young surgeon described an interesting question that had been posed that day by a Latin American visitor to the NIH catheterization laboratory.

Ross had just begun performing the "dumbbell procedure"—a technique used to determine the size of an atrial septal defect (an opening between the two upper chambers of the heart) before surgery. Atrial septal defect repair was one of the few cardiac operations that were possible at that time, and many patients with this disorder were sent to Glenn Morrow for surgery at the NIH. This was the period just before open-heart surgery was becoming common, and surgeons like Morrow would usually try to fix the defect without actually stopping the heart. To protect the patient and the defective heart during the operation, Morrow would induce hypothermia to lower the oxygen requirements of the tissues, and then briefly cut off the flow of blood into the heart. With the empty heart still beating (but not pumping blood), Morrow would slice into one of the upper chambers and sew up the defect. Blood flow to the heart would be restored, the patient would be warmed up, and the heart would never have stopped beating. In the era before stopping and restarting the heart during surgery was routine, this approach to "beating-heart surgery" was the only way to repair disorders like atrial septal defects.

The surgeon had to be quick, however, since the heart and other organs would be damaged by more than a few minutes without blood flow, even under conditions of hypothermia. Morrow was usually in and out in five minutes; but to perform the surgery rapidly, he needed to prepare in advance. Small defects could be closed with a few stitches. Larger ones might need a patch. Very large defects would be too dangerous to try to repair in this way, and could be remedied only through use of the new and still high-risk technique of cardiopulmonary bypass.

It was the job of Braunwald, Ross, and the other physicians in the cardiac catheterization laboratory to determine the size of the atrial septal defect before the patient went to surgery. To do so, they would insert a catheter with a balloon on the end into one of the veins of the legs. They would push it up through the venous system into the right atrium, and then through the atrial septal defect into the left atrium. They would then blow up the balloon—not with air, but with a liquid contrast agent that could be seen on x-ray. If the balloon was positioned correctly, they would see a dumbbell shape, with a pinched area reflecting the size of the atrial septal defect.

The dumbbell procedure was just the kind of innovation for which the surgeons and cardiologists at the NIH were becoming well known. Visitors began to flock to the NIH to see these advances for themselves, and Braunwald was aware of the organization's unique role: "There was nothing like the intramural program in the world at the time. There was its sheer size. You had maybe seventy-five full-time clinical investigators working in the National Heart Institute alone, and there were eight institutes. People came from all over the world to see us in action."

On that particular day, the day of Braunwald's dinner conversation with John Ross, a cardiologist named Emilio Del Campo, visiting from Buenos Aires, had asked Ross how often he was able to get the catheter across the atrial septal defect. With the bravado of youth, Ross had replied, "Always." It was actually the first such procedure he had ever performed.

Impressed that placing a catheter into the left side of the heart was routine for Ross, Del Campo had asked him why they didn't do the same thing in patients *without* an atrial septal defect—or at least that's what Ross believed Del Campo had said. The visitor's English was poor, and Ross was sure only that Del Campo had said something about a needle on the end of a catheter.

The appeal of the concept was immediately obvious to Ross and Braunwald. Why not use the needle to puncture the delicate wall that separates the right and left atrium in the normal heart, and push the catheter through behind the needle? The ability to get a catheter into the left side of the heart via a catheter in the right atrium would be a great advance in caring for patients with heart disease. From there, they could measure pressure waves to assess whether patients had leaking or narrowing of the mitral valve, or both. They could measure the effect of aortic valve disease on the heart. They could sort out whether patients who were short of breath or swollen with retained fluid were plagued by lung disease, weakness of the heart, or some other condition.

Back at Mount Sinai, Braunwald had watched as surgeons obtained those precious data from the left side of the heart by inserting needles directly through the wall of the heart during operations. He had watched Glenn Morrow insert rigid bronchoscopes deep into the trachea of heavily sedated patients, and thrust needles and catheters straight down into the left atrium. Now, a visitor to the NIH had suggested a way of reaching the left atrium that would be easier and safer than any of the existing alternatives. It would be virtually painless for the patient. It was an approach no one had ever tried before.

"How does that sound to you?" Ross asked Braunwald over dinner. They talked about whether it would be too dangerous, whether they could be sure the needle was pointed in the right direction, toward the left atrium, rather than backward toward the aorta or some other nearby structure.

"John, I think you should do it," Braunwald said. "I think you should take time off, and develop the catheter and needle."

Ross did just that. His boss, Morrow, gave him six weeks off, during which he worked in the industrial shop at the NIH, and tested the special apparatus in dogs. Morrow and Braunwald collaborated on the project, and soon it was ready for testing.

It worked beautifully in dogs, and in patients too. Over the next several years, Ross, Braunwald, and their colleagues performed thousands of these procedures, enabling them to reliably collect data from the left heart with only the mildest sedation and at a relatively leisurely pace, compared with the transbronchial approach. Thus was born the transseptal left heart catheterization, in which the catheter crosses the septum dividing the right and left atria. The procedure continues to be performed frequently in catheterization laboratories around the world.[6]

Today, much of the information that Braunwald's colleagues sought through transseptal catheterizations can be obtained from echocardiography, with no invasive procedures at all. Yet transseptal catheterizations are still used routinely around the world: surgeons insert catheters into the left atrium to destroy tissues that cause rapid or irregular heart rhythms, and into the left ventricle in patients with severe aortic valve narrowing or certain types of artificial aortic valves that would be dangerous to cross with a catheter coming from the other direction (from the body's arteries, via the aorta). This approach is also used for balloon valvuloplasties (procedures to open up narrowed valves). Ross, Braunwald, and Morrow thanked Emilio Del Campo in the research paper that described the procedure for the first time.[7]

⌒

NIH leaders were impressed with Braunwald's work and offered him a long-term position. But he still felt the need for more clinical training so that he could be a complete physician, and he wanted to take a year off to finish his residency training. His supervisor, Robert Berliner, understood, and offered to continue to support Braunwald if he would return to the NIH after a year away. Braunwald wanted to do that residency close to Washington, D.C., since he did not want to part from Nina for a year. He set his sights on Johns Hopkins.

: 6 :

Johns Hopkins Hospital

1957–1958

Like many immigrants, the young Eugene Braunwald was attracted to the security and acceptance that comes with affiliation with respected institutions. He had not wanted to go to just any college when he was sixteen years old, or to just any medical school when he was nineteen, or to just any internship program when he was twenty-two. When he had learned that he could not continue his residency training at Mount Sinai in 1953, he had not wanted to go to some obscure hospital just so he could complete his training requirements in 1957. His options had been limited at each stage of his life; but perhaps because of those restrictions, he wanted to do all he could to keep future options open. He wanted to finish his clinical training at a hospital that was highly respected—someplace where, if he excelled, everyone would understand that he must be first rate. Johns Hopkins Hospital more than filled the bill.

Braunwald was in the enviable position of having a job guaranteed after his residency, and having his salary covered by the NIH during his residency. But he wanted to be accepted at Hopkins—one of the most prestigious training programs in the world—on his own merits. He did not want to be a "freebie," so he did not tell anyone that he would not need salary support when he applied to Hopkins. Getting into Hopkins for training was not easy. It was at the top of every list of excellent academic medical centers—only the Harvard teaching hospitals in Boston were comparable in desirability and respect. But Boston was not an option for Braunwald geographically, and excellence was deeply ingrained in the Hopkins culture.

~

The excellence that characterized Hopkins in the 1950s was in short supply in American medicine when the hospital had opened, in 1889. Most doctors at that time were "trained" in what were essentially trade schools. Academic standards were not high; the main requirement was ability to pay the tuition. These schools provided two to three years of education that was based completely, or nearly so, on lectures by part-time faculty. Students then would become apprentices to older doctors, or simply open their own medical practice, often without any prior direct experience with patients.

Johns Hopkins rejected that model, and gradually made it obsolete throughout the United States. From the start, Johns Hopkins Hospital and its medical school took pride in maintaining the highest possible standards. The entrance requirements for medical students and house staff were rigid. The curriculum emphasized the scientific method and teaching conducted at patients' bedsides by professors like William Osler, the legendary first chairman of Hopkins's Department of Medicine. The culture demanded that everyone work tirelessly without complaint. Hopkins faculty and trainees were expected to pursue excellence in both clinical care and research.

Hopkins was founded with a bequest from a nineteenth-century investor who had died without offspring in 1873. His unusual first name, Johns, actually came from the family name of his great-grandmother, Margaret Johns. She had married Gerald Hopkins in 1700, and had given her surname to one of their children. That first Johns Hopkins was the grandfather of a second

Johns Hopkins, who earned the fortune that provided the initial funds for the hospital and medical school. His $7 million bequest was, at the time, the largest philanthropic donation in U.S. history.

The story behind that bequest unfolded over two generations, and involved an act of social conscience and a romantic disappointment. The second Johns Hopkins had a very comfortable childhood on his family's tobacco plantation in Maryland's Anne Arundel County. The plantation was highly profitable until 1807, when Johns Hopkins's father, Samuel, abruptly decided to free their slaves in accordance with the decision of their local Meeting of the Society of Friends (Quakers). The plantation was no longer adequate to support their large family, so young Johns Hopkins moved to Baltimore to learn business.

In Baltimore, he lived and worked with his uncle Gerard Hopkins, who ran a wholesale grocery business. Young Johns Hopkins fell in love with Gerald's daughter Elizabeth, but Quaker law prohibited marriage between first cousins. Disappointed, Johns Hopkins left Gerald's home and employ. He never married, and neither did Elizabeth; they remained close friends for the rest of their lives.[1] Had Johns Hopkins married and fathered children, he might not have made the large bequest that led to the formation of the hospital and medical school that bear his name.

Johns Hopkins was even more successful in business than his uncle, and ultimately became the wealthiest citizen of Baltimore. He began to ponder what he should do with his fortune, and by 1867 he had decided to establish a hospital and medical school, ultimately choosing the site of the Maryland Hospital for the Insane in east Baltimore, on what was then called Loudenschlager's Hill.[2] Hopkins died at age seventy-eight from pneumonia, on Christmas Eve 1873, before detailed plans could be formulated. But under the guidance of the trustees he had helped to select, construction be-

gan in 1877, and twelve years later, the seventeen-building structure was complete.

The domed Administration Building was flanked on either side
by men's and women's private wards, which faced west on Broad-
way. The hospital had several advanced architectural features,
including isolation wards with individual rooms and central heat-
ing. It was designed to minimize the spread of infections by restricting the flow of air from one ward to the next. It separated
patient units into pavilions, in a pattern that would be imitated
widely, including at Boston's Peter Bent Brigham Hospital.[3]

Hopkins's architecture was just one of the ways in which the
new hospital and medical school set a new standard for U.S. medicine. Hopkins modeled itself after German hospitals and universities, where medical science and research were rigorously taught
and closely integrated with clinical medicine. At the formal opening of the hospital, on May 7, 1889, the principal address was given
by John Shaw Billings, who had overseen the detailed planning for
the hospital. He said: "There is widespread hope and expectation
that these combined institutions will endeavor to produce investigators as well as practitioners, to give the world men who can not
only sail by the old charts, but who can make new and better ones
for the use of others. This can only be done where the professors
and teachers are themselves seeking to increase knowledge, and
doing this for the sake of knowledge itself."[4]

Hopkins created new models of training that revolutionized
U.S. medicine. Reflecting Osler's belief that intense and prolonged
patient contact was critical to learning medicine, Hopkins medical
students began spending their third year in clinical rotations (surgery, internal medicine, pediatrics, and so on). The students were
not passive observers; they became deeply involved in the delivery
of care. Osler also developed residency programs in which young
physicians-in-training would actually live in the hospitals.

Osler's counterpart in the Department of Surgery was William S. Halsted, the most prominent surgeon of the day. National leaders also chaired the departments of Pathology and Gynecology. They were attracted by generous support for their research, and the ability to recruit faculty with full-time salaries. With salaried faculty, Hopkins did not have to rely on teaching by part-time local practitioners. Hopkins wanted full-time clinician-researchers to serve as role models for their students and trainees.

In the decades to come, the phrase that many at Hopkins believed their institution brought to life was "heritage of excellence." The phrase was first invoked in a tribute to one of the founding physicians of the hospital, who was credited with having helped to create "something extraordinarily precious [that] comes out of the close but entirely free association of really superior people . . . persons so spirited yet so balanced, so gifted and yet so incomplete, so mature and yet so eager. . . . It is the interaction of such men that attracts great young men, leads to great living, and itself lives on long afterwards as a heritage of excellence ready at any time to burst into bloom again."[5] The phrase resonated, and subsequently was often invoked by Hopkins leaders and alumni.[6]

As audacious as such aspirations may have come to sound since then, Hopkins trainees came to epitomize excellence in clinical medicine and research, and its alumni assumed leadership roles at medical schools and teaching hospitals throughout the country. Within twenty years, over sixty American colleges or universities had three or more professors with Hopkins degrees on their staffs.[7] They spread the cultural expectation that doctors should be firmly grounded in basic science and should apply research methods to the study of disease. When the educator Abraham Flexner conducted his influential 1910 survey of American medical schools, he cited Hopkins as a model—indeed, as *the* model. "The influence of this new foundation can hardly be overstated," Flexner wrote. "It has finally cleared up the problem of standards and ideas, and its graduates have gone forth in small bands to found new institutions or to reconstruct old ones."[8]

Hopkins's reputation stemmed from respect for its legendary first chairmen of its departments of Medicine and Surgery—William Osler and William Halsted, respectively. Osler's contributions and impact became better known than Halsted's, in part because of a famous biography of Osler written by Harvard and Brigham surgeon Harvey Cushing.[9] Osler's personal charisma—he was a brilliant speaker and wit, famous for devising practical jokes—only enhanced his professional reputation.

In contrast, Halsted was a complex, even tragic figure whose long struggle with drug addiction cast a shadow over his many accomplishments.[10] After a prolonged period of study in Europe, Halsted had started his career as one of the most sought-after teachers and surgeons in New York City.[11] His problems began in October 1884, when he read about the use of cocaine as an anesthetic for eye surgery.[12] Along with his students and other physicians, he began experimenting with the drug, and became addicted. He ultimately was sent to Butler Sanatorium in Providence, Rhode Island, where physicians treated him by converting his addiction from cocaine to morphine. Around the time Johns Hopkins was opening, a close friend of Halsted's from New York Hospital, William Welch, was hired as Hopkins's first dean and its chairman of pathology. Welch pushed to have Halsted hired as the first Hopkins's surgeon-in-chief.

At Hopkins, Halsted became famous for the meticulous surgery he performed during long operations that were a marked departure from the contemporary emphasis on speed, even if that speed came at the expense of hygiene and bleeding. Halsted introduced new approaches to the control of bleeding and the reconstruction of tissue—techniques that enabled him to perform more ambitious resections of tissues for patients with cancer. And he was the creative force behind numerous other innovations, including the use of surgical gloves. Halsted also established the first formal surgical-residency program: a surgeon-in-training would complete an internship, then serve six years as an assistant resident and another two years as a house surgeon. The trainees that emerged from this program later spread around the United States, dominating institutions the way Hopkins alumnus Glenn Morrow dominated cardiac surgery at the National Heart Institute.

Hopkins's reputation for innovation went beyond clinical medicine itself. In a move that was controversial nationally and at Hopkins itself, three women were included among the fifteen students in its first medical-school class, in 1893. This progressive approach was actually forced upon Hopkins when funding from Johns Hopkins's original bequest began to run dry before the school could open.[13]

Four young women who were daughters of the original trustees offered a solution: they would raise the $500,000 needed to open the medical school if Johns Hopkins would admit qualified women. The trustees agreed, and the women began raising the funds with support from some of the most prominent women in the country, including Alice Longfellow, Clara Barton, and the wives of Grover Cleveland, J. Pierpont Morgan, and Alexander Graham Bell. They reached their goal by Christmas Eve 1892.[14]

Late in their campaign, in a letter dated December 22, 1892, the Women's Fund Committee added an additional demand: that all Hopkins students, male or female, had to meet stringent requirements, including proof of a bachelor's degree; education in physics, chemistry, and biology; and reading knowledge in French and German. The Hopkins leadership had little choice other than to accept these requirements. Thus, Hopkins's rigorous standards for its medical students, unheard of at the time (even at Harvard), came *with* the decision to include women in its classes, not despite them. William Osler thought these requirements were too rigid, and said to Welch that the two of them were fortunate to have gotten into Hopkins as professors, because they would never have been admitted as students.[15]

Of those first three women students, only one, Mary S. Packard, actually received her MD degree. One dropped out after her third year to become a Christian Scientist, and another left after she became engaged to her anatomy professor. In 1895, when Osler talked about Hopkins's experiment with women as medical students in a lecture at Harvard, he joked, "It has been a great success—33⅓ percent of them were engaged to their professors at the end of the first year."[16]

In the decades to come, however, Hopkins's openness to female medical students would enable it to recruit some extraordinary women who were unable to get into other leading medical schools. Among them were Dorothy Reed, the pathologist from the class of 1896 who played a key role in describing Hodgkin's disease; and Caroline Bedell Thomas, who helped to define the role of antibiotics in preventing rheumatic fever. There was also Dorothy Reed's less successful classmate, Gertrude Stein, who flunked out but then went to Paris and became prominent as a writer and cultural icon.[17]

The most famous of Hopkins's women graduates was Helen Taussig, who became a leading expert on congenital heart disease. Taussig was the daughter of a Harvard economics professor, who wanted her to attend the Harvard School of Public Health. Yet Taussig learned that Harvard would allow her only to take courses—it would not award her a degree.

Taussig then applied to the Johns Hopkins School of Medicine, and was admitted in 1923. She decided to become a cardiologist, which in those days was a discipline for adult medicine. But she was steered toward pediatrics because it was considered a more appropriate specialty for women physicians. Edwards A. Park, Hopkins's chairman of pediatrics and head of the Harriet Lane Home for Invalid Children, encouraged Taussig to start a cardiac clinic that would care for patients with rheumatic and congenital heart conditions. This Hopkins clinic became her base of operations.

Taussig's understanding of cardiac disease was based on insight into pathology and anatomy, and the fluoroscope was among her favorite clinical tools. (Fluoroscopy uses x-rays to provide real-time images of the body's organs; Taussig could essentially view video versions of chest x-rays to study the outlines of her patients' hearts.) Her hearing had been seriously impaired by an illness in her youth, so auscultation with a stethoscope was not her strength. But she could use the fluoroscope and correlate the findings with what she had observed in the autopsy room.

It was one thing to make the correct diagnosis in cases of congenital heart disease; it was another to do something about it. At the time Taussig entered medicine, the outlook was dismal. In the 1892 edition of *The Principles and Practice of Medicine,* Osler began his chapter on congenital heart disease by acknowledging that fact: "These [congenital afflictions of the heart] have only limited clinical interest, as in a large proportion of the cases the anomaly is not compatible with life, and in others nothing can be done to remedy the defect or even to relieve the symptoms."

Taussig would change that discouraging outlook. She and her Hopkins colleague Alfred Blalock became famous by developing an operation for "blue babies"—infants who suffered from Tetralogy of Fallot, a relatively common and serious congenital heart disease. In blue babies, defects in the heart allowed blood to "cross over" from the veins to the arteries without going through the lungs. Blood low in oxygen (venous blood) is darker, and children with such defects thus appear dusky, or blue (cyanotic). More important than their appearance was the impact of inadequate oxygen supply on their ability to function. Their survival was usually brief, and their quality of life poor.

The problem for these children was structural, and when Taussig opened her congenital heart disease program at Hopkins, there was no structural treatment. Cardiac surgery had gone into hibernation after Elliot Cutler's early adventures with mitral-valve surgery in 1923. In 1938, however, Robert Gross—a young surgeon at the Harvard-affiliated Children's Hospital in Boston—had successfully performed an operation to close a shunt connecting a child's aorta and pulmonary artery (patent ductus arteriosis, or PDA).

Technically, this operation was not really heart surgery, since the shunt was outside the heart, but it gave Taussig an idea. She thought that if a surgeon could close off a shunt to prevent the flow of blood into the lungs, why not create one to increase pulmonary blood flow in these blue babies? It might not be possible to repair the defect that allowed blood to cross from the right heart to the left without going through the lungs, but the creation of the shunt would at least push more blood through the lungs, and raise the oxygen levels in the blood.

Taussig traveled to Boston in the early 1940s to propose such a procedure for blue babies, but Gross was not interested. Taussig returned to Baltimore, where Alfred Blalock had been appointed professor and head of surgery. Together, they devised the Blalock-Taussig shunt, which carried blood from a systemic artery to the pulmonary artery for children with Tetralogy of Fallot. Because of their work, Baltimore became medicine's mecca for blue babies. And when Eugene Braunwald went to Hopkins in 1957, one of his major goals was to learn about congenital heart disease under Helen Taussig and Alfred Blalock.

~

As selective a program as Hopkins had become, Eugene Braunwald was an attractive candidate when he sought entrance to its residency program in 1957. He was now four years out of internship, and already had about thirty-five papers in high-quality journals to his credit. Some of his most important papers were not yet published, but they had been presented at cardiology meetings, and the word was out that he was going to be a force in cardiology. Leading academic medical centers had few faculty members with a comparable list of publications, let alone residents. And Braunwald came with good recommendations from a respected member of the Hopkins family: Glenn Morrow. Braunwald's major interview was with Ivan Bennett, an infectious-disease expert who was also well known in medicine as a coeditor of Harrison's *Principles of Internal Medicine*. Bennett endorsed Braunwald, and Braunwald's year at Hopkins began in July 1957.

The medical culture at Hopkins was different from those at the New York hospitals. Braunwald liked some aspects and disliked others. He greatly admired the politeness shown toward all patients, no matter how poor they might be. "My co-residents called all patients 'Sir' or 'Mr. Jones' or 'Miss or Mrs. So-and-so,' unless the patients were adolescents," he noted. "They would never address them by their first names, as often occurred with African American, poor, or alcoholic patients in New York. The culture was that you had respect for the dignity of people in real trouble, even if they might not be outstanding citizens. I found it extremely impressive. And it changed me for the better. I tried to pass this approach on to my residents when I became a chairman of medicine."

On the other hand, Braunwald was disturbed by the open segregation of patients by race. There were two separate house staff training programs, the Osler and Marburg services. The latter was for private patients, and Braunwald had applied only to the Osler service, the ward service that took all patients. This service admitted patients to four large open wards: the black-male ward, the white-male ward, the black-female ward, and the white-female ward.

Until 1958, Hopkins had a segregated blood bank. Black patients could receive blood from white donors, but not the other way around. Braunwald was astounded that white patients might be allowed to bleed to death rather than be given blood of the correct type donated by an African American. That practice was ended by Julius Krevens, who later became dean and then chancellor at the University of California, San Francisco. But segregation on the wards continued for several years after Braunwald's residency at Hopkins, until the civil-rights movement began to transform American society.

Hopkins also had a system in which residents were on call all the time. Osler had created the program, in which residents actually lived in the hospital (hence the term "residents"), the better to enhance their total immersion in patient care. Their teams accepted admissions every day; there were no days off. "We were called the Osler Marines," Braunwald recalled. "It was like you were at war. The enemy was illness and death."

The Osler residency of the 1950s was slightly kinder and gentler than it had been in Osler's day, in that the residents no longer had to live in the hospital. Instead, they lived in rented rooms right around the hospital; married residents like Braunwald could rent small houses. But Nina was doing her chief-residency year, and spending most nights in a call room at Georgetown Hospital, so they were able to see each other just once or twice a week, when Nina could find the time and energy to make what they called the "Schlep" to Baltimore.

Even when Nina made the Schlep, they had to stay very close to the hospital. In that era, there were fewer urgent crises in which the immediate presence of a physician would make a difference; hence, the pagers, or beepers, that would become ubiquitous within a decade were not yet in use. Braunwald and the other residents nevertheless had to be reachable by telephone at all times. They had to be within a few minutes of the hospital floors, in case one of their patients had a fever, or falling blood pressure, or another problem that warranted attention. And that meant they had to stay in the hospital or their rented quarters virtually all the time.

Braunwald didn't mind the total immersion. "First of all, Nina wasn't around very much. So I wasn't sitting around complaining that I couldn't go to the movies with my wife. My wife was operating on patients in another city."

The other factor that made perpetual call bearable was that the work of being on call was shared among the other "Osler Marines." Everyone was there, taking care of his or her own patients, and the new admissions were divided among the four teams. Each team might take one or two new admissions a day, instead of four to eight.

"We didn't have as many all-nighters as we did at Mount Sinai," Braunwald commented. "Somebody would crash, and you'd get called in. But there were not many nights that I didn't sleep in my bed. The pace was more leisurely, and I did not feel physically stressed—not as stressed as I did when I worked every other night as an intern at Mount Sinai."

There *was* some dissatisfaction with the system that Osler himself had created, and other leading academic medical centers had already gone to the call system. Hopkins was actually beginning

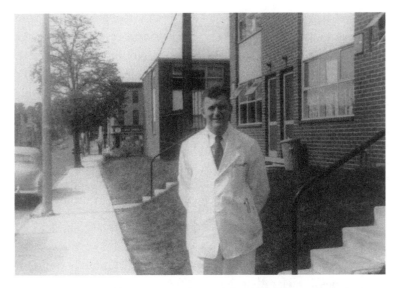

11. Eugene Braunwald at twenty-eight as a Johns Hopkins resident physician, outside housing near the hospital. *Courtesy of Eugene Braunwald.*

to lose some excellent applicants because of its approach. For example, a promising Harvard Medical School student named Burton Sobel went down to Hopkins for his internship interview, and once he understood that he would be on call the entire year, withdrew on the spot. Sobel was already married, and decided instead to remain in Boston for his residency, during which he and his wife would have their first child.[18]

Braunwald was asked to be one of three residents who went to the Hopkins chairman of medicine to request a change. "I was twenty-eight years old, and for the first time I was older than my colleagues, because they were just out of internship," Braunwald recalled. Braunwald's four-year detour into research had transformed him from boy wonder to "senior statesman" among residents.

The chairman was A. McGehee Harvey, a Hopkins trainee who had become the hospital's youngest physician-in-chief, at the age of thirty-four. The residents made an appointment to speak with him, and at the meeting proposed that Hopkins move to the Duke University Hospital system, which had residents on call five nights a week instead of seven. By later standards, the Duke system of the 1950s would be considered barbaric. But at the time, it meant asking Hopkins to take a big step in loosening up its famously rigid culture.

Harvey was not sympathetic. "So do you fellows learn something when you're on call at night?" Harvey asked.

Braunwald and his colleagues replied, "Oh, yes, sir. That's when very important things happen to patients."

Harvey responded, "Well, I think you'll learn more if you do it seven times a week rather than five."

And the meeting was over. Braunwald remained on call for the duration of his residency.

It was nevertheless a great year for him. As he had hoped, he was able to take advantage of access to Hopkins cardiology luminaries, such as Helen Taussig and Alfred Blalock. The relationship between those two was famously competitive and even tempestuous, but Braunwald knew he had a special opportunity to learn from them. He made it his business to visit Taussig's clinic and attend Blalock's lectures and conferences as often as possible.

"These were world-renowned figures," he recalled. "It was a thrill for me to attend those sessions and to hear them act and interact. I don't think they had much use for each other. But the Blalock-Taussig operation had been developed only a short period before, and it was already being done on a fairly routine basis around the world."

He met and learned from a number of other outstanding cardiologists at Hopkins, including Richard Ross and E. Cowles

Andrus, and got to know some of the upcoming young cardiac surgeons of that era, such as David Sabiston, Henry Bahnson, and Frank Spencer. In addition, he sharpened his skills in areas of medicine beyond cardiology.

His research career did not stand still during this time. There was one clinical rotation where his evenings were free, and he used to drive back to the NIH if he could get the car from Nina, or take the bus or otherwise find a ride for the forty-mile trip to Bethesda. And then he would work into the night finishing papers. He was able to complete a lot of work he had started in the first two years at the NIH. His reputation grew as these papers reached print.

～

As Braunwald was finishing his year at Hopkins, he became restless, and eager to return to the NIH—but briefly considered another possibility. He was completing his residency at Hopkins in early June 1958, and Nina continued to operate to the last day of her chief residency that same month. She had received a job offer at the NIH, and it was a rare simultaneous transition moment in their professional lives. They were excited by the future that the NIH offered, but thought they should at least be open to other options.

Braunwald was asked to consider an attractive job: head of the cardiac catheterization laboratory at the University of California, San Francisco (UCSF). UCSF was opening its now-famous Cardiovascular Research Institute, and Braunwald would be an associate professor—not bad for someone who was only twenty-eight and just completing his medical residency. The Braunwalds flew out to look around.

"On that trip, we both fell in love with San Francisco," Braunwald said. "I had been out there two years earlier to present a paper. But Nina had never been to San Francisco, and the city had an overpowering effect on both of us."

They started to think seriously about moving west. From Eugene Braunwald's perspective, the UCSF job wasn't clearly better than the role that awaited him at the NIH, but it was potentially just as good. What made the San Francisco option enticing was the city itself, and the possibility that it might be a better place for Nina to start her professional life.

"At that point in her career, Nina was primarily interested in being a cutting surgeon," Braunwald said. "Her job didn't necessarily have to be academic. But she was hesitant about going into private practice, because she wasn't sure that as a woman without 'connections' she would get referrals. So somebody suggested that she look into working at Kaiser Permanente."

Part of the appeal of Kaiser was that the staff model HMO (health maintenance organization) was growing rapidly in California, and it really needed well-trained general surgeons. They told her that she would have a full operating schedule on the day she started. She was excited.

But then Nina found that Kaiser was more controversial than she had previously realized. She learned that the American Medical Association (AMA) frowned on prepaid health maintenance organizations and that it was criticizing Kaiser as "socialized medicine." If she went to work at Kaiser, she could not become a member of the AMA or the California Medical Association.

Both Braunwalds had liberal leanings, and at that time considered the AMA to be a reactionary political force. A few years later, for example, the AMA would stridently resist the passage of Medicare. The AMA could not legally stop HMOs, but it could shun the physicians who worked for them. That gave Nina pause. "I have a problem with this," she said. "I don't want to join the AMA, but I don't want to be prevented from joining, either."

They talked it over, and decided to stay in Maryland and go to the NIH. A few decades later, Kaiser Permanente would be the largest healthcare provider in California, highly respected for demonstrating the ability of well-organized physicians and hospitals to provide high-quality, efficient care. Braunwald's younger brother, Jack, went to work as a hematologist at Kaiser, and retired after thirty-five years there. And the AMA's attitudes toward managed care evolved as well. But at the moment the Braunwalds were considering their San Francisco options, Kaiser seemed a bit too far on the fringes of medicine.

If Kaiser had been more respectable from the perspective of mainstream American medicine in 1958, the Braunwalds would have sought their future on the West Coast. Instead, they moved back to Bethesda, where Eugene Braunwald would assume leadership of the cardiac catheterization laboratory.

: 7 :

The "Golden Years" at the NIH

1958–1968

When Eugene Braunwald returned to Bethesda in 1958, the period that came to be called the NIH's "Golden Years" was in full swing. The NIH was the place to be, in part because there was nowhere else to go—at least nowhere that offered comparable opportunities. Most medical schools did not yet have the research infrastructure needed to support young investigators, or to surround them with bright people in other disciplines who would show them new techniques and give them new ideas.

External factors like the Doctor Draft were major influences on medical researchers, but something was changing in the very nature of research itself—something that made the NIH, at the time, not just the safest but also the best possible place in the country to develop one's career. By the 1960s, technological advances were making it possible to measure what had previously been unmeasurable. Researchers had a much deeper understanding of and interest in physiology, and the idea that medicine might be able to *alter* the physiology of disease processes was gaining currency. The research publications that sparked the most interest were no longer careful compilations of detailed observations on large series of patients, but experiments that stated a hypothesis, and then tested it. The new focus on experimental research required new ideas and sophisticated equipment, both of which were abundant at the NIH.

This evolution in the nature of research was accompanied by changes in researchers themselves. The tradition of William Osler, in which leading physicians were the academic version of gentle-men farmers—farmers (i.e., clinicians) first, gentlemen (i.e., re-searchers) second—was falling away. A new breed of leaders in academic medicine emerged: the Triple Threats.

This new breed was epitomized by physicians like Donald Seldin, the chairman of the Department of Medicine at the University of Texas Southwestern, in Dallas. Seldin was an accomplished nephrology researcher, but he made it his practice to do ward rounds and Morning Report with his house staff every day, reviewing the cases of the new patients who had been admitted the day before. His trainees constantly received the message that they should try to understand *why* things were happening with their patients, and if they didn't understand why, they should do research to find the answer.

This context gave rise to the Triple Threat—the physician who is an excellent clinician, researcher, and teacher. Thoughtful physicians would recognize important questions when they were taking care of patients. Teaching students and trainees forced those physicians to confront their own gaps in knowledge and understanding. Then those physicians could go to the laboratory to try to fill the gaps. Physicians like Seldin did all three things and did them all at a high level, believing that each type of work enhanced a physician's skills in the other areas. They became the new role models.

The Triple Threats soon emerged as the leaders of academic medicine. They knew how to get funding for equipment, for staff support, and for travel expenses so they could attend meetings to compare notes with other researchers. Acquiring funds required one to think strategically about the problems one wanted to solve. It was no longer enough to try to accumulate a large number of patients with a specific disease, and observe them.

"It's not that observation as an important skill disappeared, but people had to become professional researchers," Braunwald would later recall. "So a group of people emerged who did less practice. These professors had to spend significant amounts of time in research. They had the obligation to teach, but it was increasingly to teach postdoctoral fellows or graduate students, as opposed to medical students."

Braunwald noted that, in this transition phase, physician-researchers developed a form of dual citizenship. They were citizens of the community in their medical schools and hospitals, but also citizens of this other community defined by their research. "There was a brand-new culture," Braunwald noted. "Scientific and even social networks of these physician-researchers developed that had not existed before, and those networks soon became the most important relationships in their professional lives."

The new breed of Triple Threat leaders were familiar with each other's work and came to know each other's families. They socialized together in Bethesda and at research conferences, and taught each other how to play the new game. Meanwhile, the old guard faded away. "A lot of them were tremendous teachers and admirable clinicians," Braunwald said, "but they were not part of the academic network. They didn't go to the American Society for Clinical Investigation meetings; they didn't go to the Scientific Sessions of the American Heart Association."

Attendance at scientific meetings was growing rapidly (see Figure 12), and the conferences attracted actual and would-be Triple Threats. Braunwald soon became a fixture at these meetings, along with his teams of research colleagues from the NIH.

～

When Braunwald returned to the NIH from Hopkins in 1958, he was not quite twenty-nine years old and was assuming his first big job—as director of the cardiac catheterization laboratory within

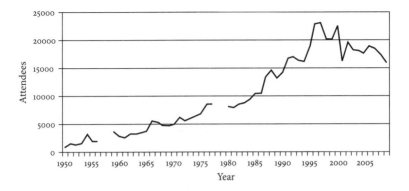

12. Attendance of medical professionals (physicians, scientists, physicians' assistants, nurses, technicians, and medical trainees) at the annual meeting of the American Heart Association. Data not available for 1957, 1958, 1978, and 1979. Courtesy of the American Heart Association.

the surgery section. In addition to leading an active catheterization laboratory staffed by several cardiologists older than him, he was to supervise medical consultation to all cardiac surgical patients. The responsibilities were considerable, but he felt ready.

He was given several positions for which he could hire promising clinicians and researchers, and immediately his ability to judge talent began to pay off. The first person he hired was Robert Frye, who had been a coresident with him at Hopkins and, after the NIH, went on to become chief of cardiology and then chairman of medicine at the Mayo Clinic. Braunwald also had three doctoral-level positions to fill. And for the first time, he could hire a secretary. He hired Mary Jackson, who would be the first of only two secretaries he had during the next fifty-five years.

His life with Nina was falling into place, too. They bought a home in Bethesda about a mile from the NIH, a choice that reflected their commitment to a long stay at the NIH. Eugene would often bicycle to work. Nina became pregnant three times and gave birth to three girls. "So now, everything was beginning to change," Braunwald said in describing those years. "We were grownup people and we were working next door to each other. And the fields of cardiology and cardiac surgery were just exploding."

About two years after Braunwald returned to the NIH, he received a tempting offer to return to Hopkins. Helen Taussig, the legendary founder of pediatric cardiology at Hopkins, was retiring, and Hopkins asked Braunwald to take her place. One Friday afternoon, he went to Robert Berliner, the director of intramural research at the National Heart Institute, to tell him the news. Braunwald said that he was probably going to accept the offer. "That's terrific," Berliner replied, "but don't make any decisions until Monday." Before the weekend was up, Berliner offered him the position of chief of cardiology at the National Heart Institute.

Braunwald was soon running the world's first truly integrated cardiology program, a group of clinicians and researchers who covered the full range of patient care and research issues relevant to adult and pediatric heart disease. The National Heart Institute had two well-equipped hemodynamic laboratories; a large, active cardiology ward; an outpatient clinic; an outstanding cardiac surgical program; a heart muscle laboratory; dog laboratories; and biochemistry laboratories—all within a few yards of each other. It became the model for modern academic programs around the world.

It was a time of plenty. In fiscal year 1956, funding for the NIH was $96.46 million; this rose to $183.01 million the next year, $211.18 million in 1958, and $294.38 million in 1959. The annual increases had begun to accelerate when James A. Shannon was appointed as director of the NIH in 1955, the year that Braunwald first arrived at the National Heart Institute.

Shannon had come with a vision and the political skills to communicate it. In discussions about science and health with members of the U.S. Congress, Shannon made the case that federal funds had previously been directed toward training medical specialists; too little had been spent on training scientists. He argued quite presciently that chronic diseases were becoming the biggest health issues for Americans, and that basic scientific research would be key to addressing them. The same public-health measures that had helped to control infectious diseases would not work as definitively for cancer, heart disease, and stroke. Shannon made the case that historic opportunities were being missed. He submitted budgets with explicit aims, including "the expansion of scientific manpower production, . . . a marked increase in the proportion of grants with long-term support, . . . and the exploitation of the full capabilities of the Bethesda, MD, facility."[1]

Marion Folsom, the U.S. Secretary of Health, Education, and Welfare, received the FY1956 budget request—and "the secretary's response was quite prompt," Shannon recalled. Folsom was not just a bureaucrat trying to control spending; he was really trying to understand what the NIH was doing, and to grasp its opportunities and needs. Folsom asked for a meeting with Shannon to discuss the requested increases, and made repeated visits himself to the NIH. Folsom was impressed by what he saw on those visits, and he became convinced that Shannon's plans made sense. Folsom backed increases in NIH funding on the order of 30 percent per year for the next few years.[2]

When Congress exceeded even those levels of support, Folsom formed a committee to review the programs of the NIH and evaluate whether they were meeting the opportunities and needs of the country. The committee was led by Dr. Stanhope Bayne-Jones, a Hopkins graduate who had been dean of the medical school at Yale. Just before Braunwald returned to Bethesda, in early June 1958, the committee sent Folsom its report, entitled *The Advancement of Medical Research and Education*.[3]

The Bayne-Jones report constituted an eighty-two-page ringing endorsement of the NIH, with support for its long-term vision. It recommended even *greater* increases—to a level of $1 billion by 1970. The Bayne-Jones report came less than a year after the United States had been stung by the Soviet Union's launching of Sputnik, the first artificial satellite to orbit Earth. It was not a good time to propose backing off from funding scientific research.

Folsom accepted the Bayne-Jones Report a few weeks before he left office, saying that it set forth "a philosophy and set of principles that will provide important guides to the development of medical education and research and the research affairs of the Department of Health, Education, and Welfare."[4] The funding for robust growth of U.S. biomedical research seemed assured, at least for the near term.

The fertile climate at the NIH made it possible for Braunwald and his colleagues to make significant advances over the next decade in four major fields: valvular disease, myocardial infarction, hypertrophic cardiomyopathy, and heart failure.

Valvular Heart Disease

Decades later, Eugene Braunwald could pinpoint the exact moment in the very early 1960s when the way he thought about valvular heart disease began to change. As is often the case with change, the shift was driven by a combination of embarrassment and necessity, and was precipitated by criticism from someone with a different perspective. That person was Glenn Morrow, who had been chief of the NIH's Surgery Branch since its inception in 1953.

The moment came at one of the regular Friday afternoon cardiac catheterization conferences, at which Braunwald and other NIH clinicians reviewed cases under their care. They were discussing a patient—a thirty-five-year-old man with severe leaking of his aortic valve (aortic regurgitation). This unfortunate man had exactly the same problem that Braunwald had created in dogs earlier in his NIH career, so he and the other cardiologists had a deep understanding of what was happening within the patient's cardiovascular system—arguably a deeper understanding than that of any other group of physicians in the world.

They just did not know what to do about it. Drugs could not fix the structural problem of the damaged aortic valve, and medications could do relatively little to alter the disastrous dynamics that Braunwald had described in his dog research. Cardiac valve surgery was still quite new—the first aortic valve replacement had taken place in 1960—and Glenn Morrow had performed only about ten such operations.

Morrow listened to the discussion, and then asked Braunwald how he thought the patient would be doing in five years if surgery was not performed. "I had to admit that I did not know," Braunwald would later recall.

Morrow erupted in disgust.

"What the hell are you guys good for?" Morrow said, referring to medical cardiologists. "You can't fix anything, and you don't know what's going to happen. If I operate on his valve, we have a pretty good idea of what his problems are going to be. But you can't tell me what's going to happen if we don't!"

At that moment, Braunwald understood that progress in cardiac surgery had rendered obsolete the medical techniques he had learned as a student and the research he had been performing. He and his colleagues had been struggling to understand the physiology of cardiac disease—that is, what was happening. Now they needed to understand what was *going* to happen—the natural history of these diseases. Because there were finally real choices to be made (surgery versus nonsurgical treatments, for example), they needed to understand the impact of various treatment strategies on that natural history. Medicine was entering an active new age, and the information needed by clinicians and patients was going to be completely different.

"The surgeons were talking about whether patients were alive or dead, and we cardiologists were talking about dP/dT," Braunwald recalled. (The term stands for "delta Pressure over delta Time," the rate at which left ventricular pressure changes with time—a measure of the velocity with which the heart is contracting.) Braunwald's point was that surgeons were focused on patients' *future* outcomes, while cardiology researchers were still describing what was occurring in the *present*. "We needed to bring the fields of cardiac surgery and cardiology together."

Braunwald was in just the right place at just the right time to integrate the perspectives of cardiac surgery and cardiology in the effort to improve the outlook for patients with valvular heart disease —and he had the right colleagues. At the NIH, he was shoulder-to-shoulder with physician-researchers like the surgeon Morrow and the surgically oriented John Ross (Ross had been a surgical trainee, but went on to become a leading cardiologist instead of a surgeon). During the late 1950s, the development of open-heart surgery had made it possible to contemplate aggressive approaches to cardiac problems that had previously been essentially untreatable. In open-heart surgery, cardiopulmonary bypass machines kept the rest of the body alive while the heart itself was stopped. Surgeons began experimenting with different approaches to correcting mitral regurgitation, including replacement of portions of the valve structure (such as the chordae tendinae, the long fibers that connect the valve leaflets to the opposite side of the left ventricle). One of those surgeons was Nina Braunwald.

Cardiac surgery in the 1950s and 1960s was not an easy world for anyone, least of all for a woman like Nina. "You must understand that the cardiac surgeons of that day had to invent everything as they went along," Eugene recalled. "They were improvising constantly, and many of their guesses were wrong. They were pushing the field forward, but they were often pretty cavalier about the lives of patients, not to mention the feelings of the people around them. They were held to a different standard. It was okay in that era for a surgeon to throw a clamp at an assistant."

Some of the most famous surgeons seemed to compete to see who could earn the most outlandish reputation. They threw tantrums and equipment, fired staff on the spot, or humiliated them by ordering them to stand in the corner, facing away from the operating field. Eugene Braunwald remembered a time at Bellevue Hospital in New York when his wife was assisting the chief of surgery during an operation. Nina's only role was to pull back on a retractor, which gave the surgeon a view of the tissues on which he was operating. She had to stand on a stool to get high enough, and lean backward for an hour or more, all the while pulling on the handle of the metal instrument.

The case did not go well, and the surgeon got angry with Nina. He kicked the stool that she was standing on, and she fell backward and struck her head. She didn't lose consciousness, but she was stunned and hurt. "There were no consequences for the surgeon, but today he would probably be arrested," Eugene later said.

Nevertheless, Nina had wanted to be a surgeon before she knew what surgery was. "She knew that she liked to do things with her hands," Eugene said. "She was just the second woman in the long history of Bellevue to be a surgical intern and resident—and she loved it." She had the psychological strength to be a groundbreaker—both as a woman going into a field dominated by forceful men, and as a physician-researcher advancing what surgery could accomplish.

When the Braunwalds moved to Washington, D.C., in 1955, Nina was not yet focused on cardiac surgery; she was actually doing extensive research on thyroid transplants. But she enjoyed, and was particularly challenged by, watching operations performed by her mentor, Charles A. Hufnagel, who had devised a valve that could be implanted in the descending aorta of patients with aortic valve insufficiency. There had not been any cardiac surgery at Bellevue, so she had never seen such procedures. Through Eugene, Nina met Glenn Morrow; he offered her the chance to get in-depth cardiac surgical training after she finished her chief residency at Georgetown, and then move into a staff position at the NIH. She leapt at the opportunity.

"He was just extraordinary to her," Eugene Braunwald said. "There were simply no other women in cardiac or thoracic surgery at the time. She was the very first woman heart surgeon. He would bring her to the annual meetings, and he was very generous in giving her prominent roles in oral presentations and on publications. It was a very, very wonderful relationship. When you look at the pictures of them together, you can see her enthusiasm."

Sharing an office at the NIH with Nina Braunwald during that period was a young surgeon from Akron, Ohio, named W. Gerald Austen. Austen was the son of an engineer, and had attended Massachusetts Institute of Technology expecting to follow in his father's footsteps. But he had been drawn to medicine, and had completed medical school at Harvard in 1955, two years after the first open-heart surgery with a heart-lung machine. For his surgical training, Austen had gone to Massachusetts General Hospital, where, during his nights off call, he had worked with his mentors on developing improved heart-lung machines. After some additional training in England and completion of his residency, Austen had been invited to the NIH, and assigned to workspace in Nina's office.

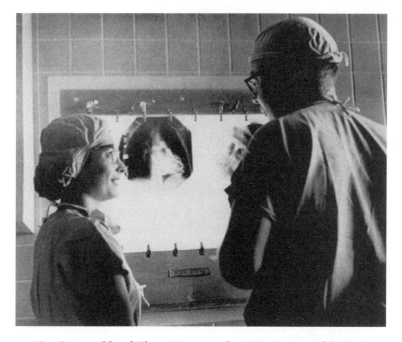

13. Nina Braunwald and Glenn Morrow at the NIH. *Courtesy of the G. V. (Jerry) Hecht Collection, Office of History, National Institutes of Health.*

Austen found Nina Braunwald quiet and shy, but determined. "She was very tough, and I mean that in the best sense," Austen recalled in later years. "And she was very innovative. She had a lot of good ideas, and she knew that valve replacement was going to be important."[5]

Working with Morrow, Nina Braunwald designed a replacement for the entire mitral valve, using flexible polyurethane flaps to serve as the valve leaflets, and Teflon ribbons to substitute for the chordae tendinae.[6] Eugene Braunwald would often see her working on the valve at their kitchen table.

Nina Braunwald tested the artificial heart valve in a large series of dogs, and soon was ready to try it in a human being. On

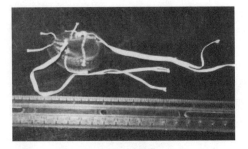

14. Braunwald mitral heart valve. *Courtesy of the Office of NIH History, Stetten Museum, National Institutes of Health.*

March 11, 1960, she used her artificial valve to perform the first total replacement for a mitral valve; the patient was a forty-four-year-old woman who was terminally ill with mitral regurgitation.[7] Glenn Morrow assisted her during the operation, and Nina stayed by the patient's bedside for the rest of the night. "She was too worried to come home," Eugene recalled. "We celebrated later, when the patient was discharged from the hospital."

The patient who received the Braunwald valve had an uneventful postoperative course, and initially did well after discharge from the hospital; but she died suddenly four months after the operation. The autopsy showed that the valve had apparently functioned well, with no blood clots; the presumed cause of death was a heart rhythm abnormality. Yet this Braunwald artificial valve never came into common use. Other valve designs led to better outcomes.

Just one day before Nina Braunwald performed the first mitral valve replacement, a Boston surgeon named Dwight Harken had performed the first successful aortic valve replacement, using a ball-valve design. Nina later helped to design another valve, a totally cloth-covered prosthesis known as the Braunwald-Cutter valve, which was implanted into thousands of patients. But the caged-ball prosthesis known as the Starr-Edwards valve became the most widely used model for many years. That design eventually gave way to newer valve replacements with better flow characteristics, greater durability, and less risk of causing blood clots.

The quest for the perfect valve prosthesis continues to this day, and will likely never end. But the question that confronted Eugene Braunwald and his NIH colleagues in the early 1960s was not which valve prosthesis to use, but which patients should get one. Now that surgery was a viable treatment option, physicians had to decide when to use it.

The opening sentence of the now-classic 1968 paper by John Ross and Eugene Braunwald on aortic stenosis captured the challenge concisely: "The advent of corrective operations for various forms of heart disease has placed increasing emphasis upon the need for accurate information concerning the natural history of patients with potentially correctible lesions."[8] The paper focused on patients with aortic stenosis—narrowing of the valve through which blood flows from the left ventricle into the aorta. Many patients with severe aortic stenosis had no symptoms at all, but some had chest pain and shortness of breath, identical to the angina symptoms of patients with coronary artery disease. Of greatest concern was that some patients with aortic stenosis would drop dead without warning, presumably because the flow of blood through their valve had abruptly become insufficient to supply their brain, heart, and other organs.

Aortic stenosis was not difficult to diagnose; it causes a loud murmur that the physician can readily detect when listening to the patient's chest with a stethoscope. Although valve replacements had become an option, the surgery itself was risky, and the artificial valves carried their own longer-term risks of infections, blood clots, and mechanical failure. Charles Friedberg, Braunwald's mentor from Mount Sinai days, used to say, "People always talk about patients with aortic stenosis dying suddenly. The most common cause of sudden death in aortic stenosis that I've seen is surgery."

Ross and Braunwald reviewed data from eleven published studies of patients with aortic stenosis. On the basis of those data, they compiled a graph which quickly became a part of every medical student's education (see Figure 15). They found that most patients had a long latent period, during which they had no symptoms; afterward, obstruction caused by the narrowed aortic valve gradually worsened. Deaths were rare during this period without symptoms, but the prognosis was dismal once patients developed symptoms such as angina, fainting spells (syncope), and shortness of breath due to heart failure. The average survival was five years after angina began, three years after initial syncope, and just two years after the onset of heart failure.

What if aortic valve replacement surgery was performed? Ross and Braunwald reviewed data on the prognosis of patients who had undergone surgery, and concluded that 50 to 75 percent of patients who had received older artificial valves for aortic stenosis were dead after five to six years. On the other hand, with more modern valve models such as the Starr-Edwards ball-valve prosthesis, the five-year mortality was only about 30 percent. Based on data from patients who underwent surgery at the NIH, they estimated that more than 80 percent of survivors had a good quality of life.

In short, progress in cardiac surgery was changing views on the "right" thing to do for patients with aortic stenosis. Ross and Braunwald's paper suggested that patients who did not have symptoms of angina, fainting, or heart failure were unlikely to benefit from surgery; but once any of those symptoms developed, patients would do best in the long term by undergoing valve replacement surgery. Ross and Braunwald concluded, "The risk of operation in

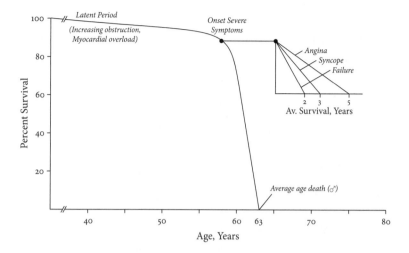

15. John Ross and Eugene Braunwald's classic figure showing poor outlook for patients with aortic stenosis, once symptoms of angina, syncope, or heart failure develop. *Adapted from J. Ross, Jr., and E. Braunwald, "Aortic Stenosis," Circulation 38 (1968): 61–67.*

this group of patients is considerably lower at present than the risk of non-operative treatment."[9]

That recommendation has stood for decades, although continued progress in surgery suggests that it will not endure forever. Advances in operating-room techniques and hospital care have reduced the short-term mortality rate with aortic valve replacement to the low single digits, and better valve prostheses have lowered the long-term complications of living with an artificial valve. Some data suggest that the mortality rate among patients who have had surgery may be even lower than that of patients with untreated severe aortic stenosis even if they have no symptoms at all.[10] And researchers have now developed devices that can replace aortic valves via catheters—without the trauma of opening a patient's chest and putting the patient on a heart-lung machine.

Hence, as medicine has progressed, the "right moment" for surgery for patients with aortic stenosis has moved to an earlier point in patients' medical histories.

Progress has also helped to redefine which patients are "too sick" for heart valve surgery. In Braunwald's very early research with André Cournand, he had seen that pulmonary vascular resistance (PVR) was "dynamic"—meaning that it could fluctuate with interventions such as drugs that dilated the body's arteries. But patients with high pulmonary vascular resistance were thought to have irreversible damage to the vessels of their lungs, and were thus generally considered to be poor candidates for heart surgery.

Braunwald led a study of patients who had high PVR but who nevertheless underwent surgery for mitral valve disease; he found that at six months, these patients almost uniformly had a marked decrease in PVR.[11] This paper showed that even marked elevations of PVR were reversible, and should no longer be considered a contraindication to surgery. Patients who had been considered beyond help were suddenly recognized as being potentially salvageable. The pool of patients for whom surgery could be considered thus expanded.

Braunwald had three coauthors on this oft-cited paper: Nina Braunwald, John Ross, and Glenn Morrow.

Myocardial Infarction

On September 23, 1955, three months after Eugene Braunwald had arrived for his first stint at the NIH, President Dwight Eisenhower suffered a major heart attack while playing golf in Denver.[12] At the time, myocardial infarctions had a special, ominous place in American culture. "Having a heart attack was like a 'bolt out of the blue'—and that was really the expression that was widely used," Braunwald recalled. "People—mostly men, because less attention was paid to women with heart attacks at the time—were struck down in their early fifties, which everyone considered the prime of life.

"So you would have the breadwinner of the family being perfectly well, and then it was like a thunder clap. They were struck down and either died or were irrevocably ill, and life was never the same. Just as it now seems impossible to predict who will be hit by a car, no one then knew who would get a heart attack. And the death rates were high, even among those patients who got to the hospital—and many did not get to the hospital."

The three words that came up repeatedly in descriptions of myocardial infarction were "unpredictable," "unpreventable," and "untreatable." Those three words faded from the landscape over the next several decades, in the wake of research progress combined with secular trends. Braunwald and his colleagues were embarking on research that would ultimately transform the understanding and treatment of myocardial infarction.

In 1955, soon after arriving at the NIH, Eugene Braunwald had begun working with Stanley Sarnoff on the question of how oxygen was consumed by the heart as it did its work, and what factors affected oxygen consumption. Later, in collaborations with Edmund Sonnenblick, Burton Sobel, John Ross, and many others, he had studied the function of myocardial cells and how they used energy. Braunwald and his colleagues found that oxygen needs were increased by three major factors, one of which was the tension developed within the left ventricle—which, in turn, was influenced by the pressure against which the heart must contract. Higher heart rate, and greater contractility induced by medications that stimulated the heart muscle, were also factors that raised oxygen consumption.

This research led Braunwald to develop a treatment for angina that briefly attracted much attention, but is now nearly forgotten:

carotid sinus nerve stimulation. In the 1960s, researchers around the world were interested in the impact of the carotid sinuses on the cardiovascular system. The Belgian physiologist Corneille Heymans had won the Nobel Prize in 1938 for showing how stimulation of nerves surrounding this swelling in the carotid arteries produced reflex responses that were the opposite of the effects of a surge in adrenaline. Massaging a patient's neck caused the heart rate and blood pressure to fall, and lowered the forcefulness of heart contractions—thus reducing the oxygen needs of the heart.

This news was not a surprise to observant physicians. Samuel A. Levine, a Harvard cardiologist at Peter Bent Brigham Hospital, had noticed that massaging the carotid sinuses could relieve symptoms for patients having angina attacks.[13] Levine taught his trainees that they could diagnose angina by rubbing on the patient's neck, and then asking a question that led the patient in the wrong direction: "Does this make the pain worse?" If the patient answered no, the pain was actually fading; there was a good chance that his or her chest discomfort was due to coronary disease. This diagnostic maneuver became known as the "Levine Test."

In the mid-1960s, Braunwald's colleagues in one part of his NIH dog laboratory were studying the effects of carotid sinus stimulation, while in another section, researchers were studying myocardial oxygen consumption. These two streams came together in 1967, when Braunwald was a visiting professor at the University of Rochester. In Rochester, he gave several lectures, one of which was on his group's research on the carotid sinus reflex and its impact on the venous side of the circulation. Up to that point, nearly all researchers had been focusing on the arterial side of the bloodstream, but Braunwald was aware that 75 percent of the blood at any given moment lay in the veins. The carotid sinus reflex caused dilation of the veins, which slowed blood return to the heart.

As he prepared to take a taxi to the airport, a young surgeon came up to him and asked if he had time to see some of the experiments in his laboratory. Braunwald went with the researcher —Dr. Seymour Schwartz, another New York native and NYU graduate. He was doing research on dogs in which he had experimentally produced hypertension (high blood pressure), and then attached pacemaker leads to their carotid sinus nerves. Schwartz had eight such dogs in his basement laboratory; when he turned on their pacemakers, their blood pressure fell.

"If they didn't have these pacemakers, these dogs would be dead," he told Braunwald.

On the flight back from Rochester to Washington, Braunwald could not stop thinking about what he had seen, and whether it might be relevant to his interest in ischemic heart disease. He wondered, "Maybe we can stimulate the carotid sinuses to reduce myocardial oxygen consumption, because it will reduce the three key determinants—heart rate, tension due to systolic blood pressure, and contractility." At the time, Braunwald and his colleagues were using a radiofrequency pacemaker to treat patients whose hearts beat too slowly. Power was supplied by a small battery pack worn on the outside of the body, on a belt, and transmitted to the pacemaker inside via antennae.

At dinner that night, after he had returned from Rochester, Eugene asked Nina what she thought about attaching those pacing wires to the carotid sinus nerves instead of to the heart. The idea would be that patients would activate the pacemaker when they developed angina pain, or do it prophylactically before engaging in exertion that was likely to cause angina. Nina's response was, "No problem."

They began to make plans for adapting the pacemaker so that it could be used to stimulate the carotid sinuses of patients with angina. Nina went immediately to the autopsy room to learn how to find the carotid sinus nerves in cadavers. She then tried the device in a series of dogs, and found that it was possible to stimulate the nerve without damaging it. Just over a month later, she and Eugene tested it in a patient.

"Well, the darn thing actually worked!" Braunwald later exulted. The pain of severe angina pectoris could be reduced or even eliminated when the patients stimulated their carotid sinuses with the device. "We published it in the *New England Journal of Medicine*.[14] And the whole time from the trip to Rochester to the first patient experiments was just about five weeks. Today it would take about five years!"

The use of carotid sinus pacing to treat patients with very severe angina drew considerable attention, because there were so few alternatives for treatment of angina at that time. Nitroglycerin tablets were available, but their effects were brief. Beta blockers like propranolol had just come along, but provided incomplete protection against attacks and were of no help once an attack began. Coronary bypass surgery and angioplasty were not yet available.

"So we thought that we had something that was pretty important for the treatment of angina," Braunwald recalled. "And then we had this one case who showed me how experience with just one patient can really change the way you look at a whole field."

As occasionally happens in medicine, this patient was one who educated his doctors by disobeying their orders. At the time, Braunwald and his colleagues had told patients with carotid stimulators not to use them if they had a prolonged episode of unusually severe chest pain. Physicians were concerned that a long episode might be a myocardial infarction in which heart muscle had died. They were afraid that a drop in blood pressure due to dilation of the arteries and veins might be dangerous, robbing the damaged heart of enough blood to supply the brain and other vital organs—including the heart itself.

One day, a man in whom they had implanted a carotid sinus

stimulator came to the NIH about four hours into the course of a myocardial infarction. The patient was placed in the small coronary care unit (CCU), where Braunwald immediately went to see him.

Braunwald saw that the patient had the stimulator on, and he told him to shut it off. The patient complied, and Braunwald departed, leaving the patient under the care of the CCU team. "But when I came back about half an hour later, he had turned it back on. I turned it off, and left again, but whenever I came back, he had turned it on again. I forget how many times we did it, but finally I took the power source away from the patient because we didn't want him to turn it on anymore." Fortunately, the patient recovered.

Shortly thereafter, Braunwald sat at the nurses' station reviewing the electrocardiographic tracings of his patient. A surprising pattern emerged. Braunwald paused and thought, "Wait a minute . . ." The electrocardiographic ST-segments were elevated above the baseline (a measure of the severity of damage) by about 4 mm, but when the stimulator was turned on, the ST-segments were only 1 mm above the baseline, signaling a marked improvement in the heart's condition. When the stimulator was turned off, the ST-segments went back up; when it was turned back on, the ST-segments came down again. Braunwald realized that the patient had somehow understood what was good for him better than his physicians had.

At that moment, Braunwald first understood that myocardial infarction was not a "bolt from the blue." The damage did not occur in an instant—it was a dynamic process that played out over hours. And he immediately began to wonder whether this dynamic process might be influenced—*hugely* influenced—by interventions that improved blood flow or lowered oxygen consumption.

Decades of research by Braunwald (and many others) would

stem from that moment. He and his colleagues began to study whether they could actually change the size of a myocardial infarction by modifying the factors that influence oxygen consumption—that is, whether they could increase the area of damage with some interventions and decrease it with others. Their findings would ultimately help to change the care of patients with acute myocardial infarction, from passive observation to aggressive intervention. But many of his key studies in this area would be performed only after Braunwald left the NIH.

Hypertrophic Cardiomyopathy

As was true with valvular heart disease, Braunwald's role in the discovery of hypertrophic cardiomyopathy was born of embarrassment, again due to criticism from Glenn Morrow. One summer day in 1958, Morrow summoned Braunwald to the operating room, where he was in the middle of an operation. "There's a terrible screw-up here," Morrow said. "I've opened this guy's heart and I just can't find anything wrong with it."

Braunwald had been called in and put on the spot by Morrow because he had been the cardiologist who had sent the patient to surgery. Braunwald had analyzed pressure tracings obtained at the patient's cardiac catheterization, and had concluded that the tracings indicated aortic stenosis—obstruction to the flow of blood from the left ventricle into the aorta. Careful examination of the pressure tracings obtained from the patient's cardiac catheterization had shown that pressures just below the aortic valve—still within the heart—were lower than pressures deep inside the left ventricle. That pressure difference had to mean that some kind of barrier was impeding the blood's exit from the rest of the left ventricle. These findings led Braunwald to suspect that this patient did not have typical aortic stenosis due to abnormalities in the valve, but was one of the rare patients in whom aortic stenosis is due to anatomical deformities just above or just below the aortic valve.

Braunwald had concluded that the patient was suffering from a rare disease known as congenital subaortic stenosis: a ring of fibrous tissue immediately below the aortic valve had narrowed the tract through which blood must flow with each heartbeat, causing a loud murmur along with the same potentially life-threatening consequences that attended aortic valve stenosis. Cut the fibrous tissue out, and the patient should be fine—that is, if the patient survived the operation.

Now that patient was on the operating table, his chest open and his heart still. Morrow had placed him on the cardiopulmonary bypass machine and had cut open his aorta, just above the heart. Morrow had peered in, expecting to see the tissue that was blocking the flow of blood. To his surprise, he had seen nothing—no fibrous ring, no deformities of the aortic valve leaflets. It was as if Braunwald had sent the wrong patient to the operating room.

Morrow had inserted his index finger into the patient's heart, but could feel no obstruction that might disrupt the flow of blood. He had made an incision into the left atrium, and inserted a finger from his other hand into the heart from that angle. He had noticed that the patient's heart was thick, but he could find no barriers to blood flow within it. There was nothing for him to cut and fix.

It was then that he had angrily summoned Braunwald to the operating room.

Braunwald never forgot that moment, and how sick he felt at the possibility that he had sent a patient who did not need cardiac surgery to the operating room. Just placing patients on cardiopulmonary bypass machines and trying to get them off after the operation was finished was still quite risky. For any physician, it is tragic to have patients die during an operation that they need, but it is horrifying to have patients die from an operation that they do not need. When Braunwald arrived in the operating room, he found Morrow looking "frazzled and angry."

Braunwald was at a loss for words. As he departed, he asked Morrow to stick a needle into the left ventricle and see if there was any evidence of the pressure gradient found in the catheterization laboratory. "And when I made that request, I said '*if* you can get him off bypass,' because in those days it was always uncertain whether you were going to be able to restart the patient's heart, especially if the surgeon had not fixed whatever was wrong with it. And then I left the room, feeling guilty of perhaps having been responsible for a young man's death by committing some inexcusable error."

Braunwald walked back to his office, shut the door, and sat at his desk. He was the director of the institute's cardiac catheterization laboratory, one of the most renowned such laboratories in the world; but he was still a young man, not yet twenty-nine years old, and he had made what seemed to be a terrible mistake. "After a while, I picked up the phone. I didn't call my wife. I called my mother."

While Braunwald was receiving reassurance from his mother ("She said the kind of things a good Jewish mother would say— 'I'm sure it's not so bad,' 'They're lucky to have you,' and so on"), Morrow was sewing up the incisions he had made in the patient's aorta and heart. Morrow *was* able to restart the patient's heart, and then, as Braunwald had suggested, he inserted a needle into the patient's left ventricle to measure the pressure.

To Morrow's amazement, he found the same large difference between the pressures inside the left ventricle and the aorta that had been noted on the catheterization tracings. Something *was* blocking the flow of blood with every beat of the heart, but the obstruction was occurring without any physical cause that Morrow could identify when looking directly into the patient's non-beating heart. Morrow was mystified; it was as if he could no longer trust his senses. He couldn't fix what he couldn't see and couldn't feel. The way in which he looked at the world was being challenged.

Morrow went down to Braunwald's office about two hours later, and told him about the pressure gradient that had reappeared once the patient's heart was restarted. "We just couldn't figure out what was happening," Braunwald said. "It seemed so very strange, and we kept talking about it every day."

Finally, after about two weeks, Morrow turned to Braunwald and remarked, "I've been in medicine longer than you have." (He was thirty-five at the time.) "Sometimes you come across something in medicine that you just can't explain. But you can't get hung up on it. You simply have to put it aside and get on with things."

"And that's what we did . . . until about two months later," recalled Braunwald. "Then another patient came along with exactly the same findings. At that point, we knew we were on to something new and that it might be very important."

As with the first case, the second patient was sent to surgery, again with the expectation that he would have some kind of physical obstruction causing his loud heart murmur and blocking his blood flow. Again, Morrow found no obstruction when he looked at and then inserted his fingers into the patient's heart. After the patient's surgical wound was closed, Braunwald rushed to the recovery room and put his stethoscope on the patient's chest. "I heard the murmur. The obstruction was there. We didn't know what the hell it was coming from."

If Morrow and Braunwald didn't know *what* was causing the murmur, they at least knew *where* it was coming from—the outflow tract of the left ventricle, just below the aortic valve. Their early uncertainty was captured in the title of the 1959 paper describing those first few cases: "Functional Aortic Stenosis: A Malformation Characterized by Resistance to Left Ventricular Outflow without Anatomic Obstruction."[15] In later years, they would be amused and embarrassed by that title. How, after all, can a patient have a "malformation" without any anatomic formation? How can a patient have resistance to blood flow without any obstruction?

The discussion section of that first paper showed Morrow and Braunwald thinking like Sherlock Holmes—eliminating all possible explanations until what was left was the truth, however unlikely it might seem. Here is the discussion's first paragraph (italics included):

> In the patients described, the hemodynamic evidence of obstruction to left ventricular outflow is unequivocal; in the first two patients a systolic pressure difference between the left ventricle and aorta was demonstrated on two separate occasions and was definitely localized to an area within the ventricle. On the other hand, it is equally evident that none of the usual forms of aortic stenosis is present since the absence of discrete supravalvular, valvular, or subvalvular obstruction was clearly proved at open-heart operation. *In these two patients it must, therefore, be concluded that the obstruction to ventricular outflow is of such a nature that it is only operative in the contracting heart and was not apparent during the diastolic paralysis induced by potassium citrate.* These features can only be explained by muscular hypertrophy of the left outflow tract of sufficient severity that flow is actually impeded during contraction.

Morrow and Braunwald had deduced that something dynamic was causing the obstruction; hence, the obstruction could not be seen in the nonbeating heart. Both of these early patients had unusually thickened ("hypertrophied") hearts; and before surgery,

Braunwald and Morrow had assumed that the hearts were thickened from the work of pumping blood past some physical obstruction. Yet these patients did not have aortic valve disease or a fibrous ring above or below the valve.

These patients' hearts were hypertrophied for no obvious reason. Instead, the hypertrophy itself seemed to be the problem. The obstruction had to be coming from muscle tissue bulging into the left ventricular outflow with each cardiac contraction. The heart was literally getting in its own way.

Morrow and Braunwald noted that there had been earlier reports of patients in whom muscular hypertrophy seemed to be the cause of obstruction to cardiac flow.[16] In later years, Braunwald made an exhaustive review of the medical literature. It revealed evidence from nineteenth-century autopsies of patients who almost surely had had this same condition, along with some prescient speculation as to the cause.[17] But such cases and speculations had been largely overlooked by physicians. After all, until the electrocardiogram came along in the twentieth century, the only way to detect a thickened heart in a patient was at autopsy.

In the late 1950s, patients with clinical profiles similar to those described in the landmark paper by Morrow and Braunwald had been thought to have cardiac hypertrophy for other reasons, such as a narrowed aortic valve or severe high blood pressure. Sir Russell Brock, a distinguished British cardiothoracic surgeon, had seen some patients with narrowing of the pulmonic valve (the valve between the right ventricle and the arteries that carry blood to the lungs) who had obstruction to flow from the thickened septum between the two ventricles. After surgery on the pulmonic valve, the thickening and the obstruction had decreased. Brock believed that the same dynamic could occur on the left side of the heart as well—a condition he described as *acquired* aortic subvalvular stenosis.[18]

But Morrow and Braunwald were describing patients who had no problem with their aortic valves or with hypertension. This meant that the hypertrophy of the heart was not a response to the need for the left ventricle to generate high pressures. The hypertrophy itself was the disease.

Other physicians began to send patients with similar findings to the NIH, and over the next eighteen months Morrow and Braunwald saw another twelve patients. They wrote a second paper in which they called their new disease "idiopathic hypertrophic subaortic stenosis"—also known as IHSS.[19] That name did not stand the test of time, because subsequent research would reveal that the disease was not idiopathic (with no known cause), but has a genetic basis in many patients.

The condition eventually came to be called hypertrophic cardiomyopathy, or HCM. (Patients with clear evidence of obstruction to blood flow, such as those described by Morrow and Braunwald, are often said to have hypertrophic *obstructive* cardiomyopathy, or HOCM.) Hypertrophic cardiomyopathy is now recognized as a common cardiac disease, occurring in about one of every five hundred live births.[20] There is a broad spectrum of disease—some patients have dynamic obstruction to blood flow, while others do not—but they all have hypertrophied left ventricles. And as became clear even from the first several cases seen at the NIH, HCM is a disease with a high risk of sudden death.

Buried in the last few pages of that 1960 paper was this comment: "It is evident that in some instances idiopathic hypertrophic subaortic stenosis may be familial." Three of those first fourteen patients were siblings. Neither of their parents had evidence of heart disease, but there had been several unexplained sudden deaths among relatives on the father's side of the family.

Braunwald and a colleague drove to West Virginia, the home of that family, where they examined seventy-five relatives, most of whom were first or second cousins of the three patients with documented HCM. Several had findings consistent with the disease. They noted that other case reports had described families with marked hypertrophy of the left ventricle. So they knew that there had to be a genetic component to this disease.

But they knew virtually nothing about how HCM might be passed from one generation to another within a family. After all, only seven years had passed since James Watson and Francis Crick had described the double helix of DNA, and another six years would elapse before Victor McKusick, the legendary geneticist at Johns Hopkins, would publish the first edition of his catalogue of all known genes and genetic disorders, *Mendelian Inheritance in Man*. Genetics had not quite arrived in clinical medicine. So, in that early description of HCM, Braunwald, Morrow, and their colleagues made that observation of the familial tendency, and then moved on to topics with which they were more comfortable: blood flow, pressures, and other things that could be measured, if not seen.

But the familial nature of this disease became increasingly compelling as more and more patients with possible HCM were sent to Bethesda. Cardiologists around the world were starting to recognize the disease, and they did not have any treatment to offer the patients. The one thing they could do was send the patients to the NIH.

At the NIH, research and the clinical care of such patients were closely intertwined, as was true for virtually all referrals to the Clinical Center of the NIH. Once, Braunwald went to the room of a patient, a woman in her fifties, to obtain her permission for him to carry out a left heart catheterization. She was thought to have aortic stenosis, and needed the cardiac catheterization as a prelude to surgery to replace her aortic valve.

Braunwald explained the procedure, obtained her consent, and then attempted to recruit her for a research protocol. He was in the middle of a series of investigations of digitalis, and asked for permission to give her the drug during the catheterization. She adamantly refused. "That's all you cardiologists know—to give digitalis. I've had it three times, from three different cardiologists, and I get much worse."

At her cardiac catheterization, she was found to have HOCM, not valvular aortic stenosis. After the procedure, when Braunwald went to her room to check on her, the woman's son was in the room, keeping the patient company. Braunwald was in his mid-thirties, was immersed in the pursuit of this new disease, and was brash enough to ask directly for whatever he wanted. He turned to the son, and asked if he could listen to his heart. The son shrugged, and took his shirt off.

Braunwald heard the same harsh murmur that was present in the mother and concluded that the son must also have HCM. He then requested permission from the son to perform a cardiac catheterization, during which he would receive drugs, including digitalis. Mother and son agreed. He, too, was found to have HCM. And the data that were obtained during the son's catheterization added an exciting new twist to thinking about the condition. The obstruction was variable—and that meant the disease might be treatable.

What Braunwald and his colleagues found when they took that young man to the catheterization laboratory was that digitalis, the age-old drug that increases the force of the heart's contractions, did not help patients with HCM. Instead, with each heartbeat, it worsened the obstruction to flow. By enhancing the "squeeze" of the left ventricle, digitalis forced more heart muscle into the out-flow tract of the left ventricle, and caused the obstruction to arise sooner in each heartbeat. The pressure gradient within the heart increased, the murmur got louder, and the output from the patient's heart actually fell. In a sense, the researchers were discovering what the mother (the original patient) already knew: that digitalis was a bad idea for people with her condition.

By 1964, Braunwald, Morrow, and their colleagues had studied, in great detail, sixty-four patients with HCM. At the time, this was by far the largest number of such cases studied at any single institution in the world. They had enough data and insight to put together the overall story in a special supplement to the journal *Circulation*.[21] The four signature features of their patients were left ventricular hypertrophy, familial occurrence, high risk of sudden death, and dynamic (variable) left ventricular outflow tract obstruction. In these and other papers they showed that the following interventions, which shrank the size of the left ventricle, all paradoxically worsened the outflow gradient in HCM.[22]

1. Less preload—that is, the amount of blood flowing into the heart. If they simply had the patient go from a squatting to a standing position, the amount of blood returning to the heart from the legs would fall for a few seconds. During those few seconds, the size of the left ventricle would decrease, the obstruction to blood flow would worsen, and the heart murmur would become louder. (In contrast, in a patient with "traditional" aortic stenosis due to a deformed heart valve, the murmur actually softens, because the amount of blood flowing across the abnormal heart valve decreases when the patient stands.) Medications such as nitroglycerin that dilate the venous system, and other maneuvers that decreased blood flow back to the heart, such as straining at stool (Valsalva maneuver), had the same transient untoward effect in patients with HOCM.

2. Greater contractility—that is, the force with which the heart squeezes with each beat. Drugs like digitalis and isoproterenol were useful for patients with weakened hearts because they made the left ventricle beat more vigorously. But as the son of Braunwald's patient had shown, a more forcefully contracting heart was a prob-

lem if the patient had HOCM. Edwin Brockenbrough, a junior colleague of Braunwald and Morrow, showed that the cardiac contraction that occurred after an abnormal heartbeat tends to be more forceful than a normal heartbeat—and that the amount of obstruction that occurred with these extra-strong "post-premature ventricular contraction" beats was greater.[23]

3. Less afterload—that is, the resistance against which the heart expels blood into the aorta. Medications that dilate the arteries (vasodilators) are helpful to most patients with heart failure, because they increase the amount of blood that gets ejected with each heartbeat. But vasodilators allow the heart to eject blood more quickly, too; and for patients with hypertrophic cardiomyopathy, that meant the muscle around the aortic outflow tract would cause obstruction earlier. The same adverse consequences occur if the patient has vasodilation due to exercise.

Knowledge of what worsened the pressure gradient in HOCM pointed the researchers toward interventions that might reduce the obstruction. Greater preload would be expected to enlarge the heart, and reduce the obstruction. Patients with HCM therefore are encouraged to avoid diuretics and other medications that reduce the amount of blood returning to the heart, and to drink plenty of fluids to avoid dehydration. Medications like beta blockers, which decrease contractility and slow the heart, can reduce patients' symptoms. The first beta blocker, pronethalol, became available in 1962, and the NIH researchers were able to obtain a small amount. They found that administration of this new medication decreased the pressure gradient and led to the first successful medical treatment of the condition.[24]

Meanwhile, Morrow was developing a surgical approach to HOCM.[25] In what became known as the Morrow procedure, he would make incisions in the septum between the two ventricles, cutting out muscle in the region that might bulge into the left ventricular outflow tract and impede the ability of the remaining tissue to contract normally. When the muscle was gone or could not contract, it could not thicken and cause obstruction. The operation led to a marked decrease in the pressure gradient in the outflow tract, and improvement in symptoms for patients with HOCM.

There were other medical centers where cardiologists did a fine job treating HOCM, but the NIH received the most patients with this condition, and it was where most of the research on this new disease was performed. Braunwald, Morrow, and their colleagues fully described the syndrome and its treatment to the extent that was possible with the technologies of the 1960s. That special supplement to the journal *Circulation* in 1964 represented the academic equivalent of an expert pool player "running the table"— that is, putting every ball into a pocket without allowing anyone else a turn.

"It was thrilling," Braunwald recalled. "There had been knowledge of a connection between cardiac hypertrophy and sudden death before, but it was all coming together. And the fact that the hemodynamics were the opposite of what one would expect with aortic stenosis was startling to most clinicians."

Almost everyone was impressed—but not everyone. One of the skeptics was J. Michael Criley, MD, who had been a resident with Braunwald at Hopkins and was a prominent Hopkins cardiology researcher at the time. (He later moved to Harbor-UCLA Medical Center in Los Angeles, where he had a distinguished career and made major contributions on a range of other topics.) In 1965, Criley published a paper questioning the importance and reproducibility of the HOCM work by Braunwald, Morrow, and their colleagues.

Criley pointed out that the correlation between patients' symptoms and the severity of the obstruction seemed weak, and that some patients with what appeared to be severe obstructions had excellent exercise capacity. Criley was also troubled by data showing that the pressure gradients were often variable and sometimes absent during the course of a single cardiac catheterization, or on repeat catheterization. He speculated that the apparent drops in left-ventricle pressure documented by the NIH group were in fact merely artifacts that were caused by entrapment of the tip of the catheter within the thickened muscular folds in the inner surface of the left ventricle. Criley's paper included data from a small number of dogs and patients showing that when the tip of a catheter was deep among these folds, the pressures measured were sometimes lower than in the rest of the left ventricle.[26]

The implication was that a tremendous fuss had been whipped up by the NIH researchers over what might just be a laboratory artifact. It was the first major academic controversy of Braunwald's career, and at stake were more than the egos of a few researchers. By this point, Morrow was routinely performing his operation to treat HOCM, and other surgeons around the world were coming to Bethesda to learn how to perform the operation by observing Morrow; they were getting important pointers from the "master" and then returning home to carry out the procedure. The procedure seemed to improve patients' symptoms—but in those early years, it still had a mortality rate of 5–10 percent. (With time, the mortality has fallen to about 1 percent.) Braunwald and Morrow were recommending the surgery in part because they had seen a startlingly high rate of death in patients with HCM and their relatives, and they hoped that the operation would reduce that risk. But if Criley was correct, patients might be undergoing a very high-risk operation without any chance of benefiting from it.

"We had quite an intellectual duel for a while," Braunwald recalled. At the 1966 meeting of the American Heart Association in New York, a full ninety-minute session focused on the HOCM controversy, attracting virtually every attendee at the meeting.[27] Shortly before that meeting, an apologetic Braunwald told a young NIH cardiac surgeon named Lawrence Cohn (later to become chief of cardiac surgery at Brigham and Women's Hospital and a major research force in his own right) that he could not present a paper on his work as planned, because the NIH group wanted its more senior "big guns" to do the talking.[28]

One of those big guns was John Ross, who had become the director of the NIH's cardiac catheterization laboratory when Braunwald was promoted to chief of cardiology. Ross provided important evidence against the trapped-catheter hypothesis by recording detailed pressure measurements obtained via a catheter that had been passed transseptally and then down through the mitral valve. This approach yielded measurements identical to those from deeper in the left ventricle, thus proving that pressure measurements were not artifacts related to catheter tips trapped in empty regions of the chamber. This finding was considered a refutation of one of the key arguments against the obstruction hypothesis.

Braunwald and Morrow never seriously doubted the validity of their findings on HCM, but Criley himself continued to express reservations.[29] The controversy faded in the late 1960s, with the development of echocardiography, which provided yet more evidence that dynamic outflow obstruction was real and a serious problem for many patients with hypertrophic cardiomyopathy.

With time, a nuanced, complex picture of the range of hemodynamic issues in HCM emerged. Cardiologists at Hammersmith Hospital in London observed that hypertrophied hearts relax more slowly than normal hearts, and that the filling of the left ventricle between cardiac contractions is therefore impaired. Less blood flowing into the ventricle meant less blood to pump out with each heartbeat. The concept of diastolic dysfunction became important in understanding the symptoms of patients with hypertrophic cardiomyopathy, but did not eliminate the role of outflow obstruction.

Braunwald and Morrow came to understand that there is a broad spectrum of HCM, with forms including:

severe obstruction *all* the time;
severe obstruction *some* of the time;
no obstruction unless provoked with medications that decreased the size of the left ventricle;
hypertrophy but with no obstruction at any time.

Within a few years, virtually all cardiologists would say that the NIH group was vindicated and had won the HCM war; but Braunwald was impressed by the fact that cardiologists whom he respected could become so personally invested in a position with which he disagreed. "I had also seen a Nobel Prize–winning scientist like Cournand hold on to an idea, even when everybody around him knew that he was wrong," Braunwald said. "This jolting experience with HCM and my observations of Cournand have been helpful to me in a perverse way. I ask myself frequently, certainly more than once a week, 'Am I doing the same thing? Why am I being so dogmatic? Is there room for another opinion?' And often I back off."

In fact, the treatments that Braunwald and Morrow first developed for HOCM in the 1960s—beta blockers and the Morrow procedure—are still frontline therapies. It is unusual for treatments for any condition to remain first choices for a half-century, and now these are complemented by some other drugs, as well as a less invasive way of accomplishing the goals of the Morrow procedure.

In a strange twist of fate, Morrow himself was to become a candidate for the therapies he and Braunwald had developed, and a victim of the disease they had discovered. "At that time, Glenn and

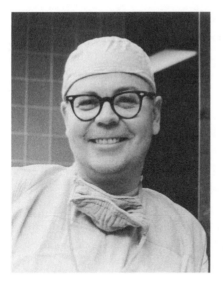

16. Photo of Glenn Morrow. *Courtesy of Lawrence Cohn, MD.*

I probably were working together in the same room at least ten hours a week, on a variety of topics, but none more frequently than HCM. We were so immersed in hypertrophic cardiomyopathy at that time, we simply referred to it as 'the Disease,'" Braunwald recalled. "We saw patients together. We participated in weekly conferences. And we sat and wrote papers together. It was a very intense professional relationship. Also, Glenn was the boss and very dedicated mentor of my wife. And we saw the Morrows socially as well.

"One day, Glenn said, 'Would you examine my heart?' He wouldn't tell me why. So I examined him, and I did a double-take. I could not have been more shocked. I said, 'My God, Glenn, your heart sounds a lot as if you have the Disease.' He had all of the features."

Morrow then revealed to Braunwald that he had been getting short of breath with minimal activities, and had at first attributed it to the effects of cigarette smoking. Many physicians still smoked at that time, and Morrow smoked at least one pack per day. Morrow reported that every morning he would have a cigarette after breakfast, and a second while driving to work. Then, as he got out of the car and walked to the NIH Clinical Center, he tended to cough up some phlegm. As he would get to the door of the Clinical Center, he would often feel light-headed, and would need to sit on a bench at the entrance to avoid fainting.

Braunwald realized that when Morrow stood up to get out of his car, the amount of blood returning to his heart briefly fell—thus shrinking his heart and worsening his outflow obstruction. When Morrow coughed, the surge in pressure within his chest also kept blood from reaching his heart, further worsening his hemodynamics. And then when he walked and pushed open the door to the Clinical Center, his arteries dilated—yet another factor that put him at risk for losing consciousness due to outflow obstruction.

By this point in their clinical research, both Morrow and Braunwald were well aware of the high risk of sudden death for patients with HCM. Braunwald told Morrow that he had to be catheterized, and then, depending on the findings, undergo surgery: the Morrow procedure, performed by one of the half-dozen or so *other* surgeons in the world who had reported favorable results with the operation. Morrow refused. Braunwald tried again a few weeks later, and over and over again during the five years they continued to work together. He begged Morrow to see another cardiologist. But Morrow wouldn't budge.

Morrow eventually developed atrial fibrillation, a common rhythm abnormality in patients with HCM. In atrial fibrillation, blood clots often form along the walls of the left atrium, and can cause damage if they break off and flow out into the body. Presumably as a result of such blood clots, Morrow had a series of strokes, and died in August 1982.

Heart Failure

At the NIH, Braunwald was able to pursue another question that had intrigued him since he first began seeing patients with heart disease at Bellevue Hospital's Thursday Night Cardiac Clinic in 1950: What is wrong with the hearts of patients who suffer from heart failure?

At Bellevue he had noticed several patients who came back every week. They looked and felt sick. They moved slowly, gingerly, because their legs were swollen and they became breathless with mild or even no activity. Their symptoms reflected the accumulation of fluid in the tissues of their lungs and their legs—congestion that resulted from their heart's inability to pump blood effectively enough to meet their body's needs. The sickest patients were clammy and cool to the touch, because the arteries supplying their bodies' surfaces had narrowed to conserve blood flow for more vital areas, like the brain and internal organs. Their pulses were rapid—ninety or more beats per minute—as their hearts tried to raise their cardiac output by pumping faster.

Braunwald wondered why the patients' hearts couldn't just squeeze harder and pump more blood, the way healthy hearts do when people walk up a hill or get excited. At the NIH, the chance to explore that question pulled him into collaborations with scientists who had expertise previously unknown to him.

Foremost among them was Edmund Sonnenblick, a 1958 graduate of Harvard Medical School who had interrupted his residency training at New York Presbyterian Hospital to spend two years at the NIH performing research. While still in his twenties, Sonnenblick began studying the function of strips of isolated heart muscle obtained from animals, and soon hit what Braunwald called "two grand-slam home runs."[30]

The first showed that the force and velocity of contraction of heart muscle cells were related to the length of the muscle cell at the time of contraction.[31] Stretched heart muscle cells contracted faster and more forcefully. This meant that high pressures due to accumulated fluid in the vessels feeding the heart would stretch out heart muscle cells—and lead to stronger contractions.

In other words, the congestion that caused patients with heart failure to have soggy lungs and swollen legs—also known as "pre-load"—was important for making their heart muscle cells pump more strongly. There was a reason that the kidneys of patients with heart failure were holding on to fluid: that fluid was maintaining the heart's output. The implication was that reduction in the congestion could actually decrease the heart's output and the supply of blood to vital organs.

Sonnenblick also showed that higher blood pressures could be expected to decrease the heart's output. In his laboratory models, he demonstrated that the force that heart muscles must generate affects the speed with which the cells can contract. Thus, if the heart has to pump against higher blood pressures, the heart muscle cells contract more slowly—so even as the rate (beats per minute) of contractions increases, each contraction is slower. The clinical implication of this finding is that the heart's output can be increased by medications that dilate the arteries—and thus reduce the afterload against which the heart is working.

The third factor affecting the force-velocity relationships of Sonnenblick's isolated heart muscle cells was their contractility—in other words, their basic strength. Medications like adrenaline and digitalis could increase the contractility of heart muscle cells (also known as inotropy).

One more factor can affect the heart's output: the speed at which the heart is beating (also known as chronotropy). Thus, after Sonnenblick's work, every medical student began to memorize the four factors that determine cardiac output—preload, afterload, inotropy, and chronotropy. This sequence rolls off the tongue of cardiologists like a Transcendental Meditation mantra.

Having hit one home run, Sonnenblick returned to New York Presbyterian Hospital to complete his clinical residency. (The home run metaphor may have been widely invoked at the time because Sonnenblick's paper was published shortly after Roger Maris's 1961 home run season for the New York Yankees.) He, too, aspired to become a Triple Threat physician-researcher. During his residency, Sonnenblick began to work with the recently developed technique of quantitative electron microscopy. With this new technology, Sonnenblick showed how the force of heart muscle cell contractions was affected by the positional relationship between the different types of filaments within heart muscle cells.

When Sonnenblick presented his electron microscopic images at the 1963 meeting of the American Society for Clinical Investigation in Atlantic City, "the audience was rapt because they sensed that something big was in the air."[32] Sonnenblick was unlocking the secrets of how heart muscle cells worked. Everyone was dazzled, including Eugene Braunwald, who was sitting in the audience.

After Sonnenblick finished his residency, he returned to the NIH, where he joined Braunwald's cardiology branch. He began working with Braunwald, Glenn Morrow, and others to investigate human heart muscle and function. They studied human muscle tissue excised at cardiac surgery, and sewed radiopaque markers onto the surface of patients' hearts during cardiac operations. After the patient had recovered from the heart surgery, the markers allowed Sonnenblick, Braunwald, and their colleagues to study the heart's contractions by measuring changes in the distance between the markers with each heartbeat.[33]

They were able to show that even mild exercise could change the force-velocity relations of the human heart, and that the heart's output could be lowered by medications that increased afterload (by causing arteries to tighten) or reduced preload. They also showed that beta adrenergic blocking medications could blunt the effects of exercise on the heart's contractility—thus demonstrating that adrenaline and the body's "sympathetic nervous system" were important factors in cardiac function.[34]

Through this work, the NIH researchers had a good idea of how heart cells and the heart itself responded to changes in its environment (such as changes in preload or afterload). But did heart failure actually change cardiac cells themselves? To answer that question, Braunwald, Sonnenblick, and their colleagues created a model of heart failure by putting bands around the pulmonary arteries of kittens. As the kittens grew, the bands remained the same size, so that the right ventricles of the cats had to pump against abnormally high afterload. Eventually, the cats developed hypertrophy (thickening of the heart wall) and then heart failure; the researchers then sacrificed the animals, and studied the force-velocity relationships of muscle strips from their right ventricles. They found that these cells showed reduced contractility, compared to those from normal cats.[35] The clinical implications of this finding were that high blood pressure not only lowered the heart's output by increasing afterload (that is, the force against which the heart must contract)—it could also lower the heart's output by weakening the cells themselves.

What was going on inside the heart muscle cells of patients with heart failure that sapped their strength? To explore this question, Braunwald and his colleagues had to develop new skills and find new collaborators. They examined issues like the availability of energy (as reflected in stores of creatine phosphate) within heart muscle cells, and found that the levels were abnormally low. The levels were probably not low enough to actually cause heart failure, but could limit the ability of the heart to respond to stress.

"In other words, there was no money in the bank," Braunwald later explained. "You had enough money in the bank to function at a reduced state, but not enough to respond to a call for more energy. You were functioning closer to the limit."

How the "bank" used the money it had available was another important question, and the exploration of that issue led Braunwald to a long-term collaboration with a young researcher named Burton Sobel.

Sobel's path to the NIH demonstrates the difference a few years and a few generations could make among researchers in this era. Like Braunwald, Sobel was Jewish and from New York City, but Sobel's great-grandparents had immigrated to the United States from eastern Europe around 1850, and Sobel himself "never had a twinge of any sense of being anything other than a totally assimilated American."[36] He grew up quite comfortably on 77th Street, between Amsterdam and Columbus avenues on the West Side of Manhattan, with several members of his extended family living in the same building or nearby. He remembered visiting Braunwald's part of New York, Brooklyn, but mainly to buy tropical fish. His father's family worked first in the clothing business, and then insurance. Later, his family moved to Westchester, and young Sobel commuted into Manhattan for piano and music theory lessons.

Sobel attended Cornell University for his undergraduate education, and graduated in 1954. By his own report, he did not feel the same kind of pressure to produce straight A's that consumed Braunwald during his college career. Sobel did work hard at topics that interested him, and he found himself drawn to the "hard sciences" of mathematics and chemistry. But, he recalled, "I did not take optimal advantage of the educational opportunities at Cornell. I was too busy doing things like playing bridge, making music, and living the social life of a college student. And my grades showed it."

So Sobel was surprised when, at Thanksgiving of his senior year, Harvard Medical School sent him a telegram offering him an interview. Sobel was assigned to be interviewed by Daniel Funkenstein, a psychiatrist who at the time was in the process of becoming legendary for his "stress interviews." In these interviews, Funkenstein created situations in which it was difficult to determine the appropriate behavior. He wanted to see how applicants would deal with the psychological pressure.

"I went into the interview, and there was no place to sit," Sobel later recalled. "So I'm standing. He doesn't say anything at first, and then he asks me to open a window. I go to open the window, and it's either nailed or glued shut. I couldn't open it.

"And then he offered me a cigarette. In those days, everyone smoked, including me. I took the cigarette, and there was no ashtray. So I was standing with a window that I couldn't open, and a cigarette that's dripping ashes all over the guy's desk.

"So I said to him, 'If you don't mind, I'd like a chair, and I'd like an ashtray, and then we can continue.' Sure enough, they materialized, and we continued and everything was very benign. But it was rather stressful, and I went home thinking that Harvard was not going to work out for me."

As it turned out, Sobel was accepted, and Harvard Medical School worked out quite well for him. (Funkenstein was later asked to stop administering such stressful interviews.) Early in his medical school years, Sobel had a research elective with a professor of physiology, Cliff Barger; and although he later recalled his performance as "inept," Sobel was sufficiently intrigued that he planned a summer doing research at the Cardiovascular Research Institute of the University of California, San Francisco.

It was an exhilarating and defining experience. Sobel and his wife loved the city, and he was inspired by working with the noted pulmonary researcher Julius Comroe on chemical receptors within the lung. Sobel decided that a career in research was what he wanted.

Following the same career game plan that Edmund Sonnenblick had used, Sobel did an internship and a year of residency, but then sought a two-year research experience at the NIH. Sobel was assigned to work in the laboratory of Donald L. Fry; but after a month, Sobel found that he was not particularly interested in the work being done there. He went to see Fry, who, without any resentment, helped Sobel to explore his more basic biochemistry interests, in the laboratory of Albert Sjoerdsma.

Sobel began to study the way in which heart failure is affected by the function of mitochondria (the components of cells in which much of energy consumption occurs). He was able to start collaborating, formally and informally, with the many established and rising research stars at the NIH, including Braunwald. Edmund Sonnenblick did the electron microscopy for Sobel's study.

These collaborations were fruitful, but not always smooth. At one point, Sobel became unhappy that Sonnenblick wanted to be a coauthor on one of his research papers. A larger number of authors would dilute Sobel's apparent contribution—after all, *everyone* always pointed out that Sonnenblick's big breakthrough had come on a paper for which he was the sole author. And Carl Wiggers's forceful message that *real* research papers should have three or fewer authors still commanded respect. Sobel felt that he was just starting out, while Sonnenblick was already established. Sobel wished Sonnenblick would remain in the background on the paper in question, and went to see Braunwald to talk about it.

Although Braunwald was only in his early thirties, keeping peace among his collaborators was already an important part of his job. He told Sobel to take the long view. "He told me that my reputation would be built on a corpus of work, on moving a field," Sobel said. "It would not be built on one paper."

According to Sobel, Braunwald said, "Years from now, you'll have a reputation as a biochemically expert cardiovascular scientist, and no one will ever think of Ed Sonnenblick as a biochemist in any way, shape, or form. He's an electron microscopist and muscle physiologist. So don't worry about it." Sobel followed this advice, and Braunwald's predictions proved correct. Sobel considered that conversation a critical one in his own maturation, and believed that Braunwald's deftness at managing potentially disruptive conflicts was a major success factor for all of their research efforts.

Creativity in research tends to occur at the interfaces between fields, and Braunwald was particularly inclined to cultivate those interfaces. He could see that Sobel had excellent skills in an area of science that could complement the skills of others around them. He knew that Sobel had specific expertise in biochemistry that could help deepen their understanding of oxygen consumption of the heart.

"I think what Braunwald found interesting about me was that I was trying to get into something about the heart that was a dimension away from what he had been thinking about up until then," Sobel later recalled. "He had not been thinking about my kind of work—but as all geniuses do, he immediately recognized the potential for that new perspective. He didn't react by thinking, 'Let's stick with the conventional.' He saw the value of a different approach."

Braunwald continued to be quite active in the care of cardiac patients at the NIH, and he knew that the technique of sewing radiopaque markers onto the surface of their hearts was never going to be useful in clinical care. He and other doctors needed some more practical way to monitor how patients with heart failure were doing. That led him to help develop a measurement tool that remains a basic tool in the evaluation of all heart failure patients: the ejection fraction, which is the percentage of the blood that is ejected from the heart with each contraction.[37]

In this research, Braunwald and a young surgical resident worked first in animals, and then in humans. They injected a liquid with a low level of radioactivity into the left ventricles, and then recorded radioactivity levels within the left ventricle before and after each heartbeat. Stronger hearts eject a greater proportion of the radioactive tracer; damaged hearts eject lower proportions.

On any given day, a patient's ejection fraction is influenced by the various factors that were illuminated by Sonnenblick's work— for example, higher afterload (increased blood pressure) leads to a lower ejection fraction. On the other hand, reducing blood pressure by dilating the body's arteries tends to raise ejection fraction. Hence, a patient might have an ejection fraction of 40 percent one day, and 45 percent the next. Nevertheless, this simple approach to making a quantitative estimate of the left ventricle's function has proven so useful to physicians caring for patients that it remains in wide use around the world today.

~

There were simply not enough hours in the day to explore all the scientific questions that were arising in cardiology. In later years, Braunwald would especially regret not pursuing one theme in heart failure research. He and his NIH colleagues began exploring whether heart failure led to increased activity of the sympathetic nervous system—the neurological and hormonal responses that help the body to respond to physical stress or danger. Osler himself had wondered about this possibility, but did not have the tools to study it. Neither did Braunwald initially, but the NIH was a place where one only needed to look down the hall to acquire new expertise. Braunwald's laboratory was just around the corner from that of Julius Axelrod, a brilliant biochemical pharmacologist who would later win the Nobel Prize for his studies of the sympathetic nervous system. Axelrod's technicians taught Braunwald's team how to measure levels of norepinephrine (a form of adrenaline) in the blood, in body tissue, and in urine.

They found that norepinephrine levels were elevated in about half of patients with heart failure at rest, but, with exercise, norepinephrine in the bloodstream rose to abnormally high levels in all of them.[38] They also showed that norepinephrine levels tended to be higher in patients with more severe heart failure. In these and other studies, they demonstrated that heart failure was not just a cardiac problem—it was a total body disorder with numerous neurohormonal manifestations. They found that the overproduction of norepinephrine occurred within the nerve fibers within the heart itself, leading Braunwald to write that the heart could actually be considered an endocrine organ.[39] This work led to a whole new concept of heart failure, called the "neurohormonal abnormality." In other words, abnormalities in the function of nerves and circulating hormones could contribute to the physiological findings and clinical picture of heart failure.

A decade later, other researchers would use this concept to make a clinical breakthrough. Swedish researchers showed that beta-adrenergic blockers—which block norepinephrine and blunt the effects of the sympathetic nervous system—could be beneficial for patients with heart failure.[40] Subsequent studies showed that beta blockers can extend survival and improve quality of life with heart failure, and guidelines today have made a trial of this class of medications a matter of routine for patients with this condition.

"I kick myself now for not trying beta blockers for congestive heart failure," Braunwald later said. "We were afraid. We were concerned that if we blocked the body's response to heart failure, the heart failure would get worse. In fact, we did studies that showed that beta blockers could worsen heart failure.

"But the Swedes showed that if they started at a low dose and slowly increased it, beta blockers could be used safely in many patients. And the benefit could be enormous, because the high sympathetic tone that we demonstrated wasn't a protective response— it was actually part of the problem."

The unpredictability of scientific progress was demonstrated on a larger and more dramatic scale during this era by the NIH's experience with its Artificial Heart Program. This initiative was launched in 1964, toward the end of Braunwald's tenure at the NIH. The mandate to begin the program came as a result of congressional action, and the goal was development and implantation of an artificial heart in a human by 1970.[41] The program's budget was in the range of $20 million to $40 million per year—a modest sum by current standards, but comparable to the entire budget for the NIH a decade earlier.

The resources were used to launch research at the NIH and at medical schools, universities, and industry laboratories around the country. Braunwald was named to the program's advisory panel, a blue-ribbon group chaired by the famed Houston surgeon Michael DeBakey. Along with leading cardiovascular experts from around the country, they met regularly to review progress toward the goal.

At first, the mood of the group was one of genuine excitement. The Artificial Heart Program issued contracts for the development of the hardware and devices that were expected to be essential for an artificial heart. Within a few years, however, it became clear that this goal was unrealistic. A 1984 analysis of the program summarized: "The first five years of work on the artificial heart proved that the initial objectives were quite naive. The scientific foundation necessary for developing the artificial heart was inadequate. The two major engineering obstacles—the development of a surface to prevent clotting and the creation of an implantable power source—could not be overcome by 1970."[42]

Researchers still needed to know more about the biology of the underlying medical problems that caused patients' heart disease, and about the body's systems for causing blood clots and fighting infections. Scientific understanding of these issues could not be mapped out on a project plan. It came in fits and starts, with bursts of new insights amid long periods of little progress.

Meanwhile, a new approach to the patient with a severely damaged heart became feasible: heart transplantation. The first human heart transplantation was performed on December 3, 1967, in South Africa by Christiaan Barnard, who had been a trainee at the University of Minnesota during those very early days of openheart surgery. Barnard and his brother Marius performed the transplant on a fifty-four-year-old grocer named Louis Washansky, using the heart of a young woman who had been killed in an accident while crossing a street in Cape Town.[43]

Washansky lived only eighteen days, succumbing to pneumonia undoubtedly worsened by the immunosuppressive drugs he received. After that, heart transplantation was performed only sporadically, until safer and more effective immunosuppressive agents were developed. By the 1990s, however, heart transplantation was being performed routinely at numerous academic medical centers throughout the world, with the main limitation being the availability of donor hearts.

Braunwald later recalled how the mood of the advisory group for the Artificial Heart Program became somber as they gained an appreciation of the formidable nature of their task. By the late 1960s, the leaders of the Artificial Heart Program decided to focus efforts on development of left ventricular assist devices (LVADs)—mechanical devices to help the heart do its work, ideally buying time for patients until their hearts recovered (for example, patients who could not be removed from cardiopulmonary bypass after heart surgery) or until they might be able to undergo heart transplantation. The budget for the Artificial Heart Program went up every year, but the real spending adjusted for inflation actually fell. The first artificial heart would not be implanted in a patient until 1982; the patient, a dentist named Barney Clark, would live just 112 days.[44]

"There was this cockiness of the Kennedy era that infected all of us," Braunwald said. "We thought that if the country set its sights on any goal, we could accomplish it. We were going to go to the moon, and we were going to develop an artificial heart. What we learned was that biological science does not move ahead with the same predictability as the space program."

~

During those NIH "Golden Years," Braunwald was in his element. There were so many ideas to explore, questions to answer. He and his colleagues had almost unlimited resources and plenty of stimulation from their patients, from each other, and from scientists in other fields. Braunwald was not one to squander the opportunities that lay before him. He worked incessantly, interacting with extraordinary people in many different disciplines.

"There were periods when he was completing a significant paper almost every week," recalled William C. Roberts, a cardiology researcher who joined the NIH during this period and who worked closely with Braunwald.[45] "No one had ever done that before. We'd work through the day, and then, nearly every evening, he would have one of the fellows over to his house. You'd sit with him at the dining-room table, and work with him through the evening. By the end of the night, the paper was essentially done."

Braunwald's nonstop approach to work was exemplified by an incident that became legendary among his colleagues. Braunwald read everywhere, even in elevators. One day, while reading, he got off the elevator on what he thought was the seventh floor. Still reading, he walked around the corner and went through the door that should have led to his office. When Braunwald looked up from his papers, he realized that he was in the wrong place. There was a woman sitting at a table, and Braunwald asked, "What is this room?" He learned that it was a new, ninth-floor laboratory within the National Institute of Arthritis and Metabolic Diseases. That lab had the technology for measuring metabolic rates in humans— the amount of oxygen that research subjects were consuming as they exercised on a treadmill, or simply sat or slept.

"I decided to stay there and watch what they were doing," Braunwald recalled. "At that time, we were doing a lot of work with digitalis, and even though the drug had been around forever, we did not really understand its actions. I thought to myself, 'Gee, this would be a wonderful way of determining if digitalis actually does something in patients with heart disease.'" Braunwald set up a research project with his newfound colleagues on the ninth floor, and studied digitalis's impact on metabolism in patients without heart failure, after exercise, to see whether digitalis actually reduced oxygen debt. The paper was published in cardiology's top journal, *Circulation*.[46]

Braunwald now ran the NIH's famous Friday afternoon cardiac catheterization conference, which met from 2:00 to 4:00 P.M. (see Figure 17). "It was by far the best conference that I have ever attended," Braunwald's colleague Bill Roberts recalled. "About eight of us would meet in this little room. Somebody would present the patient's story, and then we'd go into the patient's room and anybody who wanted to listen to the patient's heart could listen. Then we walked back to the room again, someone would present an-

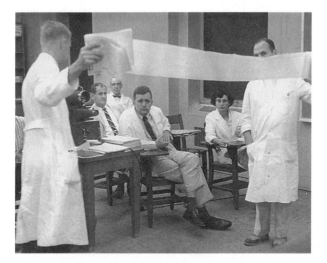

17. Eugene and Nina Braunwald at the NIH's weekly cardiac catheterization conference, 1963. *Courtesy of the G. V. (Jerry) Hecht Collection, Office of History, National Institutes of Health.*

other patient, and we'd go see that patient. It was just a wonderful experience. These patients were just mind-boggling."

Roberts also recalled that Braunwald ran a tight ship. "I remember that one of the conferences was a bit casual, and I think two of us were guilty. As soon as that conference was over, Braunwald said, 'I want to see you two in my office.' And I can tell you that there never was another casual conference."

Fifty years later, Jean Wilson, another former NIH clinical associate who went on to have a distinguished career, remembered those conferences well. "First, you have to understand the nature of the patients. The patients who were referred to that unit were all patients who had already had cardiac catheterization, most of them in university hospitals or in very good private hospitals— and they were complicated enough that the diagnosis had not been made by some very good people. Braunwald, who knew so much more cardiovascular physiology than most other people, made it a challenge to himself, a game, to figure out the diagnosis before the recatheterization.

"And most of the time he did. As far as applying physiology at the bedside, he was an absolute genius. He was really phenomenally good, and he made it fun for everyone. He was bubbly, and he had the nice ability to laugh at himself."[47]

Wilson, Roberts, and others recalled those days as exhilarating. "If you worked with Braunwald, you *really* worked, but it was fun," Roberts said. "You knew that nobody worked harder than he did, and nobody worked more efficiently than he did. But we felt like we were changing the world, and he was making all of us so much better than we would have been without him.

"Braunwald was receptive to any new idea, no matter where it came from. He couldn't care less about the source of the idea—he just cared about the idea. If you went to him, and said there was something new suggested by some of the patients we had seen with mitral regurgitation—Oh, I mean, he'd just love it!

"And what that did, of course, was stimulate me and everybody else to be thinking all the time. I know that I started asking questions. What was new about this case? If this patient had aortic stenosis and a bicuspid valve, what was different about this patient, compared to other patients with the same bicuspid valve and aortic stenosis?"

∽

As exhilarating as the progress seemed within the walls of the NIH, Braunwald at this time had his first experience with public controversy. In 1966, in the *New England Journal of Medicine,* a Harvard professor named Henry K. Beecher published an article on the ethics of human research.[48] The article did not mention Braunwald by name, but raised questions about several of the research studies described in this chapter. For Braunwald and the other researchers who had performed the studies, the Beecher paper provided a new and unanticipated type of scrutiny. In fact, in a 2012 retrospective, the editors of the *New England Journal of Medicine* singled out Beecher's piece as the very first major article on medical ethics in clinical research that the journal had ever published.[49] Thus, Braunwald's presence on the cutting edge of medical research took him into uncharted waters in more ways than one.

Beecher was an anesthesiologist at Massachusetts General Hospital who had studied the effects of pain medications while working closely with the U.S. Army during World War II, and he had been a scientific expert for human drug studies conducted by the U.S. Central Intelligence Agency during the 1950s. In the late 1950s, however, he had become increasingly interested in research ethics. In March 1965 he had delivered a talk at a conference on drug research, in which he had not named individual investigators but had discussed specific research protocols, all published, which troubled him.

The use of real-life research studies in Beecher's talk generated media attention, including major stories in the *New York Times* and the *Wall Street Journal*. Those stories led to criticism from some of his colleagues at Harvard Medical School, who called him an "irresponsible exaggerator."[50] Beecher moved to defend himself by writing an article that was reviewed and then rejected by the *Journal of the American Medical Association,* but then accepted by the *New England Journal of Medicine*.

In the paper, Beecher did not cite specific studies or researchers, but described twenty-two examples of "unethical or questionably ethical studies." His examples came from a wide range of disciplines, including Beecher's own specialty of anesthesia. He did not cite the specific research articles, but his descriptions had enough specificity that they were readily identifiable by researchers in the same fields. Many of the articles were famous studies; several were by Braunwald. Example 19 was the use of bronchoscopy to gain access to the left atrium, as Morrow and Braunwald had done in the era before development of transseptal catheterization. Example 20 was transseptal catheterization itself. Example 21 was a study of the effect of exercise on hemodynamic function in "normal" persons (patients whose diseases were not cardiovascular in nature), as well as patients with cardiovascular disease; in these evaluations, patients had catheters placed in their pulmonary arteries.

David Rothman, in *Strangers at the Bedside*, described the significance of the article: "However haphazard the selection process, Beecher was singling out mainstream science—indeed, science on the frontier. . . . These were typically protocols from leading investigators in leading institutions, working on some of the most important questions. Beecher was describing the clinical ethics of elite researchers, those already in or destined to be in positions of authority."[51]

One of the major recurring themes of Beecher's examples was that interventions were being studied that carried risk for the research subjects, and had virtually no chance of benefiting them. Normal volunteers were undergoing invasive procedures with a death rate that was only one in a thousand—but, still, greater than zero. Patients who were undergoing surgery and other medical treatments were having "extra" procedures added to their care, so that data could be collected. The risks were small, but Beecher doubted that patients had truly been informed about them.

In his conclusion, Beecher wrote: "Ordinary patients will not knowingly risk their health or their life for the sake of 'science.' Every experienced clinician investigator knows this. When such risks are taken and a considerable number of patients are involved, it may be assumed that informed consent has not been obtained in all cases." Beecher noted that the majority of these studies did not mention that consent had been obtained from the research subjects; and when it was later suggested to him that the researchers might have obtained consent but not mentioned it in the research papers, Beecher was skeptical. He simply did not believe that people would knowingly expose themselves to any risk if there was little or no chance that they would benefit.[52]

Beecher had not spoken to Braunwald or other investigators who had performed the research cited in Beecher's paper, and Braunwald began working on a case-by-case rebuttal. Braunwald later indicated that this rebuttal would have corrected some factual errors—for example, none of the subjects were "normal" controls, as asserted by Beecher; some were shown by the procedure not to have heart disease. Moreover, the patients in whom transbronchial and then transseptal left heart catheterization had been performed had benefited directly from the procedure. The rebuttal also would have emphasized that all patients who come to the NIH consent to participation in research as a condition of receiving their care, and that, despite this blanket agreement, informed consent was still obtained from all of the subjects for research protocols.

Ultimately, however, Braunwald decided not to respond; he could recognize a no-win situation when he saw one. Although he felt unfairly criticized, he saw that Beecher had made two points that were impossible to refute: first, that truly informed consent was difficult to obtain, and, second, that potential research subjects who had no chance of benefiting from an invasive procedure should be made to understand that they were undergoing risk solely for the greater good of humankind.

The furor generated by Beecher's lecture and then his paper lasted decades, as did speculation about Beecher's motivations. In a 2009 paper, George A. Mashour, of the University of Michigan Medical School, wrote that Beecher's interest in the ethics of human experimentation may have stemmed from his own studies during the 1950s. In research presumably supported by the U.S. Army, Beecher and colleagues evaluated subjects' responses to Rorschach tests before and after they were administered lysergic acid diethylamide (LSD). Mashour noted that Beecher had undertaken the research even with the knowledge that a Swiss psychiatrist had committed suicide after being administered LSD.[53]

In retrospect, Beecher's article and the ensuing controversy were considered an important "growing pain" for clinical research. In interviews for this book, Braunwald and several of his colleagues observed that Institutional Review Boards (IRBs), also known as Human Subjects Committees, had not yet been instituted at the time the research described by Beecher was conducted. Indeed, at the time, many innovations were being tested in cardiovascular surgery without pause to consider whether the clinicians were performing "research." It was a time of transition, and research ethics needed to catch up with research itself.

~

"As I look back on it, I think that decade at the NIH was probably the best period of Nina's and my life together," Braunwald later recalled. "We were totally fulfilled, personally and professionally.

Until those years at the NIH, life had been quite a struggle. Even though things worked out, it wasn't exactly fun. I had always felt like an outsider, and Nina had her own hurdles, being Jewish and having two X chromosomes. But during this decade, we felt relieved."

Their first daughter, Karen, was born in February 1959. Their other two daughters, Allison and Jill, were born two and six years later, respectively. Nina Braunwald approached motherhood with the same discipline she had applied to her work. "She was very

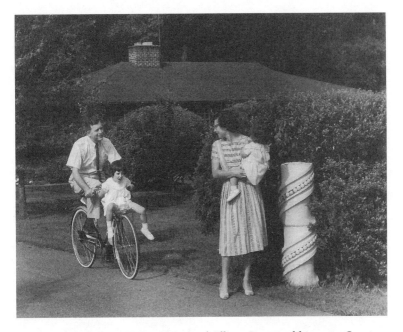

18. From left: Eugene, Karen, Nina, and Allison Braunwald in 1963. *Courtesy of the G. V. (Jerry) Hecht Collection, Office of History, National Institutes of Health.*

compulsive about getting up extremely early and being with the children at breakfast," Braunwald recalls. "We lived only a mile and a half from the Clinical Center, and surgery did not begin until 8:00 A.M. in those days. She was virtually always there for their dinner and tucking the children into bed. Not infrequently, she had to return for an emergency in the middle of the night."

Despite the challenges of having three young children, Nina Braunwald was determined to master the new field of cardiac surgery and to pursue her own career as a Triple Threat. During her pregnancies, she continued to operate through the eighth month, until she could not reach the operating table comfortably. Eugene

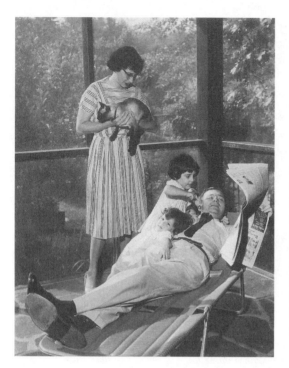

19. The Braunwald family with their cat, named for cardiovascular physiologist Carl Wiggers. *Courtesy of the G. V. (Jerry) Hecht Collection, Office of History, National Institutes of Health.*

Braunwald recalled she would say at that point, "Okay, this is great. Now I can concentrate on the laboratory." She would return to work about a week after each delivery, first doing paperwork, and then resuming surgery a couple of weeks after that.

Eugene and Nina Braunwald were ahead of their time in yet another way: figuring out how to make family life work when both parents had consuming jobs. In the 1960s, few other researchers at the NIH were facing this challenge, which would become commonplace a generation later. Eugene Braunwald had to plunge in and do his share of the parenting—and sometimes a little more.

"We went through a whole series of nannies," Braunwald recalled. "They each had a problem. One was stealing. Another was drinking alcohol. And the third one was simply unreliable—just failing to show up and not letting you know. Nina would have a patient on the operating table, and I would have to do double duty because no one's life was going to be in danger if I wasn't there in the next two hours."

Eventually the Braunwalds hired a nanny from Scotland named Rena Stark. She came for one year, and ended up staying until their youngest daughter, Jill, went off to college twenty-one years later. "She made an enormous difference in our lives," Braunwald said. "To have someone totally reliable and totally devoted to the children, but somehow knowing just when to step back and let the mother be the mother. And she was just seventeen at the time."

Braunwald remained extremely close to his parents through-out this period, and as the years went by, his appreciation for them only deepened. He recalled an episode during the mid-1960s, when his mother was deeply troubled by the health issues of her oldest sister, who had no appetite and was losing weight. She had been seen by several leading physicians in New York City, but no cause could be found. Braunwald arranged for her to be seen by his old role model from Mount Sinai, Charles Friedberg, but even Friedberg could not explain her deteriorating health.

One day, during one of their almost daily phone calls, Braun-wald's mother pointed out that her sister was taking digitalis, the same cardiac medication that Braunwald had been studying for several years. "Could this be responsible?" Claire Braunwald asked her son.

"Gosh, Mom, you may be right!" Eugene answered. He knew that excessive levels of digitalis could cause loss of appetite, weight loss, and a general failure to thrive. Braunwald's mother told her sister to stop taking the medication—and within two weeks, her health had returned.

After the crisis had been resolved, Eugene Braunwald said to his mother, "Mom, that was absolutely brilliant. How in heaven's name did you figure that out?" Braunwald's mother answered that she had been in the habit of looking at his medical textbooks in the days when he was attending medical school and living at home. "I've gotten a little education on the side," she said.

～

As magical as that decade at the NIH was, Braunwald understood it would not, could not—and, indeed, should not—last forever. The Doctor Draft remained a major force pushing young researchers toward Bethesda, but conscription of physicians had been rare in U.S. history, and it would end in 1973 when the United States went to an all-volunteer military. Of greater long-term significance was James Shannon's robust support for extramural research —grants that funded research outside the NIH. This research support was doing just what Shannon intended, which was to cultivate a generation of excellent researchers at medical schools around the country.

The NIH Bethesda campus remained a national treasure where important research was performed. But for the best and brightest of medical researchers, the sense that the NIH was the *only* place to be would not last through the 1970s. The intramural NIH program would become a victim of its own success, as the advances that occurred in Bethesda whetted the nation's appetite for even more investment in research. The U.S. medical research enterprise outside Bethesda became so robust that other options for building a career eventually evolved. As funding for NIH-sponsored extramural research grew, universities and other institutions encouraged their most promising investigators to build laboratories and supported them until they could secure sufficient grants. The best and the brightest no longer needed to go to Bethesda to become Triple Threats. They could develop these skills and build their careers at their own institutions. "Shannon understood what the funding for extramural research would do to the intramural program," Braunwald said, "but he believed it was the right thing to do for the country. But it was the end of our version of Camelot."

Still, it was a shock to his NIH colleagues when Braunwald announced that he was leaving to become chairman of a new Department of Medicine at the University of California, San Diego. "I think Braunwald saw the changes coming before the rest of us," Bill Roberts said in a 2010 interview. "He knew the action would be elsewhere, and he laid the groundwork for his move years before he actually left the NIH."

: 8 :

Building a Medical School in San Diego
1968–1972

Late in 1966, Braunwald was contacted by Joseph Stokes III, who had become the first dean of the medical school at the University of California at San Diego (UCSD) two years before. Stokes was a Harvard-trained epidemiologist who had a strong background in cardiology, and could thus appreciate the importance of Braunwald's work at the NIH. He invited Braunwald to San Diego, where Braunwald met with the university's basic-science researchers. UCSD was building a new medical school and creating a brand-new Department of Medicine. Its administrators had an ambitious vision for the way in which clinical and basic sciences could be integrated—a vision that resonated deeply with Braunwald.

Stokes offered Braunwald the job as UCSD's first chair of medicine, and Braunwald accepted. "It was an 'A' match," Braunwald recalled. "San Diego was a long way from home, but Nina and I had vacationed there once, and we loved it." He agreed to move to San Diego in July 1967, to prepare for the first class of students who were scheduled to start in 1968.

Braunwald's announcement that he was leaving the NIH to help start a new medical school in San Diego surprised many observers. Colleagues saw him as a young man who seemed completely in his element doing research in Bethesda. At the NIH, he was at the center of a whirlwind of activity that was changing cardiovascular medicine, pursuing fifteen or more projects at a time. He had virtually unlimited funding, and was attracting extraordinary patients and extraordinary colleagues.

Yet Braunwald had been getting restless. "I love steak, but I was eating steak three times a day, seven days a week," he would later say when looking back on his NIH years. "Things were going extremely well—but I began to feel, around 1965 or 1966, that it was going to become repetitive." Although still in his thirties, he felt that he needed more of a challenge, that he was getting a bit stale.

Braunwald's concern was that if he stayed at the NIH, his forties and fifties might feel like a reenactment of his thirties. He had decided that he did not want to pursue an administrative path at the NIH, such as becoming director of the National Heart, Lung, and Blood Institute or of the NIH itself. "I was not interested in testifying in front of Congress and probably would not have been very good at it. I wanted to stay closer to the ground, nearer to patient care, and to be personally involved in research. That's where I was most comfortable."

Braunwald had gradually become convinced that his personal future would be in institutions whose goals included patient care, teaching, and clinical research, along with basic science. "At the NIH, I was surrounded by people who were drawn to pretty basic laboratory research. I was confident that I could do that kind of work—study what happens in cardiac cells, for example. But my 'specific gravity' was at a different level. I liked research that was closer to patients and their diseases."

Braunwald was watching the era of the Triple Threat unfold, and he saw that an increasing amount of the action was outside the NIH, at medical schools. "The people who were rising to the top were people like Donald Seldin and Holly Smith," Braunwald recalled. (Seldin was chairman of the Department of Medicine at University of Texas Southwestern in Dallas, and Lloyd H. Smith headed the Department of Medicine at the University of California San Francisco.) "They were a half-generation older than I was, and by the end of the 1960s these people had taken over, and were changing the whole landscape of academic medicine. I admired so much what they were doing—a combination of teaching, research, and clinical medicine, all in synergy.

"I was particularly wowed by Don Seldin, and what he was doing in Dallas. I watched what he did, and thought, 'Now I know what I want to be.' Like him, I wanted to create an environment in which talented young physicians could become Triple Threats.

"I wanted to be one of them. I realized that I wanted to become a chairman of medicine. For a long time, I didn't even tell Nina."

~

A different world existed outside Bethesda—one in which obtaining research funds required writing and winning grants from the NIH, foundations, and industry. Braunwald was better informed than most NIH researchers about how that outside world worked, in part because, several years before, Robert Berliner, then director of intramural research at the National Heart Institute, had recruited him for a "Study Section" that evaluated grant applications to the NIH from researchers in pharmacology.

The first meeting he had attended was in Tucson, Arizona, in January 1961. Braunwald would later recall how they paused in their deliberations to listen to John F. Kennedy's inaugural address. The room had no TV set, just a radio. Kennedy talked about the torch being handed to a new generation, exhorting young people to ask not what their country could do for them, but what *they* could do for their country. Braunwald was awed by Kennedy's speech, which reminded him of how the forces of history had shaped his own life, and how—despite his growing success within the worlds of the NIH and cardiovascular research—there was a larger world of which he was a citizen. This perspective contributed to a restlessness that made him open to leaving the NIH, despite his success and comfort there.

As a member of the Study Section, Braunwald read dozens of

research proposals every year, and participated in intense critical discussions of them. He learned what made a strong research proposal, and what constituted fatal flaws. He also came to understand what sorts of backgrounds defined credible investigators, and who some of the most promising ones were. When he began to recruit faculty for his Department of Medicine, all these types of knowledge proved invaluable.

In addition to research and patient care, Braunwald had also been cultivating his expertise and credentials on the third skill of the Triple Threats: teaching. This area was certainly less important at the NIH than the other two—but Braunwald had never completely abandoned his desire to be a master internist and professor like Isidore Snapper at Mount Sinai, who could care for any patient and teach clinical trainees how to think. After returning to the NIH from Johns Hopkins in 1958, he had secured an appointment on the physiology faculty of George Washington University's medical school. In the early 1960s, he had decided that he wanted to focus his teaching time on clinical care rather than physiology, and he started attending in internal medicine at Georgetown University. By the mid-1960s, Braunwald was a full clinical professor of medicine at Georgetown. He attended on the medical service two months each year, during which he would get up at 5:00 A.M. each day to work at the NIH, and then head downtown at 8:30 A.M. He would see patients and teach at Georgetown until about 12:30 P.M., and then return to Bethesda to resume his NIH work.

While still at the NIH, he also began to establish his presence in another major aspect of medical education: the development of the textbooks from which trainees learn medicine. His entrée was his research on valvular heart disease with Glenn Morrow, Nina Braunwald, and others. In the mid-1960s, Braunwald was asked to write the chapter on valvular heart disease for the twelfth edition of one of the textbooks his mother had consulted, the *Cecil-Loeb*

Textbook of Medicine.[1] The invitation was a significant honor for an academic physician only in his thirties. It was a sign that Braunwald had "arrived."

A year later, though, Braunwald was puzzled when he received an invitation to write not a chapter, but a review of the entire cardiovascular section of Harrison's *Principles of Internal Medicine.* In every edition of *Harrison's* to date, that section had been written by Tinsley Harrison himself. *Harrison's* was by then *Cecil-Loeb's* rival—the young upstart that resonated more with the Triple Threat generation. *Cecil-Loeb* was tremendously respected, but was described as "an encyclopaedia rather than a textbook."[2] *Harrison's* was recognized from the start as something different, with aspirations to integrate clinical science and medicine, as demonstrated in this review of the first edition: "The chief aim of the authors is to integrate the pertinent content of the preclinical sciences with clinical medicine and to approach the subject not only from the standpoint of disorders of structure, but also by way of abnormal physiology, chemistry and disturbed psychology. This follows the modern trend in medical education. It makes for a rational understanding of the how, the why and the wherefore of diseases and their management."[3] *Harrison's* was in fact the textbook Braunwald had admired most since medical school. Since its debut in 1950, it had been shaping the way a new generation of physicians looked at medicine. It was the way *he* looked at medicine.

So when Braunwald received that invitation, he was a bit intimidated. Who was he, after all, to be critiquing the work of the great Tinsley Harrison? On the other hand, he was flattered and intrigued. In addition, the publishers were offering a stipend of $2,000—a sizable supplement to his salary, which was about $16,000 per year at the time.

Braunwald worked intensively on the review, reading every

sentence of the cardiology chapters carefully, pondering what might be done to improve the material. He submitted a ten-page single-spaced assessment, hoping that he had done something to improve an already great book, and reminding himself that he had at least earned $2,000 for his efforts.

Shortly thereafter, Braunwald got a second mysterious message from the publishers—a request for an interview. Now the solicitation of the review began to make sense: Braunwald was being auditioned for something, but he did not know what.

Braunwald went to a Washington hotel, and met with the editors of *Harrison's*, minus Harrison himself. The interviewers included George Thorn, from Peter Bent Brigham Hospital, and Raymond Adams, the famous chairman of neurology at Massachusetts General Hospital. Like Thorn, several had roots at Johns Hopkins, including Maxwell Myer Wintrobe (a distinguished hematologist who, like Braunwald, was a Jewish immigrant from Austria), Ivan Bennett (who had interviewed Braunwald for his Hopkins residency a decade before), and cardiologist William Resnik.[4]

They told Braunwald that they had read his review with interest, and now could reveal why they had asked him to write it: Tinsley Harrison was retiring, and they were considering several people to take his place as the editor in charge of the cardiovascular, pulmonary, and renal sections. Braunwald did his best to act comfortable with this notion, but he did not feel that way. "They were the acknowledged leaders of academic medicine in the country, and I was just a young whippersnapper from the NIH. Strictly speaking, I wasn't even in academic medicine, and I was twenty years younger than the youngest of them."

The interviewers asked Braunwald a long series of questions. Where did he see cardiology going? Did he know anything about pulmonary and renal disease? Braunwald assured them that he had indeed learned a great deal of pulmonary medicine while working in André Cournand's cardiopulmonary laboratory at Columbia-Bellevue, where he had personally performed many pulmonary-function studies and had also worked in a lung disease clinic. He confessed that he was less expert in renal diseases.

There was one final question from Ivan Bennett: "Have you ever seen a patient with carcinoid heart disease?" This particular question was a "lucky break," Braunwald thought. Yes, he had seen such patients before—in fact, he had seen many patients with this rare condition, which is caused by tumors that secrete high levels of serotonin and kallikrein. Such patients often develop scarring of the endocardium (lining of the heart). A senior scientist at the NIH, Albert Sjoerdsma, was perhaps the world's leading expert on carcinoid syndrome; hence, many patients with this disease were sent to the NIH, and Braunwald had frequently been asked to evaluate their cardiology problems, which were often their most devastating complication.

Bennett noted that *Harrison's* did not have anything on carcinoid heart disease, and asked Braunwald his opinion about this. Braunwald replied that he thought the book should include a short chapter on the disease. Bennett then asked what section he would put the carcinoid material in. Braunwald surprised the editors by saying it should be not in the cardiac section, but with the chapters on metabolic diseases. He told them that although carcinoid syndrome had important cardiac clinical manifestations, the disease was not primarily a cardiac disease.

Braunwald later learned that this answer won the job for him. He showed the other editors that he was not just another cardiologist—that he had a broader vision of medicine, and that he thought about diseases based on their mechanisms, not merely on the organs that were affected. He was one of the new breed of Triple Threats. A month later, he was offered the position as an editor of

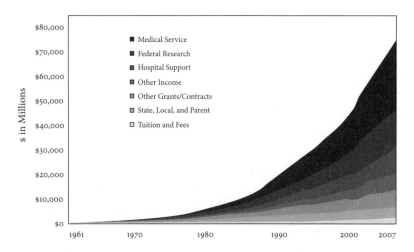

20. Growth in revenue at U.S. medical schools. *Courtesy of the Association of American Medical Colleges.*

Harrison's—right around the time he was leaving the NIH to become chairman of the new Department of Medicine at UCSD.

Just as Braunwald's timing in going to the NIH had been impeccable, he departed for UCSD at just the right moment. Braunwald was leaving the intramural program of the NIH as its Golden Years were coming to an end and as income and faculty recruitment at medical schools were about to rise (see Figures 20 and 21). The growth in number and in size of medical schools was accelerated by the passage of Medicare and Medicaid in 1965, and by the expansion of NIH funding for research outside the NIH's Bethesda campus.

UCSD was a new general campus of the University of California. It had been founded in 1960 during a period of ambitious expansion of California's higher-education system. In a sense, the opening of UCSD's medical school was a long-term consequence

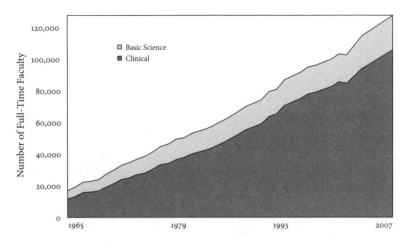

21. Increase in full-time faculty at U.S. medical schools. *Courtesy of the Association of American Medical Colleges.*

of the opening of Johns Hopkins in the late nineteenth century, and of the influential Flexner Report that had celebrated it in 1910. Abraham Flexner (1866–1959) was an educator who had been asked by the American Medical Association and the Carnegie Foundation to study U.S. medical education. He had visited all 155 medical schools in North America, and had been appalled by what he saw. He documented the variability and general inadequacy of the admissions and educational processes at most schools. The report concluded that the nation had too many medical schools, that too many doctors were being trained, and that most of them were being trained poorly. It singled out Johns Hopkins as a model worth emulating, and also offered praise for Harvard, Western Reserve, Michigan, and a few other schools. But other than these select schools, Flexner was scathing in his assessments.

The bluntness of his final report became famous. For example, he called Chicago's fourteen medical schools "a disgrace," and wrote that "the city of Chicago is in respect to medical education the plague spot of the country. . . . With the indubitable connivance of the state board, [standards for applicants] are, and have long been, flagrantly violated. . . . There is absolutely no guarantee that the candidate accepted on the equivalent basis has had an education even remotely resembling high school training."[5] He made specific recommendations for the requirements to be met by medical-school applicants and for the length and content of medical education, and urged that stand-alone for-profit medical schools be closed or incorporated into existing universities.

In the wake of the Flexner Report, the number of degree-granting U.S. medical schools fell from 160 to 85 by 1920, and declined to 66 by 1935. A quarter-century later, in 1960, only 86 U.S. medical schools were accredited by the Liaison Committee on Medical Education.[6] Flexner had achieved his goal of cutting away the weakest parts of the medical-education system; but as a result, a physician shortage loomed just as the American body politic was getting increasingly interested in health. So as Braunwald was beginning his NIH career, plans were launched for 40 new medical schools in the 1960s and 1970s, and a 50 percent increase in the number of young physicians being trained. One of those new medical schools was at the University of California, San Diego.

It was a time of remarkable optimism and growth throughout the University of California system. From the start, UCSD was planned as a graduate school of science and engineering, and its founders hoped that it would one day rival California Institute of Technology (Caltech), which was located just 120 miles to the north, in Pasadena. Large gifts were donated by industry, enabling recruitment of outstanding faculty, such as Harold Urey, who had won the Nobel Prize in Chemistry in 1934, and Maria Goeppert-Mayer, whose research proposing the nuclear shell of the atomic nucleus would make her the second woman (after Marie Curie) to win the Nobel Prize in Physics, in 1963.

When the graduate division of UCSD opened, in 1960, its classes initially met in the nearby Scripps Institute of Oceanography, a branch of the new university. Graduate training was offered in physics, biology, chemistry, and earth science. Within a few years, new facilities had been completed for the School of Science and Engineering, and buildings were under construction for the social sciences and the humanities. The first undergraduates were accepted in 1964.

But UCSD did not have a medical school. Its leaders seized the opportunity to create one that would be fully integrated with the rest of the university, in particular with its graduate schools. The Yale biologist David Bonner, who was the founder of UCSD's Department of Biology, articulated a vision in which graduate- and medical-school faculties would be merged, thus ensuring a free flow of information and ideas among researchers, teachers, and physicians.[7]

"UCSD had a plan for its medical school that had me very, very excited," Braunwald later recalled. "The basic premise was that this was going to be very different from any organization and from any medical school that existed at the time. Everywhere else, the various departments were very powerful, and run like fiefdoms. There were very few interdepartmental interactions, and virtually no interaction between schools within the university."

Elite institutions such as Hopkins and Harvard had superb clinicians and excellent basic scientists, but in the 1960s collaboration among them occurred by accident, not by design. In UCSD's vision, research was going to be a powerful part of the educational program, and there would be no basic-science departments at the medical school. Instead, the basic-science teaching was going to be divided among the clinical departments, which were integrated with the rest of the university's campus. Collaboration between basic and clinical scientists was as fundamental to the plan as the recruitment of outstanding individuals.

The UCSD School of Medicine was poised to train a generation of Triple Threat physicians like Braunwald and his NIH colleagues, a generation that would be fully comfortable moving from basic-science laboratory bench to the bedside, and back. The term "translational research," later invoked to refer to the translation of basic laboratory research into clinical advances, was not used in the late 1960s but actually was at the core of the UCSD approach to research. (The phrase first appeared in medicine's leading journal, the *New England Journal of Medicine,* in a 2003 article on the use of stem cells to repair injured tissue.)[8] At the NIH, Braunwald had seen the intellectual energy that could be generated by the juxtaposition of different disciplines. He had been able to discuss fundamental muscle biology with Edmund Sonnenblick, while actual patient care was being delivered on the clinical cardiology unit just four doors away.

"The philosophy behind UCSD was perfect for me," Braunwald said. "At the NIH, I was deeply involved in research, and now I could make that next step to lead a large research enterprise that was broader than my own work. I could use approaches that I had been exposed to at the NIH to develop research in other medical specialties, such as endocrinology and infectious disease."

The plan made perfect sense for someone whose view of medicine had been shaped by *Harrison's Principles of Internal Medicine,* and who had found his stride as a clinical associate at the NIH. Still, it was an audacious move. Braunwald would have to hire the entire faculty for a new department and play a major leadership role in developing a curriculum for the medical students. He was comfortable with the role of being a research director—but for him to create and run educational and full clinical-care programs was a huge leap.

There are advantages to having a grand vision and a blank slate, but there are disadvantages, too. For starters, UCSD's medical school did not have a hospital. It leased the county hospital in Hillcrest, a densely populated, diverse neighborhood just northwest of the city's Balboa Park. Braunwald's Department of Medicine was to have 10,000 square feet of renovated space in the basement of that hospital immediately, and then, within a year, additional space would be made available as new facilities came on line at the university's campus in La Jolla. Braunwald began recruiting faculty, including six researchers from the NIH, such as Burton Sobel and John Ross. He lured away many of the NIH's rising stars. "My former bosses at the NIH were not happy with me," Braunwald recalled, "but they understood."

Braunwald started going out to San Diego once a month, beginning in January 1967, and quickly became concerned that the renovations needed for a July 1967 move were not progressing rapidly enough. "I was getting more and more nervous," he recalled. "I felt a tremendous obligation to the people I was going to bring. They were all married, and they had children. I had moved their appointments through the university. They were changing their lives because they believed in me, but there was no place for them to go."

As the months went by and the July 1967 date loomed, Braunwald's agitation increased. He felt like the leader of a band of pioneers who were supposed to cross the continent to provide the intellectual energy for a new medical school. Within his family, the uncertainty was a huge problem. Nina Braunwald had her own career, after all. They had purchased property in La Jolla on which to build a house, and decisions needed to be made about the start of construction. Braunwald had to act.

"I had many sleepless nights," he recalled. Still, his pleas for more progress did not seem to be yielding results. In late spring, he finally said to the dean, Joseph Stokes, "This isn't going anywhere. I'm not coming."

As Braunwald expected, a crisis ensued. He went to San Diego for a meeting with the chancellor, who previously had met Braunwald for only a single forty-five-minute conversation. The chancellor did not want to lose Braunwald and risk a ripple effect that would give other recruits cold feet. The result was the forced resignation of Stokes as dean, and the appointment of Clifford Grobstein as his successor. Grobstein was a highly respected developmental biologist, and David Bonner's successor as chairman of biology. He was not a physician and was thus an unusual choice to be dean of a medical school. But he was an effective administrator who could get things done.

Braunwald helped the chancellor to create a new role for Stokes as the head of the Department for Community and Family Medicine. After all, Stokes was the person who had hired him, and Braunwald felt a sense of obligation toward Stokes even though he had been unhappy with Stokes's inability to implement their plans. In addition, in the late 1960s, Community Medicine was an important emerging area, and Stokes was well equipped to lead this new department. Braunwald then made plans to delay his own move for one year, and turned to calming down and trying to retain the outstanding young researchers whom he had worked so hard to recruit.

One of those recruits who had a family was Burton Sobel, the young physician from New York and Harvard who had so impressed Braunwald with his ability to bring biochemistry expertise to research on heart failure. After his two-year stint at the NIH, Sobel had returned to the Peter Bent Brigham Hospital in Boston to complete his residency training. He was offered a position with Richard Gorlin, a highly respected cardiovascular researcher at the Brigham, at the same time that Braunwald invited him to come to San Diego.

"I was really conflicted," Sobel recalled in a 2009 interview. "On one hand, if I stayed at the Brigham with Gorlin, I felt like everything would be secure. The Brigham and Harvard were the Holy Land of academics, after all. San Diego was a long way away, and I had never been anywhere near there. I knew that there were palm trees and all sorts of other things about which I didn't have the faintest idea. But I also knew that San Diego would have Braunwald."

Sobel did not know what to do, and finally sought advice from William Reddy, a physiology researcher at Harvard. The resulting conversation helped Sobel to make up his mind, and changed the way he looked at life itself. Reddy had been a promising student in high school and had won a scholarship to Harvard, with plans to go to medical school. But he developed muscular dystrophy, a severe variant that would limit his life expectancy and eliminate any chance of his becoming a physician.

Clifford Barger, a Harvard physiologist who was likewise Sobel's mentor, had taken Reddy under his wing and encouraged him to get a PhD in physiology. Sobel would often see Barger and his wife helping the wheelchair-bound Reddy negotiate flights of steps. Reddy turned out to be a brilliant biochemist, and played a critical role in the research on steroids in the laboratory of George Thorn, chairman of the Brigham's Department of Medicine.

Sobel recalled his conversation with Reddy. "He was sitting behind his desk, and he could barely move because he was so disabled. I told him about my dilemma—whether to stay at a great place with friends that I loved, or go chasing out to San Diego with this fellow Gene Braunwald. I told him that I knew Braunwald a little bit and thought that he was very inspiring, but I didn't think it was a sure thing that he was going to be able to run this medical school at all."

Reddy reflected for a moment, and then, according to Sobel, said that it didn't really matter what decision he made: "What is going to determine whether you're successful is not where you are, but what you accomplish. If you're good, and do good work and advance knowledge, you'll be fine. And if you don't, you can be in the finest citadel of excellence, and it's not going to matter."

Sobel took a deep breath, and thanked Reddy. "I think I'm going to San Diego," he said. In retrospect, Sobel's assessment was that Reddy had a perspective on life and work that was shaped by his disease and prognosis. Reddy understood that a person's sense of security should not be based on the reputation of the institution with which he or she was affiliated. What mattered was making an important contribution to knowledge, not being at a famous place like Harvard. And Sobel's instincts told him that working with Gene Braunwald was the path most likely to lead to that contribution.

~

Braunwald met no objections when he told the NIH that he needed to stay in Bethesda one more year (a year that turned out to be another extremely productive one for his group's research program). Meanwhile, he was flying back and forth to San Diego each month and helping to recruit additional faculty for UCSD, including new chairmen for the departments of Pathology and Radiology.

During that last NIH year, UCSD had a five-day curriculum planning retreat in Borrego Springs, California, and Braunwald knew that he had to be there. Since everything about UCSD's curriculum was being invented for an organizational structure that had no precedent, the faculty had to address fundamental questions, such as who would teach anatomy (the Department of Surgery, they decided) and who would teach biochemistry (the university's Department of Chemistry). Braunwald had never served on a medical-school curriculum committee, and had to come up with plans for basic issues such as how to teach students the skills of physical diagnosis.

Two days before leaving Bethesda for the Borrego Springs meeting, Braunwald fell off his bicycle and fractured part of his pelvis (the iliac bone). He was in considerable pain and confined to a wheelchair, but was nevertheless determined to attend. In those days, passengers could enter airliners only by climbing stairs, and a special motorized apparatus was employed to get Braunwald on and off the plane. An ambulance was used for ground transportation. Braunwald's thinking was clouded by the codeine he was taking for pain, but he did not miss the meeting.

The assembled faculty leaders were making decisions such as how many hours were going to be devoted to specific courses, and Braunwald knew he needed to fight to get enough time for courses essential to the practice of medicine, especially those that would be taught by his faculty. Ronald Reagan had just been elected governor of California, and immediately fired the president of the University of California, Clark Kerr.[9] Reagan then asked for 10 percent funding cuts across the board in the state's university system. The UCSD to which Braunwald had been recruited was not going to be the one in which he had to build a department and a new medical school.

The "coin of the realm" in the system was the FTE (full-time equivalent) position, and each FTE faculty position came with permanent "hard-money" funding for a full-time salary for the faculty member, office and laboratory space, some research support, and the salary of a technician or secretary. Braunwald had told the dean that he needed 40 percent of all the FTEs for the medical school, because, in addition to teaching internal medicine, his department was charged with teaching physiology, pharmacology, and microbiology. As Braunwald later recalled, the dean said the request was "ridiculous" and offered 25 percent. They compromised at 32 percent. Braunwald had not even started his tenure at San Diego, but he was building the case that, if cutbacks occurred, his department would have at least 32 percent of the FTEs, and would not be reduced in greater proportion than the rest of the school.

Braunwald also had to go out and fill those FTE positions. He was a search committee of one, recruiting faculty who were his senior by a decade or more. He did his homework—closely reading the papers written by the prospective faculty members, so that he could figure out which ones had the real "goods." And then, when he set his sights on someone, he was often successful, luring distinguished faculty from the NIH and prestigious universities like Yale and Columbia to a new medical school that didn't really have a hospital or space.

Sobel remembered Braunwald's effectiveness as a recruiter: "He was charismatic. He conveyed so much intelligence, so much energy, so much optimism, that you just did not want to miss out on the chance to work with him. And he was just brilliant in knowing what buttons to push for each individual."

In later years, Braunwald described his recruiting strategy. "I'd pick them up at the airport personally and drive them around. I'd take them up to Mount Soledad in La Jolla, with its incredible view, and give the message: 'This can all be yours. It just takes somebody like you, with imagination, with drive, and with enthusiasm. For example, you can develop a course in microbiology and run an infectious-disease program the way you like it. We have the resources to do it, and you are the one who can do it. I want you, and I'm going to support you. I have a track record of supporting people, and I never let people down.'"

That approach worked, Sobel said, because Braunwald did indeed have a reputation for never promising something he couldn't deliver, but also for delivering everything he had promised. Braunwald would mention the six colleagues who had left the NIH and brought their families to San Diego because of their faith in him. Those NIH colleagues would join Braunwald and the recruits for dinner. The recruits would spend an evening in a beautiful setting, surrounded by brilliant people who seemed to be changing the world and enjoying each other's company as they did so. Who wouldn't want to be part of that group? And then, more often than not, the recruits would commit to coming to San Diego.

In May 1968, Braunwald finally made the move to San Diego, ahead of his family. (Nina would come a month later, when Karen and Allison, now nine and eight, had finished their school year.) There was a warm goodbye party at the NIH hosted by Bob Berliner, at which Berliner's executive officer presented Braunwald with a big briefcase. She said, "Come back here three times a year and fill it up with money." Braunwald needed little encouragement —he and his recruits had already applied for substantial grant funding from the NIH, and his new department would get off the ground with plenty of financial support.

Braunwald did not go directly to San Diego; he first went to research meetings in Atlantic City, and then flew to Los Angeles to visit his brother, Jack, who was now a hematologist at Kaiser Permanente. The next day, Braunwald took the train south to San Diego, and moved into a double patient room in the hospital.

"It's not that I couldn't afford an apartment," Braunwald said, "but I wanted to get a real feeling for how the hospital worked. I walked the halls in the middle of the night. I hung around the

Emergency Department and visited with the radiology technicians. I learned what was working, and what needed fixing. There was a little of the former, but plenty of the latter."

Braunwald was unimpressed by the interns and residents in the hospital, and hit the road to start recruiting new ones. He got a set of Kodachrome slides of La Jolla that Joe Stokes had compiled when he was recruiting Braunwald, and started going from medical school to medical school, asking to meet with the senior class. On those trips, he was also recruiting faculty members. "I was like a traveling salesman. I was selling medical students, selling young researchers and everyone else up to the level of distinguished professors."

One month after his arrival in San Diego, Braunwald was reunited with his family. He picked them up at the airport, along with their nanny, Rena Stark, who moved with the family from Bethesda. He took all five of them to the two-room apartment that he had rented on La Jolla Shores, where they would live for a week until larger accommodations were available. Shortly after midnight, Nina and he turned on the television and learned that Robert Kennedy had been killed. It was June 5, 1968.

Just two months before, Braunwald had been shaken by the assassination of Martin Luther King, and Kennedy's death added to his distress. "There were race riots in Washington, and tremendous tension around the country about Vietnam. My feelings about Vietnam were shaped by my childhood. I thought of the Communists as being like the Nazis—evil people who had Gulags, who imprisoned and killed many millions of people. I felt—naively—that you have to draw a line in the sand with the Communists. The world could not afford another Munich. So in 1968 I was still defending the war in Vietnam, but, like everyone else, I was deeply troubled by how things were going. It took me another year to make a 180-degree turn on the war."

But Braunwald did not have time for politics—there was too much work to do at UCSD. Sobel joined him in midsummer, and later recalled their first conversation after his arrival. Braunwald greeted Sobel with real warmth, and then said, "You know, it's very lonely at the top." It *had* been lonely, in part because no one else was there to work with him; but with the arrival of Sobel and others, he at least had some trusted and familiar colleagues with whom to share the responsibilities.

Braunwald's early plans and actions at UCSD were deeply influenced by his observations of the way Donald Seldin, in Dallas, was building a great Department of Medicine from virtually nothing. Like Braunwald, Seldin had been lured to the West by the opportunity to help build a new institution. And, as was true with Braunwald's time in San Diego, the early years were anything but smooth.

Seldin had arrived in Dallas on January 8, 1951, at the invitation of Charles Burnett, a Harvard-trained endocrinologist who had just assumed the role of chairman of the Department of Internal Medicine at the University of Texas Southwestern (UTSW). Seldin was a promising researcher in kidney disease at Yale, and Burnett told him that he could start his own nephrology program if he came to Dallas.

Seldin was only thirty-one, and nowhere in the traditional medical schools of the East could he have had such an opportunity. "At Yale, there were so many first-rate faculty members crowded into one section of the department that the chances of my setting up a program of my own or advancing along academic lines were very slim." Seldin also sensed that "concern over the fact that I was Jewish" might limit his career at Yale.[10] So he agreed to go to UTSW, though he had never seen the medical school or the city of Dallas.

Seldin packed his wife and baby in their Kaiser and drove south. He found Maple and Oak Lawn avenues, the Dallas address he had been given for the medical school. At the intersection, he found a gas station, and the attendant told him that the medical school was down the street, near the railroad crossing. Seldin followed the directions, and saw only a row of shacks, strewn with garbage. He returned to the gas station, and learned from the attendant that the row of shacks was, in fact, the medical school. The shacks were prefabricated army barracks that were being used by UTSW, which did not have the resources for either permanent buildings or a new hospital.

From that inauspicious start, matters got worse. In April, Seldin was invited to give a presentation on the main program of the Atlantic City meetings of the American Society of Clinical Investigation (ASCI)—a high honor in those days for a young researcher. Excited, he went to tell Burnett, and Burnett said, "Oh, that's wonderful, but I should tell you that I'm considering an offer in North Carolina." A few months later, Burnett was gone, after less than one year in Dallas, and UTSW had no chairman of medicine. Then the chairman of pediatrics left for Rochester, the chairman of surgery left for Washington University in St. Louis, and the chairman of obstetrics and gynecology left for the University of Illinois. By the end of 1951, there were no full-time chairmen in any clinical department at UTSW.

Seldin weighed his options. He had an offer to return to Yale, and another to join Burnett in North Carolina. He'd also received a feeler from Harvard. UTSW was desperate, though, and offered the thirty-two-year-old the chairmanship. Seldin refused, and his wife went back to New Haven to look for a house.

But then Seldin reconsidered. There was a new dean, George Aagard, and Seldin liked him. And funds were found for the construction of a new Parkland Hospital and for breaking ground on a permanent medical school, so UTSW would eventually have a modern hospital. He decided to stay on as chairman of medicine.

Seldin had an impressive title, but no money, no full-time faculty, and no funding for research fellows. He decided that he had to make the best of the only real resource he had: the medical students, about a hundred per class. He began making rounds with students and the house staff as often as possible, and he took Morning Report (in which the admissions from the prior day were discussed) virtually every day. He hoisted the burden of teaching onto his own shoulders, and, over time, onto the shoulders of full-time faculty he attracted or who came up through the UTSW system.[11]

Through teaching, he found exceptional students. Some were diamonds in the rough, like Jean Wilson (from a small town in Texas) and Joe Goldstein (from a small town in South Carolina). He would invite them to do research in his own laboratory, and then send them off to the NIH for a couple of years, in hopes that they would come back. More often than not, the ones Seldin really wanted did return, and eventually made UTSW one of the leading academic medical centers in the country. Wilson became one of the finest endocrinology researchers of his time, and Goldstein won the Nobel Prize for his research on cholesterol metabolism.

Braunwald adopted Seldin's approach of recruiting Triple Threats—faculty who were willing and able to do research, teaching, and patient care, all at a very high level. "We all did everything," Sobel recalled. "And it worked, because we had all just come out of training. I knew all about the kidney because I had just had my own education in kidney disease. So I could teach that material. But I'm not so sure it would have been sustainable if we'd been older and further along in our careers."

Like everyone else in the department, Sobel also worked intensely as a clinician. Within a short period after his arrival, he became director of the coronary care unit—which meant he was on call twenty-four hours a day, seven days a week. Meanwhile, Braunwald was attending on the hospital wards, teaching general medicine and later clinical cardiology to the medical students and house staff.

Like any proprietors of a new business, they had to drum up customers. Sobel joined Braunwald on trips around southern California to towns like El Centro and Calexico, and across the Mexican border to Mexicali and Tijuana, to seek referrals for their clinical services. Sobel recalled driving at reckless speeds down to Tijuana, with Braunwald at the wheel of a dilapidated car. They would visit the Tijuana Medical Society, which consisted of eleven physicians, one dentist, and two nurses.

"I don't know how the hell we lived through this," Sobel said. "He would go down there to cultivate a very busy practitioner named Dr. Ramirez, who had a big network of referring doctors. Gene would give a lecture on angina. What was amazing is that, even though this was such a foreign environment for us, his talks were always pitched at just the right level for the audience."

〜

As September 1968 approached, Braunwald and the dean, Clifford Grobstein, wanted to open the new medical school with a splash. They wanted to send a message about UCSD's vision to the new students and the several new department chairs and other faculty members who were just arriving, many of whom Braunwald had played a critical role in recruiting. They wanted to demonstrate that UCSD stood for integrating clinical medicine with the most fundamental biological science.

They decided to open the year with a Saturday session built around the famed chemist Linus Pauling, the only person to have won two unshared Nobel Prizes (Chemistry in 1954, and Peace in 1962). Pauling was spending a year as a visiting professor at UCSD, and agreed to discuss his brilliant work on sickle cell anemia, the first genetic disease that had been dissected biochemically. As the new chairman of the Department of Medicine, Braunwald was responsible for finding a patient with the disease, and for discussing clinical aspects of the case in a session he would conduct along with Pauling. Braunwald found a young man who had developed complications of sickle cell disease, including a permanent erection (priapism) because of the sickling of his red blood cells in the venous plexuses of his penis.

To share the stage with Pauling would be one of the highlights of Braunwald's developing career. Thus, on the day of the session, Braunwald wanted to get to the auditorium well before the 9:30 start time, so that he could make sure his slides were ready to project. He was so anxious that he was stopped by police and given a ticket for speeding on the newly opened Interstate 5. He arrived in time despite that delay, and the session came off flawlessly.

"Pauling was incredible—he gave a lecture that I will always remember," Braunwald said. Pauling talked about his basic-science insights into the abnormality that causes sickle cell disease, but he also discussed how sickle cell anemia provided protection from malaria, a fact that explained why the genetic abnormality was so common in people of African ancestry. He described the frequency of the gene in various populations, and concluded that the mutation had probably arisen in Africa, and spread eastward, through India.

The sweep of Pauling's lecture was dazzling. "Talk about bigness!" Braunwald exclaimed. "Remember—this was 1968. It was like the Middle Ages, and he was lifting the discussion of this disease up to an amazing level."

The auditorium was filled with the new medical students, professors from UCSD and other faculty members, along with the new house staff. As the thirty-nine-year-old Braunwald looked around the room, he saw Nina and the faces of many individuals whom he had personally recruited. He was making good on his promises to them.

"It was one of the great moments of my life," he said.

$\sim$

The clinical enterprise was as chaotic as any other startup business, but the research environment was as vibrant as Braunwald had promised those recruits it would be. "It was an incredible time, because Gene had attracted all these great people," Sobel said. The group included John Ross, Jim Covell, Bill Friedman, and Peter Pool from the NIH, of course—but also John West, an internationally known pulmonary expert from Australia; Dan Steinberg, a lipid expert from the NIH; Jay Seegmiller, a world-renowned authority on gout; Leonard Garren, a molecular endocrinologist from Yale; and many more.

Braunwald himself remained a research catalyst, even though he devoted only one or two half-days per week purely to research, and focused his efforts on one topic: myocardial-infarct size reduction. Sobel would later recall many occasions on which he showed Braunwald some data, and walked out of the room energized by the excitement Braunwald had expressed at their potential importance. For Braunwald, too, these sessions were a source of joy.

"I thought I had basically said goodbye to research. I thought I had entered a new period of my life. I was going to be a leader of a new school, and a chairman of the Department of Medicine. I was going to worry about the quality of the curriculum, about the house staff, and about helping new faculty put their programs together."

But Braunwald did have a grant from the NIH to continue research on infarct size reduction, stemming from his observation of the patient with a carotid-sinus nerve stimulator who had developed a myocardial infarction and had limited the damage by stimulating the carotid sinus nerve. He found space for a dog laboratory at nearby Mercy Hospital, and worked with research fellow Peter Maroko to open a research facility there. Maroko, Burton Sobel, John Ross, and Braunwald performed studies in which they placed electrocardiographic leads directly on the surface of dogs' hearts, and then occluded one of the major coronary arteries. The size of the resulting myocardial infarction was estimated by measuring the amount of change in the S-T segment of the electrocardiograms, as well as the release of an enzyme (creatine phosphokinase) from dying heart cells into the blood.

Maroko would often come to Braunwald's office to go over data, but Braunwald would also slip away from his administrative duties a couple of times a week or more to visit the lab. "I wanted to see the dogs, to see the research actually happening. I felt like I was being pulled there. And when I got to the lab, I would feel this incredible happiness."

Braunwald's research team found that they could change the size of the infarction by giving different drugs before the coronary artery occlusion, or up to three hours later. Medications that increased the heart's oxygen consumption (such as isoproterenol and digitalis) increased infarct size. In contrast, the beta blocker propranolol reduced oxygen consumption—and infarct size. Infarct size also fluctuated with interventions that changed blood pressure.

The results were published in the paper that Braunwald would eventually consider his most important, one that he referred to as simply the "Factors Paper."[12] It was the 471st paper on his curriculum vitae (out of more 1,200), but it would become widely quoted, and perhaps more influential than any of his papers before or after. Braunwald and his colleagues had shown that the size of a myocardial infarction could actually be *changed* by modifying the factors that influence oxygen consumption. The area of damage could be increased with some interventions, and decreased with others.

The Factors Paper was a study performed in dogs, however, and probably few practicing physicians noticed the paper when it was published in the journal *Circulation* in 1971. But Braunwald and his colleagues understood the potential implications. Their last sentence in the paper was: "This suggests that measures designed for reduction of myocardial oxygen demands and improvement of coronary perfusion, when effected promptly after a patient has been brought to a hospital, might potentially reduce the ultimate size of the infarction." They had opened the door to the possibility that the future for patients with heart attacks could be changed.

"It's hard to appreciate now just how revolutionary a concept this was at the time," Burton Sobel said in a 2009 interview. "Physicians were just not thinking this way."

Braunwald and his colleagues were providing the scientific base for the coming era of activism in cardiology—an era in which physicians could do much more than aggregate patients with heart attacks in one part of the hospital, give drugs to prevent arrhythmias, and try to resuscitate people if they had cardiac arrests. From the 1970s on, medicine could try to change the long-term natural history of heart attacks by reducing the amount of muscle lost and protecting the heart muscle that remained.

⌒

For a short period after they moved to San Diego, the Braunwalds continued to work with Medtronic, a Minnesota-based medical-device company best known at that time for its pacemakers, on development of a carotid sinus stimulator as a potential treatment for coronary artery disease. They were just about to start a long-term clinical trial of the stimulator in 300 patients (a large clinical trial for that time), when an even better treatment strategy for coronary disease came along, rendering carotid sinus stimulation to a relative cul-de-sac of medical history.

That better intervention was coronary artery bypass surgery, and the key steps to develop it were made 360 miles to the northwest of the NIH, at the Cleveland Clinic. The Cleveland Clinic was not a diverse academic powerhouse in the mode of Johns Hopkins or the Harvard teaching hospitals, but it had busy cardiology and cardiac surgery programs that were led by innovative physicians.

One of those physicians was Mason Sones, the cardiologist who developed selective coronary angiography—the procedure in which a catheter is inserted into the opening of a coronary artery, and radiocontrast dye is injected so that blockages and narrowings in the artery can be revealed on x-ray.[13] The story of how the first coronary angiography case occurred is yet another illustration of the role of chance—indeed, of error—in medicine.

During the 1950s, the insertion of catheters into the heart and the major blood vessels was an increasingly common procedure, performed by physicians such as Sones, Braunwald, and many others at leading institutions. But no one wanted to put a catheter into the opening of a coronary artery. First, the openings of those arteries are small—finer than a pencil—and physicians twisting and thrusting a plastic tube from outside the body would have had a difficult time finding them. More important was the belief that if fluid was injected down a coronary artery, the interruption of the blood supply could cause a fatal heart arrhythmia. That traditional reluctance to touch the beating heart was so strong that no serious scientists were proposing coronary angiography. And there were no Werner Forssmanns ready to do the procedure on themselves.

So the big step forward had to occur by accident. On October 30, 1958, Sones was performing a cardiac catheterization on a twenty-six-year-old patient with aortic valve disease. He wanted to perform a "root shot"—injection of a large amount of radiocontrast into the aorta just above the aortic valve, so that the severity of leakage back into the left ventricle could be assessed. (Today, that leakage can be assessed via echocardiography, without the need to insert anything into patients, to expose them to radiation, or to inject any contrast agent.)

On that day, however, the tip of the catheter wandered out of the middle of the aorta, and accidentally flipped into the opening of one of the coronary arteries. To the horror of Sones and the others present, the radiocontrast dye was all injected down the coronary artery. They paused, waiting for the expected fatal cardiac arrhythmia. This mishap was occurring before Bernard Lown had developed the direct-current defibrillator, so the chances that they could resuscitate the patients from an arrhythmia were low.

Nothing happened. Instead of a dead patient, they had a beautiful film revealing the patient's coronary anatomy. For the first time, physicians did not have to guess which patients had coronary artery disease, its location, and its severity. Sones made comments that might have made William Osler squirm, such as: "Clinical acumen and indirect information are not as good as thirty feet of motion picture film."[14]

Listening to patients did not go completely out of style in the years that followed, but coronary angiography improved as researchers developed special catheters that were shaped to "find" the coronary arteries, and the technique spread throughout the world.[15] Within one to two years, Braunwald and his colleagues at the NIH had learned coronary angiography and were performing it routinely. When Mason Sones died of lung cancer in 1985 (he was a heavy cigarette smoker, like so many physicians of his era), one of the tributes to him was made by René G. Favaloro (1923–2000), a cardiac surgeon at the Cleveland Clinic. Favaloro said, "Without the work of Dr. Mason Sones, Jr.—the most important contributor to modern cardiology—all our efforts in myocardial revascularization would have been fruitless."[16]

Favaloro's perspective on Sones was noteworthy, because Favaloro was the surgeon credited with performing the first series of coronary artery bypass graft (CABG) operations. Favaloro was a native of Argentina who had arrived at the Cleveland Clinic in 1962. He had finished medical school in 1948, shortly after Juan Perón came to power in the aftermath of a military coup d'état. Favaloro was interested in becoming a chest surgeon, and was offered a staff position at the University Hospital in Buenos Aires. First, however, he was told he had to sign a document indicating his support for the government. Favaloro hesitated. "This was very difficult for me; I had always believed in freedom," he later recalled. "I went home to think this over."[17]

The next day, Favaloro returned and told the director he would not sign the document. Soon he learned that he could not get any position in Argentina where he could pursue surgical training. He left for the rural southwestern pampas of Argentina for a twelve-year self-imposed exile, during which he worked as a country doctor. He and his brother started a small clinic, and provided general medical care to their patients. But, he said, "All this time I was thinking of resuming my training in thoracic and cardiovascular surgery."

Favaloro's exile ended in 1961, when one of his old professors introduced him to George Crile, Jr., son of a founder of the Cleveland Clinic, and the head of the General Surgery Department. Favaloro was told that he had none of the various certifications necessary to become a surgical fellow or other type of trainee in the United States—but that he should come anyway. He could observe patient care while securing the needed qualifications.

Favaloro became a resident physician, and started working with Sones, as well as with Donald Effler, the head of cardiovascular surgery. His goal was always to return to Argentina to raise the quality of healthcare in his native country; and after finishing his chief residency in 1965, he went back. He spent a few months trying to set up an open-heart surgical program there, but the process was frustrating. Meanwhile, Effler was writing to him with invitations to return to Cleveland as a staff physician.

Favaloro did go back to the Cleveland Clinic, where he joined Effler in performing an operation developed by the Canadian surgeon Arthur Vineberg for patients with intractable angina. In the Vineberg procedure, an artery from the chest wall (internal mammary artery) was implanted directly into the heart muscle, with the hope that blood would make its way into tiny vessels within the heart to supply the threatened myocardium. It seemed to help some patients, but its benefits were modest and inconsistent.[18] The Vineberg procedure and several other operations aimed at improving blood flow to the heart were used in desperate circumstances, mainly because little else was available. (The Braunwalds had not yet described carotid sinus stimulation.)

Favaloro began trying some new approaches, using segments of vein obtained from the legs of patients (the saphenous vein). He did no experimental work in animals—he simply tried his ideas in patients.[19] First, he tried cutting out diseased segments of arteries, and replacing them with vein grafts. Then, in 1967, he performed the first CABG operation, in which he plugged one end of a saphenous vein graft into the aorta, and the other into a diseased coronary artery beyond its atherosclerotic obstruction.

The ability of bypass surgery to relieve symptoms of angina was dramatic, and the procedure spread rapidly. CABG was an idea whose time had come. Some other surgeons can legitimately claim to have performed earlier variants of bypass surgery, but credit for the first series of CABG procedures is usually given to Favaloro, Effler, and their colleagues.

Once the Braunwalds heard about CABG, they decided to give up on their plans for a large trial of carotid sinus stimulation. Nina Braunwald had learned how to perform CABGs, and they could see the impressive results firsthand. The dean of students at the UCSD School of Medicine had severe angina, and Nina operated on him. "It was if he could suddenly start dancing again," Braunwald recalled. "We knew the carotid sinus stimulator was dead."

∼

When Eugene and Nina had moved to San Diego in 1968, they expected to be there for the remainder of their professional lives. They bought a beautiful house on a cliff overlooking Black's Beach, in one of the most spectacular sections of La Jolla, and Braunwald's parents began looking for a place to live somewhere between their two sons' southern California homes. Braunwald's three daughters had quickly adjusted to West Coast life.

But problems were brewing even before the Braunwalds arrived. When Ronald Reagan ran for governor in 1966, he had targeted the University of California system for reprisals because of its perceived leniency in dealing with protests against the war and with the Free Speech movement. One of Reagan's standard campaign refrains was a promise to "clean up the mess at Berkeley," and he fired Clark Kerr within days of taking office. Soon thereafter, he began pushing for greater budget cuts across the board for the University of California system, and even proposed that Berkeley raise funds by selling some of its rare-book collections. Most of these measures were not approved by the legislature, but lesser cuts were imposed.[20]

As a result of those cuts, building at the three new medical schools in the university system (Davis, Irvine, and San Diego) was put on hold, including the planned construction of a new university hospital on the La Jolla campus at UCSD. "Now, that was a real blow to the midsection," Braunwald said. "That hospital was a central part of the vision for UCSD. The vision came together later—but decades later."

Braunwald made multiple trips to Washington, seeking funding from the Veterans Administration for a hospital and research facility. These were approved, and the hospital's construction began. But he came to realize that the "incredible dream" of UCSD's plan was not going to work out—at least, not in a time frame that he could tolerate.

Another major problem was that Nina's professional situation was terrible—in part because she was married to him. The chairman of surgery viewed Eugene Braunwald as his rival for power, and was far from welcoming to the first woman cardiac surgeon in his department. The environment for her was hostile from the start, and Nina became progressively more unhappy. Eugene felt guilty that he had dragged his wife away from the NIH, where her career had been on a brilliant trajectory, to UCSD, where she had become a pawn in a medical political battle.

After a few years, the combination of disappointingly slow progress for the medical school and an increasingly hopeless situation for his wife persuaded Braunwald that he should be open to leaving San Diego. As his sense of desperation increased, George Thorn offered him an opportunity to exit UCSD. Thorn was a Hopkins-trained endocrinologist who had become chairman of the Department of Medicine at the Peter Bent Brigham Hospital in 1942, when he was thirty-six. Thorn was a major leader in academic medicine and one of the founding editors of Harrison's *Principles of Internal Medicine.* He had interviewed Braunwald as a potential editor for the textbook's cardiovascular disease sections in 1967, and had played an important role in the selection of Braunwald for that position.

According to Harvard rules, Thorn had to retire as chairman after age sixty-six in 1972, so the search for his replacement became serious in 1971. That fall, Braunwald was invited for a visiting professorship across town at Massachusetts General Hospital, at the invitation of its chairman, Alexander Leaf. Leaf was a member of the search committee for Thorn's replacement—so now, two key Boston medical leaders had met Braunwald and were impressed with him.

Braunwald made three visits to Boston in the fall of 1971, and by November the search committee had agreed that he was their first choice. The committee was chaired by Francis "Franny" Moore, the legendary chairman of the Brigham's Department of Surgery. It included many of the most prominent leaders of Harvard Medical School, including Judah Folkman, who in 1971 was beginning to publish extraordinary research findings on the relationship between cancers and the growth of the blood vessels that supply them; Gustave J. Dammin, who played a key role in the first successful human kidney transplant, performed at Peter Bent Brigham Hospital in 1954, and who helped to describe Lyme disease; Robert Ebert, the dean at Harvard Medical School; and Howard Hiatt, who had been chief of medicine at Harvard's Beth Israel Hospital and was about to become dean at the Harvard School of Public Health.

They offered Braunwald the job. He agreed to become the tenth Hersey Professor of the Theory and Practice of Physic (Medicine) at Harvard Medical School—the oldest "named" chair at an American medical school—and the fourth physician-in-chief at the Peter Bent Brigham Hospital, effective July 1, 1972.

"It was not really a difficult decision for us," Braunwald later recalled. "I only have one life to live, and I wanted to be in a place where I could make a difference. I could see that San Diego would not become great for a very long time. And I also thought San Diego was not going to work, because Nina was not going to be able to stand it."

Braunwald left UCSD in 1972. In marked contrast to the warmth of the farewell party when Braunwald had left the NIH, the departure was uncomfortable for all. He stayed long enough to see the graduation of that first class of medical students who had entered with him in 1968, but he had no official role in the proceedings. He stood in the back at the outdoor ceremony.

The faculty whom he had recruited understood the personal and professional reasons behind Braunwald's departure, but were deeply saddened. "When Gene left, the glue was gone," Sobel said.[21] "It was like a death. But during those four years, it was spectacular. I never worked any harder, and I've never learned more. I've never had a more rewarding time."

: 9 :

Rebuilding the Brigham

1972–1980

In 1972, as Eugene Braunwald prepared to come to Boston, the United States was in social and political turmoil. The previous decade had witnessed the assassinations of John F. Kennedy, Robert F. Kennedy, and Martin Luther King, Jr., and the eruption of riots and widespread protests in American cities. The escalating Vietnam War had aroused skepticism about the policies and pronouncements of U.S. leaders. That skepticism became even stronger after June 16, 1972, when a security guard foiled a break-in by supporters of President Nixon at the Democratic National Committee headquarters in Washington's Watergate Hotel.

Although Braunwald did not cultivate a public profile outside academic medicine, his family experiences made him keenly attuned to the impact of the forces of history. His interest in sociopolitical events had intensified during the JFK years, a natural inclination reinforced by the fact that he and Nina were living in the Washington area during this period. He remembered lying in bed with the flu, in 1960, watching the Kennedy campaign on a portable TV that Nina had wheeled into their bedroom. She told him to stop reading medical journals and just watch some TV to relax, and he became entranced by Kennedy's ideas and charismatic performance. Braunwald was in his early thirties at the time, and saw himself as part of that new generation of leaders to which Kennedy so often referred.

During his four years in California, he had seen firsthand the impact of politics on UCSD, and he knew that academic medical centers were unlikely to be untouched by the social upheaval of their times. In May 1972, shortly before his arrival in Boston, he published an article in the *New England Journal of Medicine* called "Future Shock in Academic Medicine," in which he made wide-ranging predictions about trends that would play out over the next several decades. The title of Braunwald's article alluded to the book *Future Shock,* published in 1970 by Alvin Toffler, who argued that the world was undergoing a transition from industrial to "super-industrial" society. Toffler said this cultural change was overwhelming people, to such an extent that they felt disoriented, shattered, and stressed: "future shocked."[1]

Braunwald read Toffler's book while on a family vacation in Arizona. One night, he stayed up late reading the book while his family slept. He was struck by the fact that his own field was being altered by trends similar to the ones Toffler described. In his *New England Journal* article, he summarized the "profound changes that have taken place in academic medicine since World War II," specifically

> the flowering of the full-time system in clinical departments; the progressively increasing penetration of the fundamental biologic, physical, behavioral, and social sciences into clinical medicine; the effect on every aspect of medical education, first, of the exponential growth of federal support for research and research training, and, more recently, of the drastic slowing of this growth; the increasing fraction of federal resources devoted to goal-oriented research and the correspondingly growing role of administrators, of representatives of the public, and of nonscientists in defining these goals; the cry for relevance in medical education begun by the students, but more recently joined by house staff and faculty; and the resulting loosening of the rigidities of the post-Flexnerian curriculum.

He quoted a comment by John W. Gardner (U.S. Secretary of Health, Education, and Welfare under Lyndon Johnson)—"Most

organizations have a structure that was designed to solve problems that no longer exist"—and argued that the healthcare delivery system was about to change.[2] He described the importance of
primary-care physicians, and predicted that "the future system of
health-care delivery will be more formally tiered than today's non-
system: primary care offered by adult and pediatric generalists or
primary-care physicians; secondary care offered by organ-system-
oriented specialists operating in groups and utilizing community
hospitals; and tertiary care for the gravely ill and for the most
complex problems, offered by subspecialists trained to utilize the
most advanced technology, usually within university hospitals."

Braunwald was describing a future in which integrated delivery
systems would be structured to deliver coordinated, high-quality,
efficient care to a broad population of patients. "As such a system
of delivery becomes more sharply defined and operational, the
pressure on medical schools to reorganize their structures so that
their educational products are most appropriately equipped to operate successfully within it will become irresistible."

Braunwald's article created a modest tempest. In its issue of August 10, 1972, the *New England Journal of Medicine* published six
long Letters to the Editor, a sampling of those it had received. (In
that era, publication of this many letters, and at such length, was
the *Journal*'s way of acknowledging an important controversy.)
The letters all sounded similar themes, decrying the potential impact of the changes Braunwald described.

Braunwald's response, published in the *Journal* with those letters, was empathetic but relatively short and blunt:

> Lest my personal opinion in the matter be misunderstood, I am
> anxious to indicate that I agree with the correspondents that many
> of the aspects of "Future Shock" are very undesirable, so far as aca-
> demic medicine, as we have known it, is concerned. Nonetheless,

simple nostalgia for the past is unlikely to retard the rapidly changing values and behavior patterns occurring in all sectors of society,
including academic medicine. Although the suggested treatment
for "Future Shock" admittedly may be merely symptomatic and
less effective than prevention, perhaps the first step in the control
of the condition is its recognition; the major purpose of my essay
was to call attention to the existence of "Future Shock," with the
hope that it might elicit the thought and dialogue that will allow us
to cope with it.

Braunwald's article had been published when he was a "lame
duck" in San Diego, marking time before his arrival in Boston. His
response to the letters was written from Peter Bent Brigham Hospital. He had a sense of how the Brigham and Harvard would need
to evolve in the coming decades, but once that paper and its ensuing controversy were behind him, he had to adopt a shorter-term
perspective. He could not be looking at the horizon when there
were icebergs in the water straight ahead. The Brigham had serious problems that needed immediate action.

⌒

When Braunwald arrived at Peter Bent Brigham Hospital in 1972,
it was a well-known and highly respected Harvard teaching hospital, famous for medical advances that included Harvey Cushing's creation of a new specialty, neurosurgery, early in the twentieth century; the development of kidney dialysis in the late 1940s;
Dwight Harken's pioneering heart valve surgery; and the first successful organ transplant (kidney) in 1954. That kidney transplant
won a Nobel Prize in 1990 for Joseph Murray, the transplant surgeon. The 1934 Nobel Prize in Medicine had been shared by the
Brigham's George R. Minot and William P. Murphy, along with
George H. Whipple of the University of Rochester, for their development of an effective treatment for pernicious anemia. Bernard
Lown had been the first to use direct-current (DC) cardioversion

to restore a normal cardiac rhythm. Past and future Nobel laureates walked the Brigham's halls every day.

But those halls were in terrible shape, as was the rest of the physical plant—so bad that planning focused less on fixing the existing Brigham than on building a new one. The hospital had opened in 1913, funded with a bequest from a Boston restaurateur and real-estate baron. It had been designed by John Shaw Billings, who was also the driving force behind the creation of Johns Hopkins Hospital. Billings had created a hospital with two-story brick and wooden buildings spread over a long block adjacent to Harvard Medical School. Those buildings were connected by a 250-yard walkway called "the Pike," the south side of which was open to the elements to ensure a constant flow of fresh air. Infections like tuberculosis, which thrived in stagnant air, were not likely to spread from ward to ward in this hospital—and in 1913 such contagion was of great concern.[3]

In warm weather, the design worked beautifully. Wisteria vines hung on the open-air side of the Pike. Patients could be pushed in wheelchairs or beds from their wards onto open-air porches, and could bask in the sun as they convalesced. The design worked less well during cold weather, however, and snow would sometimes pile up along the Pike.[4] An oft-told joke was that the hospital had been designed by a man who had never spent a winter in New England.[5]

Many physicians considered the structure to be out of date almost immediately after it was built. Soma Weiss, MD, who had preceded George Thorn as the Hersey Professor of Medicine, had complained forcefully about the facility in his annual physician-in-chief report to the hospital.

> The problems of the Peter Bent Brigham Hospital are numerous, and in some cases grave. . . . The physical plant of a hospital is only

of secondary significance as compared with the quality of the [medical] work done. In fairness one must point out, however, that there is a "minimal" standard of facilities below which the physical and mental comfort of the patient suffer and standards in technique cannot be maintained. . . . Most candidates, old or young, for positions in surgery, medicine, pathology, social service, nursing, or hospital administration will be influenced if the physical standards reach a level below that of other institutions.

Weiss wrote that report in 1939, and the physical plant had hardly changed at all by the time Eugene Braunwald arrived in 1972. "It was a hovel," Braunwald recalled. "There was no place to sit down during rounds, the rooms were tiny, and the place was smelly. I was embarrassed to bring people here."

Yet Braunwald took the Brigham job, because he knew that a new hospital was being planned, and because the Brigham had a precious asset: young talent, a "farm system" as good as any in academic medicine. Most of the trainees had been among the top students at Harvard and other leading medical schools, and, even by Braunwald's exacting standards, they were smart, hardworking, and ambitious. If one of Braunwald's major long-term personal goals was to emulate Donald Seldin, and train a generation of Triple Threat physician-scientists, he would be working with first-rate raw material at the Brigham.

He had had an extended look at that young talent four years before. In the winter of 1968, he was invited by George Thorn, who had been impressed by his interview with the editors of *Harrison's,* to be the Brigham's visiting physician-in-chief pro tempore. Braunwald was still officially at the NIH, and he had already accepted the chairmanship of the Department of Medicine at UCSD; his mind was three thousand miles southwest of bitterly cold Boston. But, as the Brigham's visiting physician-in-chief pro tempore, he lectured at Grand Rounds and research conferences, and saw patients with the house staff and medical students. He lived in the hospital for a full week, sleeping in the accommodations for residents—small on-call rooms that overlooked the noisy intersection known as Brigham Circle. Still in his thirties, Braunwald felt comfortable mingling among the trainees, even if they might feel nervous in his presence.

One of those residents was John Mendelsohn, who would later become a leading cancer researcher and chief executive officer at Houston's MD Anderson Cancer Center. Mendelsohn recalled meeting Braunwald while they were shaving at adjacent sinks, in the lavatory for the house staff on-call rooms. Mendelsohn had been on duty the night before, and Braunwald had just arrived. Braunwald introduced himself and asked Mendelsohn if he could follow him around while he did his work.

Braunwald liked what he saw in Mendelsohn and the other house staff he met. "I knew that building a good house staff program was going to be a long, uphill struggle in San Diego," he later recalled. "But here they were just terrific, fully as good as the group I'd trained with at Johns Hopkins a decade earlier. Actually, the young house staff were better than many of the faculty I encountered at the Brigham."

Toward the end of the week, Braunwald went to dinner with the seven senior residents at the Tavern Club, a private social club just off the Boston Common where men (in that era, only men) gathered to have dinner, smoke cigars, and talk. Braunwald would later recall feeling out of his element in that setting, but feeling at home amid the residents. He asked them about their backgrounds and aspirations, and spoke about his own. Mendelsohn was there, as were two other residents who would later play major roles in Braunwald's career and the Brigham's future: Joseph Dorsey and Marshall Wolf.

"He talked about how fortunate we all were to be residents at the Brigham," Dorsey recalled.[6] "He talked about what a great place it was, and how important it was in American medicine. He was very positive, very upbeat."

Dorsey and the other residents glowed with pride, both institutional and personal, as Braunwald plunged into discussions with each of them about their future plans. "I remember thinking, 'What an intellectual force!'" Dorsey said. "Even though he was known as a hard-ass scientist, the breadth of his interests was obvious in the way he would ask questions and wanted to hear about different things that people were going to be doing."

As they left the Tavern Club, Dorsey turned to his friend Robert Blacklow, the chief resident: "I know he's heading to San Diego, but I think he wants to come to the Brigham and be chief here someday. And I hope he does."

Four years later, Dorsey got his wish, in part because of Braunwald's frustration that construction plans for a new hospital in San Diego were not moving forward. During his courtship by the Brigham, Braunwald had been assured that a new Brigham was about to be built. Shortly after he accepted the job, an architect had even flown across the country to go over the plans for Braunwald's office suite in the new hospital. Braunwald was asked to make detailed design decisions, such as whether the restroom outside his office would be on the left or the right side of the waiting area. (He chose the left.)

Banking on a state-of-the-art hospital, Braunwald—even before his arrival in Boston—began working on one of his most ambitious goals: he wanted to make the Brigham the very best place in the country to launch a career in academic medicine. He was tough-minded enough to acknowledge that the Brigham was probably in the top ten departments of medicine in the country, but not in the top two or three. It frequently lost candidates for its training programs to its crosstown rival, Massachusetts General Hospital—where any sense of rivalry was barely acknowledged.

Braunwald understood the factors that had been important in his own development as a Triple Threat at the NIH, and the strengths and weaknesses of training programs he had visited around the country. He wanted to make the Brigham a place that trained physicians who epitomized excellence both in research and in patient care. It was a goal that resonated with the "heritage of excellence" theme so closely associated with Johns Hopkins, where Braunwald had trained fifteen years before.

He knew he needed help, and he thought he knew just the right person to help him: John Mendelsohn, the resident he had met while shaving in the Brigham bathroom back in 1968, and who had then come to San Diego to work in his department. Braunwald asked Mendelsohn to return to Boston and run the house staff program. Mendelsohn considered the offer, and then turned it down. He wanted to build a cancer research program more than he wanted to train residents, and thought he could make a bigger splash in San Diego. But Mendelsohn had another idea. He suggested Marshall Wolf, a young cardiologist who had likewise been at the Tavern Club dinner in the winter of 1968.

Wolf's parents, Jewish immigrants from the border region between Poland and Russia, had arrived in Chicago as children shortly after the turn of the century. One grandfather was a tailor, the other a mattress stuffer. The latter grandfather died of chronic lung disease when Wolf's father was only in elementary school, forcing him to quit school to help support the family by delivering telegrams and performing other odd jobs. Eventually Wolf's father built a modest business distributing merchandise to small stores. He married a young accountant and had three children, the youngest of whom was Marshall.

Though far from well-to-do, Marshall Wolf came of age in the safe and secure 1950s, rather than in the hazardous 1940s, and the pressures to move quickly from Point A to Point B in one's life were not as intense as they had been for young Eugene Braunwald. Wolf took his time finding his way.

Wolf's intelligence was obvious as he progressed through Chicago's Hyde Park High School. He won an award as the top mathematics student in the city, and received a full scholarship to the University of Chicago. He expected to live at home and attend the "U of C," but a chance encounter led to a change in his plans.

One weekend a man who sold his father LePage's Glue struck up a conversation with young Marshall, who was working in his father's store. "He was very mean," Wolf recalled in later years.[7] "He gave my father a hard time about some business things right in front of me. And then he turned to me."

"So what are you going to do, kid—spend the rest of your life in this dinky little store?" the salesman asked, as Wolf's father stood by. Wolf told him that he hoped to go to college, and the visitor said, "Before you go to college, you have to get into college." Wolf said that he had in fact been accepted at several—the University of Chicago, and also Harvard, Yale, and MIT.

The visitor said to Wolf's father that if Marshall had really gotten into Harvard, he should go there. The father then turned to Marshall and said, "Okay, you're going to Harvard." That decision meant considerable financial stress for Wolf's family, since he had only minimal financial aid from Harvard, but off to Cambridge he went.

He excelled academically in college, but he still did not know what he wanted to do with his life. Though he had done some research as an undergraduate, he didn't enjoy it enough to commit to graduate school. Instead, after graduation, he obtained a travel fellowship and went to Europe. In keeping with the goals of the fellowship, he did not enroll in any formal educational program; he simply traveled, and learned about music, poetry, and literature.

When he returned to Boston, he entered Harvard Medical School, and on the first day of classes met Katharine (Katie) Poole. She was his lab partner in gross anatomy, and their relationship deepened as they dissected their cadaver. They married after their second year, and graduated from medical school in 1963, just as U.S. involvement in the Vietnam War was escalating. Wolf had just begun his internship at the Brigham when he and the other interns were told by the program director that they should apply for a job at the NIH or the Centers for Disease Control; otherwise, they could expect to be drafted into the military. "There were fourteen of us in that internship group, and eleven went to the NIH," Wolf later recalled. "Of the other three, one went to the Centers for Disease Control, one was 4F [received a military deferment for medical reasons; this was Dorsey], and the last person was thirty-one years old. He figured he was too old to be drafted—and he got drafted."

So after his junior residency year, Wolf headed to Bethesda. His wife, Katie, was at Johns Hopkins, training in pediatric cardiology, and they would occasionally socialize with Helen Taussig, who was in her final years. Wolf did not, however, cross paths with Braunwald. He worked in a laboratory elsewhere at the NIH, and did not have the same exhilarating experience that Braunwald had had as a clinical associate. The intense immersion in research convinced Wolf that he was not cut out for that line of work.

When he returned to the Brigham to complete his residency training, Wolf decided to become a cardiologist. He admired several of the hospital's cardiologists, including Samuel Levine, Bernard Lown, Richard Gorlin, Lewis Dexter, and David Littmann. After residency, he spent one year as a fellow under Littmann, and then three years as a fellow under Lown.

These four years as a cardiology fellow were four years more than Braunwald, Sobel, and many other famous cardiologists from that era had spent in formal cardiology training. But Wolf was still not sure where he was trying to go, and thus was in no big hurry to move on to a permanent staff position. He simply liked being a doctor, and enjoyed the process of learning more and more about medicine. As 1972 began, however, Wolf knew he could not be a fellow forever. He and Katie had two young sons, and, while their tastes were inexpensive, he knew he had to take an actual job.

He was offered one as chief of cardiology at an innovative health maintenance organization called Harvard Community Health Plan (HCHP). HCHP had been started in the late 1960s by a group of progressive Harvard physicians whom Wolf admired, including the dean of Harvard Medical School, Robert Ebert; H. Richard Nesson, a nephrologist and general internist at Beth Israel Hospital; and the other young resident who had gone to dinner with Braunwald in 1968, Joe Dorsey. Wolf had worked as a moonlighter at HCHP, and shared the conviction that prepaid managed care could be as good as traditional fee-for-service medicine, or even better. He thought HCHP was potentially important for the country.

But Wolf was still ambivalent. "The problem I had with HCHP was that it wasn't very academic. HCHP wasn't worried about increasing the skills of the people who worked there. They gave the message that clinicians come here to practice and that they can go back to the teaching hospitals to get skill improvement. I was interested in always improving my skills, so I didn't like that."

Wolf was still contemplating his options in the spring of 1972, when Braunwald started coming to Boston for one or two days every two weeks. "The word was out that he was interviewing everyone to see how they would fit into his idea of a department," Wolf recalled. "I got a message that Dr. Braunwald wanted to meet with me. I went in there prepared to describe my research and tell him my options, and ask him what I should do next."

Braunwald had done due diligence, and had talked to people who knew Wolf personally and professionally. He liked the idea of filling the role of director of the house staff training program with someone like Wolf—smart, open-minded, and exhilarated by learning and teaching clinical medicine. So at that first meeting, after a few pleasantries, Braunwald immediately cut to the chase, offering Wolf the job.

Wolf was surprised by the proposal; it was an important role, and as far as he could tell, Braunwald barely knew him. The director of the house staff program during his internship had been Eugene Eppinger—a godlike figure to Wolf. Eppinger was considered one of the very best physicians in Boston, the doctor to whom other doctors turned when they themselves, or members of their family, were seriously ill.[8] And he was beloved by generations of house staff, for whom he played the role of teacher, friend, and, at times, disciplinarian. He had strong organizational skills, and emerged as the right-hand man for George Thorn, who let Eppinger handle administrative challenges.

The idea that he might be considered for "Epp's job" startled Wolf, but he did not hesitate. "Okay, I'll take it!"

Now it was Braunwald's turn to be taken aback: "What do you mean?" Wolf repeated that he'd like the job. Braunwald asked, "Don't you want to talk about salary or anything?"

"No, I'm sure you'll pay me enough," Wolf said. "Why don't we talk about what we're going to do together?"

So just a few minutes into their first meeting, they began discussing their goals for the house staff program. They talked about adding a primary-care residency and a research track. And they talked about getting more women into the program. Both of them were married to women physicians, and knew how sexism could affect women's careers. They agreed at that first meeting that they were going to make the Brigham a different kind of institution.

Braunwald said to Wolf, "Your job is the most important job at the Brigham, because you are going to pick tomorrow's faculty."[9] That meeting initiated twenty-four years of collaboration on house staff training, during which they never once discussed Wolf's salary. Braunwald always decided on what seemed fair, and Wolf never found reason to complain.

Wolf left that meeting, and picked up a bottle of champagne on the way home. He walked into the house, told Katie that he had "Epp's job," and said he was absolutely thrilled.

∽

Braunwald was relieved that, even before his arrival in Boston, he had found the perfect director for the training program. But he could not wait for his residents to "grow up" before he had a faculty to match. He needed dynamic researchers, space to put them in, and resources to support them. And he could not afford to postpone working on this problem until he actually took office in Boston.

He knew how to find first-rate Triple Threats for the faculty, drawing on skills and contacts he had developed at the NIH and honed at UCSD. He would study the curriculum vitae of each potential recruit in detail, and would read two or three of the candidate's papers closely. He would speak to his growing network of colleagues about the person's work and about his or her promise of future achievement. He gained additional perspective on the work of researchers through his involvement with academic societies like the American Society for Clinical Investigation and with medical research journals such as the *Journal of Clinical Investigation* and the *New England Journal of Medicine,* and through serving as a senior advisor to the NIH's extramural grants program. He came to know how their work was regarded by colleagues and how likely they would be to obtain grant funding. He would visit recruits at their own institutions, both to demonstrate the seriousness of his interest in them and also to get a firsthand look at their facilities and their work methods.

He usually could sense the best way to approach those he wanted to persuade—that is, he knew which "buttons to push." For example, in January 1972, after he had agreed to go to the Brigham but six months before actually arriving there, he sent a two-page handwritten letter to a well-known Brigham physician who was being recruited by another institution and whom he did not want to lose. He made a highly personal appeal to the physician's sense of loyalty. The letter read in part:

> I have just returned after a very hectic week in Boston. I think that I'm beginning to get a much clearer picture of the situation that we confront at the Brigham. I don't need to tell you the problems— they're evident even to a relative outsider like myself, and must be distressing to someone like yourself, who has given the hospital so much for so long. . . . You are in a position to influence the future of the Dept. of Medicine at the PBBH very profoundly. This is *not* an exaggeration.

Braunwald went on to describe the work that would be needed to bring the Brigham's Department of Medicine to greatness, and then wrote:

> I know that I can't do it alone. As I look around the Department, you are literally the *only* senior person who is widely respected and shares my values. If you leave, I am convinced that I'll be licked before I start.
>
> I know that you have withdrawn from the PBBH in the last couple of years, but I interpret this as a symptom of the problems.

More than anything else, I want to turn this around and ensure that you become a part of *all* significant decisions. . . . Maybe it's unfair of me to pressure you, but by the same token, it would be equally unfair of me not to tell you, in all candor, how I see the situation.

In marked contrast was a letter he wrote soon thereafter to a prospective division chief, someone who was not particularly sentimental, and who wanted every administrative detail spelled out. Braunwald's letter to him was typed, three pages single-spaced, with sixteen numbered points. It described exactly how many square feet of research space would be provided to the physician, and where the space would be located. It described in detail financial arrangements related to the physician's salary and research funding, remuneration for expenses on his visits to Boston prior to his move, and a sundry fund of $7,500 for his use ("consistent with hospital policy") after his arrival. It was a no-nonsense letter that did not tug at any heartstrings, but anticipated every question that the physician might have.

The physician who received the first letter stayed at the Brigham, and the one who received the second letter decided to come to the hospital. Both became major figures in Braunwald's department.

In those months just before and after his Boston arrival, Braunwald had no clear idea of how much money he would have to recruit faculty, but he knew resources were surely going to be a problem. At UCSD, he had known exactly how many FTE faculty positions were available to him, and how much of the state government's support for the University of California system was available to fund them. But at Harvard and the Brigham, the flow of funds was cloaked in mystery. George Thorn, the patrician gentleman researcher who preceded Braunwald, had been uncomfortable discussing the mundane details of running the department, and financial matters had usually been handled by Eppinger and others. Throughout Braunwald's interview process, there had been vague references to a budget for new faculty from Harvard Medical School, but budgets were always in flux, and he was told that his would be reviewed "later."

So in his last months in San Diego, Braunwald formulated a plan for generating more income at the Brigham. He conceived a faculty group practice in which *all* full-time members of the Department of Medicine would need to be members of a new "Brigham Medical Group" (BMG), and *all* of their payments for clinical services would flow through the BMG. Two-thirds would go to the division chiefs, who would use the funds to pay faculty salaries and invest in people and other programs. One-third of the revenue they generated would go to the Department of Medicine, to provide the resources Braunwald needed to rejuvenate and grow the department. He could redistribute the other money as he saw fit, and would return more than the one-third he had taken from divisions (such as infectious disease) that were essential to clinical care but could not generate much clinical income.

Although this model spread widely in subsequent decades, it was unusual—possibly unique—at the time. The BMG model would give Braunwald the resources, flexibility, and influence to recruit, retain, and support the people he needed to move the Brigham to the first ranks of academic medicine. Many of the faculty thought the Brigham was already in that elite group, but Braunwald did not. He believed that he needed to recruit excellent people in almost every field—and to do so, he needed these resources.

He would later realize that his UCSD experience had been crucial training: "If I had gone directly from the NIH to the Brigham, I would have fallen flat on my face. I would have lasted two years at best." His four years at UCSD had taught him what a department chairman had to do, and by 1972 he was ready to use the freedom of the Brigham's unstructured environment to his and the department's advantage.

~

On July 1, 1972, Eugene Braunwald took office at the Brigham. He hit the ground running—and by the end of the day, the ground would hit back.

At 8:00 A.M., he stood before the faculty in the Brigham's Bornstein Auditorium to describe his plan for the Brigham Medical Group. Braunwald was not really sure that he had the authority to impose the BMG model on the faculty (he later concluded that he probably did not), but he was determined to bluff his way through the furor that surely would come. He knew he had to start his tenure with a clear and tough message, and he let the faculty know that "it was a new ballgame."

Braunwald explained to the faculty that there simply weren't sufficient resources to take the department to the very front ranks of academic medicine without major changes in the rules by which the department was run. He reassured them that he was not going to reduce anyone's salary, but stated that he thought they could do a better job of collecting payments and creating other efficiencies if they all worked for the yet-to-be-formed BMG.

He did *not* bring up something else he had learned from his many trips to Boston before starting the job: that some faculty members were actually earning considerably more from their private practices than they declared to the medical school, and were thus making more than was allowed under medical-school salary caps. Braunwald did not need to say that fully transparent bookkeeping would lead to a fall in their take-home pay; the physicians in the amphitheater were making their own silent calculations of the impact of the BMG on their personal incomes. Those calculations quickly led to others in which physicians reassessed whether they wanted to stay at the Brigham for the Braunwald era. More than a few would eventually depart.

Also on the agenda that first day was a meeting with the hospital's lead administrator, William Hassan, Jr. In the course of their conversation, Braunwald made a comment about the impending start of new construction. He later recalled that there was a pregnant pause, after which Hassan said, "Well, we have a little problem." About two months earlier, the Brigham had received bad news: the Certificate of Need for the new hospital had not been approved by Massachusetts officials, and construction could not begin. Apparently, no one had had the courage to tell Braunwald that the new hospital was now an uncertainty. Hassan told Braunwald about the Certificate of Need ruling, then rushed to explain that an appeal was already under way, and that he was sure everything would work out. But the fact was that no one knew when the situation would be resolved.

Braunwald was stunned. "I had moved my family, our nanny, my secretary, and her family across the country, along with three horses we had bought for our daughters to soften the blow of the move. I had made commitments to a lot of people back in San Diego, and I had really upset them when I left. And then to discover, on the first day, that one of the major reasons I had left and come to Boston was not actually happening was beyond belief."

That evening, as Braunwald headed home on the Massachusetts Turnpike, his thoughts in turmoil, he had the only major automobile accident of his life. The one-car crash destroyed his car and left him deeply shaken, though unhurt. The Boston phase of his career was not off to a good start.

Before things got better, they would get worse. After he dusted himself off from his car accident, Braunwald made an appointment with the dean of Harvard Medical School, Robert Ebert. He was worried because he had been reviewing documents related to the finances of the Department of Medicine, and he could find virtually no evidence of funding from Harvard. It was mid-July in a gentler era, however, and Ebert was out of town until after Labor Day, in September. The same was true of Henry Meadow, the associate dean who handled financial affairs.

Labor Day came and went, and Braunwald finally met with Meadow to ask about the medical-school budget for funding new faculty. Meadow gave him a quizzical look. Braunwald pressed on, asserting that it was time to get clarity on the budget. He reminded Meadow that he and Dean Ebert had developed a plan for rejuvenating the Brigham, and that there were twelve to fifteen division chiefs who had to be recruited.

Meadow then gave him the bad news: there was no budget for expanding the faculty beyond the modest funding (about $60,000 per year) that currently flowed to the department for teaching third-year medical students. Stunned, Braunwald was asked how he was supposed to find the funds to recruit the new faculty. "Doctor, I don't really care where you get your money from," Meadow said. "If you want to sell pretzels in front of Children's Hospital, that's okay with us."

Braunwald understood the implications of Meadow's joke. "I knew I had to raise money, and to do it quickly," he recalled. The future of his department depended on the success of the BMG and its audacious 33 percent tax on all clinical revenues. Every morning, even when traveling, his first phone call was to Richard Harris—the administrator whom Braunwald had hired to run the Brigham Medical Group—to ask about revenue collections from the previous day. For the first several months, the numbers he heard were terrible—often just a couple of thousand dollars, or even less. Collections had to be about $20,000 per day just to meet the payroll.

But on one occasion, the number rose abruptly. "I was a visiting professor at the University of Chicago, and called Richard, who told me that we had collected $12,500 on the previous day. I knew that the dam had finally been broken." Harris and his team had figured out how to bill effectively and quickly, and they were finally making progress in their efforts to teach the physicians how to submit bills for their services accurately and on time. "I breathed a sigh of relief," Braunwald said. "After all, I was hiring new division chiefs, and I had to find the money to pay them."

Those new division chiefs—and the departures of the people that they were replacing—were another source of turmoil. Braunwald wanted to clean house and bring in new talent. The research of most of these old-guard division chiefs was not cutting-edge; they tended to come from the gentleman-farmer school of medical researchers, not the Triple Threat generation. "I didn't throw anyone out on the street," Braunwald recalled. "But they got the message that I was bringing in someone new in their field, and I strongly urged them to pursue other opportunities."

The next several months, for many people, became known as the "Slaughter on Shattuck Street" (named for the street that runs between the Brigham and Harvard Medical School). After the first eighteen months, thirteen division chiefs had departed. During these transitions, Braunwald acquired a reputation for toughness as an administrator that was unsurpassed in academic medicine. Braunwald did not relish that reputation, but felt that he could be successful only if he transformed the department quickly during a "honeymoon" that he knew would be short. That meant asking several people to make room for their replacements.

Direct and decisive management and blunt recommendations to leave were something new in the genteel world of academic medicine, particularly at Harvard in the early 1970s. Braunwald was no longer perceived as the practical joker known to Jonathan

Uhr back at Mount Sinai, or the electrifying research colleague from the NIH. Objectively, everyone knew that tough decisions had to be made, but Braunwald was seen as all too comfortable making them and carrying them out. Decades later, rumors persisted that he had taken away telephones from faculty members who were not leaving quickly enough. ("Not true," Braunwald said. "But I did tell some people to forget my phone number.") The personal and professional strengths of the young stars he was recruiting were not yet appreciated, but nearly everyone was ready to mourn the loss of the friends who were on their way out the door.

Braunwald kept just one of the old regime's division chiefs. The other divisions were taken over by a succession of outstanding young physician-researchers in the Triple Threat mode, many of whom had spent time at the NIH during or shortly after Braunwald's time there. Thomas W. Smith was hired to run cardiology; Roland Ingram, pulmonary; Frank Bunn, hematology; Barry Brenner, nephrology; Bernard Fields, infectious disease—and so on. And these young stars recruited even younger faculty, some of whom would become even brighter stars.

Like the general manager of a sports team, Braunwald also hired some experienced veterans to mix with his up-and-coming talent. Over the years, he provided a home for a series of prominent figures, such as Howard Hiatt, Arnold Relman, and Louis Weinstein, some of whom had already completed the phase of their careers for which they had earned their fame, but who added depth and perspective to the teaching program. Medical students and house staff would go to Grand Rounds in Bornstein Amphitheater, and see in the first row these faculty members and others whom they knew as the authors of key chapters in their textbooks —Braunwald, Robert Petersdorf, Daniel Federman, and so forth.

Many of those trainees would think, "I want to be one of them someday." Within just a few years, the Brigham had become a hot spot of academic medicine.

~

Braunwald knew from his long study of Donald Seldin's success in Dallas that many of that next generation of young stars could and should come from the Brigham's own house staff program. Thus, even as he recruited division chiefs, Braunwald worked closely with Marshall Wolf on development of the house staff program. They knew that they were not going to attract top talent with their outmoded hospital—they needed to recruit them *despite* the physical plant. They needed to build the brand, make the case that the Brigham was the ideal place to launch one's academic career—and the attractions were Braunwald himself, those terrific young division chiefs, Marshall Wolf, and a flexible training program that could be tailored to meet trainees' ambitions and needs.

Moving quickly, Wolf and Braunwald created a primary-care residency program—one of the first in the country. That two cardiologists should make primary care one of their initial emphases was surprising to many at the time, particularly since Braunwald was best known as a cutting-edge cardiology researcher. The concept of primary care was just emerging in American medicine, and no one associated Braunwald's name with it.

Yet Braunwald had never completely given up his aspirations to be a complete physician in the mode of Isidore Snapper, his hero from Mount Sinai days—thoughtful, thorough, able to care for patients with practically any medical problem. The idealism of the Kennedy era and the political turmoil of the late 1960s and early 1970s had likewise made their mark on Braunwald, who was more attuned to the healthcare needs of the community around medical schools than many in the prior generation of department chairmen at teaching hospitals.

In San Diego, Braunwald had been quietly appalled by the quality of many of the physicians in the community. Many of them had had only a single year of training beyond medical school, and Braunwald found their care to be spotty at best. "I would hear terrible stories at morning report, day after day, and then I would try to track down the doctors who were responsible. I'd look them up. They were people who had never done a residency." In San Diego, Braunwald had needed the referrals of not-so-great community physicians to keep his department's specialists busy. In Boston, however, he saw the chance to create a residency track that would train first-rate primary-care physicians.

Precisely because he was so well known as a cardiovascular researcher, Braunwald's support for the development of a primary-care program was conspicuous and effective. He joked that it was like "Nixon going to China"—a visit that had taken place the year Braunwald arrived at the Brigham. In his 1975 physician-in-chief report to the hospital, Braunwald wrote: "After a period in which most progress in medicine was made by examining, in great depth, individual organs and organ systems, it is time to 'put the patient together again' and to build up a strong cadre of general internists capable of seeing the patient as a whole and serving as models for students and residents."

Marshall Wolf, for his part, had stumbled into primary care without any plan to do so. He had been responding less to the forces of medical history than to the patients sitting in front of him. Before Braunwald had arrived, he had worked for the Harvard Community Health Plan, where the leaders believed that subspecialists should all practice general medicine in addition to their specialty—a view that was based on practical considerations as well as ideology, since the startup organization did not have enough patients to keep specialists busy. Wolf quickly realized that he did not know how to address many of the problems that his patients had, so he started spending a couple of half-days per week in clinics in other specialties. He learned how to inject joints, diagnose rashes, and do pelvic examinations. "I essentially crafted a primary-care residency program for myself."

As Wolf assumed his role as director of the house staff program, he opened a private practice in which he provided cardiology and general medical care. He was joined by three other general internists, including his close friend William Branch. Wolf soon became the "doctor's doctor" for the Harvard Medical School community, much as his predecessor, Eugene Eppinger, had been, and his reputation as a charismatic teacher grew as well. He and Branch developed a series of lectures and rotations, and then created a primary-care residency track in which trainees would spend substantial portions of each year practicing under faculty supervision in an outpatient setting.

The Brigham primary-care residency and similar programs that arose around the country in the 1970s and 1980s attracted many young physicians who were idealistic and highly politicized, and who wanted to provide care to underserved communities. It attracted others who wanted to develop new methods of studying the delivery of healthcare itself and to become influential in health policy, or leaders in improvement of quality and efficiency. Suspicions that Brigham's primary-care residents were second-class citizens who were not good enough to get into the "traditional" program faded away within a few years, and the track became the preferred destination for many applicants.

~

While Braunwald and Wolf were developing the primary-care track, they were also creating another track for trainees with strong commitments to research. Braunwald had been brewing the idea for this program since his first days at the NIH. During the short walks between his laboratory and the clinical facility, which he made several times a day, he became convinced that highly motivated physician-researchers could learn clinical medicine and perform research at the same time, if the physicians and the environment were right.

Braunwald and Wolf devised a program in which carefully selected trainees spent half of each year performing clinical work with the rest of the house staff, and the other half working on their research. Among the first interns selected, two were from Harvard Medical School: Jeffrey Drazen, who would go on to become an outstanding pulmonary researcher and the editor of the *New England Journal of Medicine,* and Thomas A. Musliner, who became a major leader of research at the pharmaceutical manufacturer Merck. A long line of other outstanding researchers followed, including Edward Benz, who became chairman of medicine at Johns Hopkins and then president of the Dana Farber Cancer Institute, and Gary Nabel, leader of the NIH's program to develop a vaccine against HIV.

Not all of the "Hemi-Docs," as they were called, were smashing successes in both laboratory and clinical work, and some did not succeed at either. The phrase "Hemi-Doc" itself was a bit of an insult in the minds of full-time clinicians, and Wolf monitored the clinical performance of the residents in this program especially closely, to ensure their competence. But with that support and supervision, many of the Hemi-Docs became Triple Threat physician-researchers who assumed leadership roles in academic medicine. The Hemi-Doc path allowed them to save a few years and get a jump-start on their careers, as Braunwald had done by taking the New York State Regents exam and entering college early. The shortening of their training period allowed them to assume major roles at an earlier age than otherwise would have occurred.

At first, the Hemi-Doc program focused on laboratory scientists; but with time, young physicians who were also economists, anthropologists, and other types of researchers were attracted to the Brigham because of the chance to pursue their research while learning how to take care of patients. Openness to new ways of making a contribution to medicine, and flexibility in structuring an individual's training, began to emerge as the hallmark of the Department of Medicine under Braunwald and Wolf. Their trainees later assumed unconventional leadership roles. For example, physician-economist Mark McClellan went on to lead the Centers for Medicare and Medicaid Services, and physician-anthropologists Paul Farmer and Jim Yong Kim founded the non-profit organization Partners in Health.[10] Kim later became president of Dartmouth College, and then president of the World Bank.

Although two cardiologists who had spent time at the NIH might be expected to have a laser-like focus on laboratory research, both Braunwald and Wolf enjoyed cultivating these unconventional researcher-residents. ("Not too bad for a Hemi-Doc," was Braunwald's reaction when Kim was named president of the World Bank.) Their broad concept of professional success made sense in the context of their own experiences. Braunwald was a European war refugee who understood how his social context had affected his life and work; he had wide-ranging cultural interests, including a love for opera. And Wolf was a Renaissance man of sorts who had spent a year bumming around Europe and was married to a psychiatrist. They both appreciated nonlaboratory intellectual life, so it was natural for them to be supportive of emerging researchers in health policy and clinical epidemiology, such as Lee Goldman, Anthony Komaroff, and Arnold Epstein, and to steer young trainees their way.

The culture of the program changed in other subtle but important ways. Wolf dropped the arduous oral examination that had been a traditional part of the Brigham's interview process. During these examinations, applicants would be asked to discuss a patient they had seen, or to give an impromptu discussion of a scientific topic. (One Brigham researcher used to start a metronome on his desk, and ask applicants to name as many causes of low blood calcium levels as they could during the next thirty seconds.) Wolf decided that nothing valuable was being learned about the applicants from these examinations, and that the Brigham was losing good people who considered the examinations humiliating. Interns and residents were also added to the house staff selection committees. These changes helped to set a new tone, and the Brigham Department of Medicine became known as a serious but happy place. It was an attractive message for a generation of house staff who were Baby Boomers raised during a time of peace and prosperity, in contrast to the Braunwald generation of survivors of the Depression, the Holocaust, and World War II.

Braunwald and the faculty conveyed another message to young applicants: that the Brigham was a place where hard work paid off. One Asian-American applicant for an internship recalled a conversation in December 1978 with Victor Dzau, MD, the Brigham's chief resident (later Braunwald's successor as Harvard's Hersey Professor, and subsequently chancellor for Health Affairs at Duke), in which the applicant noted that Dzau was the first chief resident of Chinese extraction that he had met in his tour of leading academic medical centers. (In that era, virtually all chief residents were still Caucasian males.) In response, Dzau said that there were no perfect meritocracies, but the Brigham came close— and that Braunwald set the tone. "You don't get ahead here by playing golf with the chairman, because the chairman doesn't play golf," Dzau said. "Dr. Braunwald doesn't care what color you are— he wouldn't care if you were purple. What he cares about is whether you're smart and work hard. If you are, and if you have any kind of luck at all, things tend to work out well here."

With increasing frequency, the Brigham got the people it wanted, and by the late 1970s it was among the top few training programs—arguably even Number 1. There was no formal ranking system, but Brigham advocates could now assert that it was a premier program.

~

Braunwald had made progress with getting the right people and with finding the funding to support them—but there was still the unmet need for a new hospital. The moment to move that agenda forward came a few years after his arrival, when Braunwald was asked to chair the search committee for a new chairman of the Department of Surgery. This new chairman would replace Francis Moore, a giant in his field.[11] Moore had played a crucial role in assembling the team that performed the world's first successful kidney transplant, and his textbook, *The Metabolic Care of the Surgical Patient,* was considered essential reading for surgeons-in-training.[12] He was one of the great names at the Brigham that helped to distract the world from the hospital's outmoded facilities.

When Braunwald learned that he was to lead the search for Moore's successor, the first thing he did was to meet with Moore and ask him to reconsider his retirement. Braunwald knew that Moore was in excellent health, and argued that his departure would jeopardize the Brigham's very existence. "You know better than I do that we can't survive without a new hospital," Braunwald told him. "We don't have the money, we don't have permission, we don't even have the plans. This just isn't a good time for you to go."

Moore would not change his mind, however, and the search committee soon focused on John Mannick, chairman of the Department of Surgery at Boston University. Mannick, a vascular surgeon, was a year older than Braunwald. He had attended Harvard College and Harvard Medical School, trained at Massachusetts General Hospital, and made major advances in surgical treat-ment of abdominal aortic aneurysms and peripheral vascular disease. He was a highly respected researcher and surgeon who had successfully run a major department of surgery—a prime can-didate for the Brigham, as well as for every other institution in the country looking for an outstanding surgical chief. Mannick was interested in the position, but he told Braunwald that there was no way he was coming unless he was absolutely certain a new hospital was going to be built.

The Certificate of Need for a new hospital had been denied in 1972 for two reasons. One was the terrible relationship between the Brigham and its surrounding community. The second was that the proposed construction was to serve three affiliated but non-merged hospitals: the Peter Bent Brigham Hospital, the Robert Breck Brigham Hospital (a small hospital, focusing on joint dis-eases, that had been started in 1914 with a bequest from Peter Bent Brigham's nephew Robert), and the Boston Hospital for Women. Massachusetts government officials thought that the new facility would be more efficient if the hospitals merged into one.

Progress was being made on both of these issues, but only slowly, and Braunwald did not feel confident that a new hospital would be built any time soon—at least, not without some political maneuvering that forced definitive action. Braunwald knew that he had to extract a real commitment from the Brigham's Board of Trustees, and asked for a meeting with the chairman and two other members of the board.

"How does a great hospital die?" Braunwald asked them. "It dies when it is unable to fill a key position. And that's where we are." Braunwald told them that the search committee had found a candidate, John Mannick, who was interested in the position and who had the qualities and experience to do a terrific job—but Mannick was not going to come without assurance that a new hospital would be built. Braunwald himself was not threatening to leave, but he said that he would resign from the chairmanship of the search committee unless the commitment to a new building was made, and that he was certain his resignation would not go unnoticed.

Shortly thereafter, while the board members were still digesting Braunwald's message and implied threat, Mannick called Braunwald to say that he was now under serious consideration for chairman of surgery at UCLA Medical Center. Braunwald told him that progress was being made on demonstrating a commitment to building the new hospital. Mannick replied that he needed something concrete.

Braunwald met with the three trustees again. "This is it," he said. The trustees decided they would show Mannick that they were serious about a new hospital by clearing out a parking lot next to the Brigham as a prelude to construction. They still did not have the Certificate of Need, but nothing prevented them from excavating their own parking lot. They arranged the work order for the excavation, and showed it to Mannick. That was sufficient proof of commitment: Mannick decided to accept the hospital's offer.

The Brigham closed the parking lot and began preliminary excavation for the foundation of the new hospital, even though it did not have permission to build. "Parking became terrible," Braunwald recalled. "It was very bad before, and then it became impossible." But at least the Brigham had its replacement for Franny Moore.

Mannick became chief of surgery in 1976, and Braunwald and he were effectively running the hospital soon thereafter. Of course, the new hospital that had been promised to Braunwald and now to Mannick did not spring up right away. The hole for the foundation was dug—but without the Certificate of Need, construction could not begin. Soon, the hole filled with water, and children would occasionally canoe in it. One Saturday night, a drunk driver careened through the surrounding barriers into the hole, and had to be fished out of his car and brought to the Emergency Department. Braunwald joked to the house staff that the drunk driver was the new hospital's first patient, even though the new hospital did not yet actually exist.

$\sim$

Eventually, permission to build was granted, and the new hospital, known as Brigham and Women's—a merger of the Peter Bent Brigham, the Robert Breck Brigham, and the Boston Hospital for Women—finally opened, in the summer of 1980. Braunwald now had new facilities and a top-tier department of medicine. But as he celebrated his fifty-first birthday, he looked back on a decade that had been difficult both professionally and personally.

During the mid-1970s, William Braunwald had been diagnosed with malignant melanoma. Eugene was painfully aware of the endless sacrifices his father had made for the family—when referring to his parents, he would frequently say, "After all they went through . . ." Showing his parents that those sacrifices had been worthwhile was an important motivation for him. William had died in 1977, at age seventy-three, and his premature death meant that he would never see the full extent of his son's success. Eugene had painful, vivid dreams for two years after the loss of his father.

His parents had been extremely close and dependent on each other, and Claire grieved deeply after her husband's death. Eugene felt responsible for his mother—after all, he was the elder son, and his brother, Jack, lived in Los Angeles. Eugene made frequent trips to New York to see Claire, as often as weekly during some periods, adding to the stress of his "crisis-of-the-week" professional life. About a year after William's death, Eugene took his mother on a trip to Israel. Six months later, he took her to London. Braunwald had been invited to deliver the keynote lecture at a celebratory meeting at the Royal College of Physicians, where he was able to introduce his mother to Prince Philip, the Duke of Edinburgh and the husband of Queen Elizabeth II. Claire was thrilled.

Despite these moments of pleasure, the decade was a difficult one. Braunwald was concerned about his mother, but he needed to devote tremendous amounts of time and attention to the hospital, to ensure the survival of the institution and his department. Later, he would admit that there were times during the 1970s when he'd felt overwhelmed by the challenges, particularly with the construction of the new hospital.

During that difficult period, leaving his position did cross his mind. "But I didn't quite know where to go. Everybody thought the Brigham was a destination job, a place you would never leave by choice. So I was not getting other feelers for chairmanships. And my children were getting used to their new schools and friends, and moving again would have been too hard for them. It simply was not an option."

Braunwald stayed, and by the end of the 1970s, survival was no longer an issue: his department was flourishing, by all conventional standards. Yet Braunwald knew that maintaining the new status quo was not a sound strategy. It was a time to contemplate growth—across Harvard's many hospitals, and in the Brigham's research enterprise.

: 10 :

Growth and Integration

1980–1996

As the 1980s began and the Brigham's Department of Medicine was hitting its stride, Eugene Braunwald might have turned back to his research with greater intensity, or he might have given more time and energy to his roles as a clinician and teacher. Instead, in that decade and beyond, his work as a department chairman and as a researcher changed in ways he had never anticipated.

When Braunwald left the NIH in 1968, he knew he was entering the "real world"—a world in which there were "normal" patient populations, not just the rarefied few who were referred by their stymied physicians to Bethesda. But, by 1980, he knew from experience that it was also a world in which hospitals competed for market share; where battles for space and resources within hospitals were especially intense because funding was so difficult to obtain; where there was a growing need to integrate care provided by many clinicians, often in many institutions. It was a world in which the nature of research was changing because the questions that needed to be answered were evolving. Braunwald was living through many of the changes he had anticipated in his 1972 article "Future Shock in Academic Medicine."

The issues seemed anything but academic, once he was ensconced in his new role at Harvard. One year after he arrived at the Brigham, he wrote his first physician-in-chief report, and gave considerable space to the hospital's need for rapid evolution. "Radical changes are likely to take place in health care delivery. The skyrocketing costs of inpatient medical care are forcing a fundamental reexamination of the necessity and duration of hospitalization. Alternate means of care, particularly ambulatory care, will be used to an ever-increasing extent. . . . This nation is faced with a shortage of skilled, well-trained primary care physicians. . . . A major direction for the Department will be to increase its contributions to the solution of the health problems faced by the local community."[1]

In these efforts, Braunwald wrote, he expected that the Department of Medicine would work closely with the Harvard Community Health Plan. In making this assertion, Braunwald was mapping out a strategy unusual among leaders in academic medicine, for whom managed care was new and suspect. But Braunwald was more than open to collaborating with this new HMO. Throughout the 1970s, and then in the 1980s, when HCHP's growth accelerated, Braunwald cultivated HCHP as an important partner for his department's expansion.

∼

HCHP was the brainchild and obsession of Robert Ebert, the dean of Harvard Medical School, and a group of his associate deans, including Henry Meadow. Several academics, including John Kenneth Galbraith and Howard Hiatt, lent their support to the country's first managed-care organization sponsored by a medical school—an organization that had opened its doors only three years before Braunwald's 1972 arrival in Boston.

In retrospect, the initial HCHP vision was just what one would expect from a group of 1960s idealists who wanted to serve their community, who looked askance at healthcare providers motivated by money, and who thought they could control healthcare costs through more effective prevention of disease. It was a vision unsullied by the skepticism about managed care that would become common in the decades to come, when large, for-profit health maintenance organizations became prominent as insurers.

This vision was to replace fee-for-service medicine with a pre-paid group practice, which would use salaried physicians and other clinicians to deliver comprehensive, coordinated care. The practice would emphasize prevention and teamwork, and when patients needed to be hospitalized, it would refer them to two respected Harvard teaching hospitals: Beth Israel and the Brigham.

Ebert and his associates planned their initial staffing for an anticipated membership of 10,000 people, but scaled their projections back to just 1,000 members in the weeks before HCHP opened its doors. Even that figure turned out to be overly optimistic. By opening day, October 1, 1969, only eighty-eight people had signed up, most of whom were employees of Beth Israel or the Brigham. The first patient to seek care was a man with chest pain, and the physician who evaluated him could not find a stethoscope. Just thirteen patients came in for visits during that first month.[2]

At least for a while, HCHP's doctors and nurses had time on their hands. "So the Harvard Plan quickly became one of the greatest donors of health care in the Greater Boston area," wrote H. Richard Nesson, the HCHP medical director at Beth Israel, in 1970. "We made arrangements for the medical staff to work in neighborhood health centers and other places where people needed help—and for free, because we were paying them a salary. They just needed things to do."[3] One of those locations was the Mission Hill–Parker Hill Health Center, just a few hundred yards from the Brigham.

During one of his earliest trips to Boston before formally moving into his role at the Brigham in 1972, Braunwald had visited HCHP and had met with its medical directors at the two Harvard hospitals—Nesson at Beth Israel and Joseph Dorsey at the Brigham. Nesson and Dorsey had been surprised that their HMO was so prominent on Braunwald's radar screen, as he gathered information about the position he was about to assume. HCHP was still a small organization, and in those days most leaders in academic medicine were just learning about health maintenance organizations; the abbreviation "HMO" had appeared in the *New England Journal of Medicine* for the first time only in 1971. In fact, many leaders of academic medicine were actively opposed to managed care—but Braunwald was not among them. His brother, Jack, was a Brigham-trained hematologist in the Kaiser organization. Through him, Braunwald was quite familiar with the quality of medical care delivered at Kaiser, and his reaction was positive.

Nesson and Dorsey were, at first glance, an unlikely team. Nesson was an affable Boston native from a Jewish family, and a Harvard College graduate; he had trained in nephrology at Beth Israel and then focused his energy on primary care. He possessed extraordinary interpersonal skills, and a knack for getting people to work together. He exuded warmth, and seemed to have done a favor at some point for every person in Boston. He thought acts of generosity were good strategy, and would often say, "I really do believe that every good thing you do eventually brings something good back to you. It may take a while, but it does." With countless small acts and some big ones, Nesson built an enormous web of supporters.

Dorsey was a devoted Catholic, the grandson of Irish immigrants. He had grown up in Pennsylvania's coal country without his father, who had died when Dorsey was four years old. He was an outstanding student and basketball star in high school, and he'd won a scholarship to the University of Scranton. But just as Marshall Wolf was pushed to look beyond the University of Chicago and apply to Harvard, Dorsey was encouraged to apply to Holy Cross (in Worcester, Massachusetts) by the headmaster at his Catholic school. That headmaster had come across Dorsey in the library, where the teenager was looking at catalogues from nonlocal schools, and said: "Well, if you're going away, you're going to

Holy Cross—it's the best Catholic school in the country. And put those non-Catholic-school catalogues away right now."

After Holy Cross, Dorsey went to Dartmouth Medical School for two years, and then finished his medical education at Harvard. He started his internship at Peter Bent Brigham Hospital, and began to make plans to apply for a two-year stint at the NIH, along with his fellow interns. Dorsey did not need to worry about avoiding the Doctor Draft, because he had developed diabetes and was thus ineligible for the draft—he was the one intern in Marshall Wolf's group who was granted a 4F deferment. But the NIH was where virtually everyone he respected sought to go, so Dorsey did, too.

Another plan materialized, however. Around this time, Robert Ebert was assuming his role as dean of Harvard Medical School, and was drumming up interest in his idea of a prepaid staff model HMO. George Thorn suggested to Dorsey that he get some further training in public health, and then come back to be the Brigham person in Ebert's organization. Since Dorsey was 4F, he was the one person in that residency group who would not be exposing himself to the Doctor Draft by doing so.

Dorsey liked the idea, and got a Master's in Public Health at Yale before returning to the Brigham for his senior residency. Dorsey turned down an offer from Eppinger to be chief resident at the Brigham; instead, at the end of the year he moved into Dean Ebert's offices at Harvard Medical School, and worked on getting HCHP off the ground.

Almost immediately after becoming chairman of the Department of Medicine, Braunwald scheduled frequent meetings with Dorsey and Wolf. Dorsey would give updates on how the HCHP's relationship with the Brigham was going, and Braunwald would ask what he could do to help. If there was a complaint from the house staff about the HCHP physicians, Braunwald would ask

Dorsey to look into it. And if one of the Brigham physicians had treated Dorsey's colleagues with disrespect, Dorsey would ask Braunwald for his help.

"At the end of our meetings, he would tick through the list of issues," Dorsey recalled. "He would let me know that *this* problem was on my side, and I needed to go fix it. But *that* issue was on his side, and he would take care of it. And when he said that, I could just scratch it off my list, because I knew I could count on him. You could put money in the bank that it was going to be fixed."[4]

Braunwald needed HCHP's patients for the Brigham, in order to have a vibrant medical service, but he also knew that was impossible if HCHP's physicians were seen as second-class citizens at the Brigham. Thus, Braunwald and Dorsey devised ways to integrate HCHP's staff with the Brigham faculty. Braunwald had originally proposed to Dorsey that Brigham specialists provide all inpatient specialty care for HCHP patients, but Dorsey said that HCHP would never be able to recruit its own specialists if he made that concession. In fact, Dorsey said, HCHP needed all its primary-care physicians to be credentialed as Brigham physicians.

At many places in the country, relationships between academic departments of medicine and staff model HMOs foundered on such issues, but Braunwald was determined to find solutions that would enable the Brigham to capture HCHP's patients for the good of the training program and the hospital. They agreed that Dorsey would talk to Brigham division chiefs when he was recruiting specialists, so that the roles might be filled with physicians loyal to both organizations. And one of Braunwald's most trusted internists, Tony Komaroff, would review the credentials of all the HCHP primary-care physicians who were being proposed for admitting privileges at the Brigham, and let Braunwald and Dorsey know if there were any problems.

Dorsey got credentials at the Brigham for his doctors, but

Braunwald made sure he knew that the stakes were high for both of them. Dorsey recalled one meeting at which Braunwald said, "Joe, I can see to it that your people will get privileges. What I can't guarantee is that they will have the respect of the house staff. That they have to earn."[5]

Braunwald told Dorsey that the HCHP physicians didn't have to participate in research; they needed to do just two things. "One, they have to take very good care of their patients, and, two, they have to be good teachers—and that's in your court to take care of."

Marshall Wolf and Richard Nesson worked closely with Braunwald and Dorsey to make the Brigham-HCHP relationship a model for the way HMOs and academic medical centers could collaborate. As with any complex relationship between two large groups of physicians, there were bumps in the road, but Braunwald, Dorsey, and Wolf were able to work most of them out. Wolf was quite familiar with HCHP from having worked there as a cardiologist, and the fact that Wolf and Dorsey had been residents together was another major positive factor. And when Dick Nesson came to the Brigham from Beth Israel in 1977—first as chief of the Division of General Medicine and then as president of the hospital—he used his special genius for cultivating relationships to become an effective fourth member of that group.

Dorsey remembered one day when he and Nesson were having a disagreement over a staffing issue. Dorsey told Nesson that he had to cut the discussion short, because he was going to a weekend retreat at St. Joseph's Abbey, a Trappist monastery in Spencer, Massachusetts, about fifty-five miles west of Boston. Nesson asked, "Do you think they'd ever let a Jew come along?" Dorsey replied that he wasn't sure, but they could find out.

Nesson went with Dorsey, and they shared a room during the retreat. The quiet, contemplative weekend turned out to be full of conversation—conversation about *everything*, not just healthcare but their personal lives as well. "From that moment forward, there was never anything difficult between us," Dorsey said. "What I saw was a man who was willing to do something like that to forge a friendship and to break through some barriers between us. He turned out to be the best friend I ever had."

During the 1980s, those close relationships among Dorsey, Nesson, Braunwald, and Wolf made it possible for HCHP to close a small hospital it had acquired on nearby Parker Hill, and consolidate their hospital admissions at Brigham and Women's. The Brigham charged HCHP rates for secondary care that were comparable to what it would cost HCHP to put the patient in a community hospital. This enabled the Brigham to fill beds that might otherwise have been empty, generating no income at all. And it enabled HCHP to market itself as an HMO that hospitalized patients in one of the most respected hospitals in the country.

There were several perpetual sources of discontent, and the Brigham-HCHP relationship required constant management. The HCHP physicians wanted to perform procedures in the cardiac catheterization laboratory and operating rooms of the Brigham. Giving those slots to HCHP physicians was beneficial for the hospital, but took them away from other Brigham physicians. The deal that gave HCHP low rates for routine care was a smart one when Brigham beds were empty, but was less attractive when the Brigham was full and could not find room for patients who would bring the hospital higher reimbursement. And HCHP was constantly tempted to move profitable services (such as radiology) outside the hospital and within its own walls (eventually it did so).

Yet the Brigham likewise derived benefits from the HCHP relationship. Because Dorsey and his HCHP colleagues were working relentlessly to improve efficiency, the Brigham tended to have a shorter average length of stay than other hospitals in the region— shorter by a full day or more. That was a "spillover" effect, through which the care of HCHP patients made the care of all Brigham patients more efficient. And Dorsey was a clear, unshrinking, and persistent "voice for the customer," pushing the Brigham to deliver what he needed to provide good and efficient care.

For example, in the early 1980s, the chief of radiology, Leonard Holman, proudly told Dorsey that his department was now able to get transcribed radiology reports into the charts of hospitalized patients within two days. A delay of several days had been common in the past; the medical chart was used more to create a permanent record than to capture the "news" for clinicians caring for a sick patient. If you really needed to find out what an x-ray had showed, you walked down to Radiology and looked for the film, and tried to grab a radiologist to review it with you.

Dorsey appreciated the improvement in turnaround time that Holman described, but was not embarrassed to suggest what he actually wanted. "That's very nice, Len," Dorsey said. "But the truth is that I need that information in about two hours." Holman was taken aback, but then helped to create a system through which radiology reports could be heard by telephone as soon as they had been dictated.

The Brigham primary-care residency was expanded by placing some house staff in HCHP centers for their ambulatory experience, so trainees who were steeped in the culture of a high-quality HMO began making their way onto the faculty. And HCHP began to produce its own diaspora of physicians, who went on to lead major change in the healthcare system elsewhere. Influential exports from HCHP included Donald Berwick, who started the Institute for Healthcare Improvement and became director of the Center for Medicare and Medicaid; Lawrence Shulman, chief medical officer at Dana Farber Cancer Institute; Louise Liang, who became chief operating officer of Group Health Cooperative of Puget Sound and then the leader of Kaiser Permanente's ambitious national quality agenda; and Glenn Steele, the former Brigham-HCHP surgeon who became CEO of Geisinger Health System. These HCHP alumni were known as physicians who understood that excellence and efficiency were not in conflict, and that they often came together. With time, Brigham residents realized that their colleagues who were assigned to the HCHP track were not getting a second-class experience; they were getting a different one—in fact, an experience providing certain strengths that the traditional Brigham tracks did not.

Not all of Braunwald's initiatives beyond the walls of the Brigham worked out as well as the partnership with HCHP. In 1980, he took on a second job as physician-in-chief at Beth Israel, the Harvard teaching hospital adjacent to the Brigham. For most of the next decade, when he was in his fifties, Braunwald did something no one in academic medicine had done before: serve simultaneously as chairman of two major departments of medicine. It seems unlikely that anyone will attempt to do so again. Asked later why he took on this dual role, Braunwald said, "I look back and wonder."

At the time, the chairman of medicine at Beth Israel was Franklin H. Epstein, a highly respected and well-liked nephrologist who had started his tenure as chief at Beth Israel on the same day in 1972 that Braunwald had started at the Brigham. Like Braunwald, Epstein was from Brooklyn; he'd graduated from Brooklyn College in 1944. He'd attended Yale for medical school and clinical training, and had done research under Dr. John P. Peters, who was also a mentor to Donald Seldin.

Epstein had not really sought the role of chairman of medicine; he essentially fell into the position in the aftermath of some local academic and political upheavals. He was a pleasant man and a clinical scholar, much loved and respected by his colleagues, and someone who did not particularly enjoy the hiring, firing, and politicking that dominated the life of a Harvard department chairman. By the end of the decade, he was ready to give up the chairmanship and resume his more natural role as researcher, physician, and teacher.

Braunwald was on the search committee for Epstein's replacement. Some very good external candidates had turned down the job because they believed that Beth Israel was dominated by part-time physicians who were in private practice and that the hospital would never be able to compete with its two major Harvard rivals, Massachusetts General Hospital (MGH) and the newly strengthened Brigham. To Braunwald, it seemed foolish to have two Harvard hospitals, the Brigham and Beth Israel, competing so fiercely within a few blocks of each other. He thought that eventually the Longwood Medical Area should become the Harvard Medical Center, and that the two hospitals should merge.

As the conventional search process sputtered along, another idea began to take shape. Braunwald could not remember who first proposed that he might serve as chief at both the Brigham and Beth Israel; he was quite sure it wasn't his idea. Yet when Beth Israel's leadership asked Braunwald to succeed Epstein, Braunwald agreed to do so. He thought he could move the two hospitals toward becoming a single institution and forming the clinical core of the Harvard Medical Center, even though he knew that such a merger was not a motivating vision for most people at either institution. He first needed to show the trustees, physicians, and administration at Beth Israel that he was "one of them," so he took pains to emphasize that he was physician-in-chief at two hospitals, not one.

Braunwald used the two campuses as an opportunity to try different things. He introduced the "firm system," in which Beth Israel's inpatient medical service was divided into subunits. Braunwald had seen the firm system in action while serving as a visiting professor in leading London teaching hospitals, and had observed that it created a culture akin to that of the multiple colleges at Oxford and Cambridge universities. Braunwald thought that Beth Israel's medical service was too large and diffuse, with dozens of patients admitted each day by different private practitioners, who would come by the hospital briefly and then return to their offices. Under the new system, the house staff was divided into "firms," each of which was headed by a respected academic leader who was responsible for teaching the trainees. The firm chief was on service for the entire year, and, for the most part, house staff performed all their clinical work with the same group of colleagues within their firm.

"And, by George, it worked!" said Braunwald. "People identified with the firms, and they wanted to be firm chiefs. They took those roles seriously—so seriously that I had to come up with firm associate chiefs because it became such a heavy responsibility." Many other academic departments of medicine, including those of Johns Hopkins and Massachusetts General, soon adopted the model, albeit each with its own distinct flavor.

Braunwald brought a number of up-and-coming physician-researchers from the Brigham to Beth Israel, even though such moves created anxiety on both campuses. But Braunwald was beginning to see that one of the problems of having such young stars as division chiefs at the Brigham was that there was no room for even younger rising stars to move upward. Now Braunwald had an outlet for them. Thus, he appointed William Grossman, who had been leading the catheterization laboratory at the Brigham, as the new chief of cardiology at Beth Israel. And he recruited a young Brigham transplant expert named Terry Strom to be Beth Israel's chief of immunology. Both had been considering major posts at other institutions, and Braunwald knew that their days at the

Brigham were numbered. By giving them leadership roles at Beth Israel, he was keeping them at Harvard.

Braunwald gave some people roles at both hospitals. Jeff Drazen, the first Brigham Hemi-Doc resident, had become an outstanding pulmonary researcher; he and the Brigham's pulmonary chief, Roland Ingram, worked at both institutions. Jack Rowe, who would later go on to be president of the Mount Sinai Medical Center, in New York, ran geriatric units within both departments. And Lee Goldman, who had emerged as Braunwald's other lieutenant at the Brigham along with Marshall Wolf, took on comparable management responsibilities at Beth Israel. Braunwald's plan was becoming apparent: to replace one person at a time with someone from the other hospital, or appoint one person to do the same job at both institutions until the two departments were virtually one.

Yet that plan would not come to fruition. As the 1980s progressed, managed-care organizations began to appear, and they started to steer patients to preferred hospitals. The Brigham and Beth Israel found themselves in direct competition for those patients, particularly those enrolled in the Harvard Community Health Plan. And in that competition, both organizations wondered aloud which side Braunwald was on.

To try to alleviate concerns at the Brigham, Braunwald put together a summary of progress at its Department of Medicine, citing the fact that its NIH research support had more than doubled during his years at both hospitals. His point was that similar progress at Beth Israel did not come at the expense of the Brigham's success. He acknowledged that the departures of physicians like Bill Grossman and Terry Strom were losses for the Brigham, but said those staff members would have departed to other places if Braunwald had not created an option for them within the Harvard system.

His diagnosis: "I don't think people at either hospital saw themselves as being part of a system, and that was the problem." They were not particularly worried about the future of Harvard—this they took for granted—but they were quite concerned about the competitive status of their hospital programs. When stars like Grossman and Strom left, many Brigham people privately acknowledged that they would have preferred to see them go across the country, rather than across Longwood Avenue to Beth Israel.

The incident that made Braunwald surrender his vision of bringing the two hospitals together occurred as he was leading a search for a joint chief of neurology for the Longwood Medical Area. The neurology chief at Beth Israel had died suddenly—a loss that created an opportunity to form a single neurology program that would serve the Brigham, Beth Israel, and Children's Hospital. An outstanding Canadian researcher—an expert in Alzheimer's disease—was identified, and he was poised to bring a terrific group of researchers with him. Everyone thought he would be a fine addition to the Harvard community, even MGH neurologists who would be his crosstown competitors.

The neurology researcher needed space, however, and that's where the deal fell apart. To start, he needed 5,000 square feet; later, he'd require 15,000. And he insisted that the laboratories couldn't be spread all over the Longwood area—they had to be contiguous. The demand made perfect sense if one wanted a great neurologist to lead a great laboratory and a great neurology program for the Brigham, Beth Israel, and Children's Hospital. But space was owned by the hospitals individually, not collectively, and Braunwald could not get any of the three hospitals to come up with that much space for someone who would be leading work at all three campuses. The deal unraveled, and the researcher stayed in Canada.

"At that point, I could read the writing on the wall, and I threw in the towel," Braunwald said. He could see that the integration of the Brigham and Beth Israel would take decades if it was accomplished one physician at a time, with every joint appointment comparable to giving birth to a baby. He did not want to spend the rest of his academic career fighting those fights, trying to find space at hospitals whose leaders wondered why they were asked to allocate resources to someone who was not completely "theirs." Braunwald announced that he was leaving Beth Israel, and gave the hospital one year's notice. A search committee for Braunwald's successor chose Robert Glickman, who at the time was chief of the medical service at Columbia-Presbyterian Hospital in New York.

In a sense, the Braunwald experiment as chief at two hospitals was a success for Beth Israel. The institution's inability to attract anyone outstanding in 1979–1980 was exactly what caused it to turn to Braunwald. Over the next decade, he improved Beth Israel to the point where it could lure an outstanding academic leader such as Glickman away from a top position at another first-rate institution.

Braunwald, though, regretted the experiment. Trying to manage two departments of medicine had turned out to be more than psychologically demanding—it had been physically painful as well. One winter day in 1987, Braunwald had slipped while walking between the Brigham and Beth Israel, breaking his shoulder. At the moment he fell, he was on a sidewalk beside Children's Hospital and was looking up at Dana Farber Cancer Institute. The four institutions were so close that they all figured in Braunwald's injury, but cooperation among them was a daunting challenge.

"In retrospect, I gave up a lot, and I feel that it was a professional mistake. I was fifty years old when I started, and it was energy-draining being in overdrive for nine years. What did I give up? I gave up my growing personal practice, because I had lots more administrative work. Being physician-in-chief at two hospitals meant twice as much of going to innumerable staff meetings, dinners with trustees, fundraising, et cetera.

"I did some things I was proud of, but I was so busy that I missed the chance to do research in heart failure that I was poised to do if I hadn't been at Beth Israel. And I was less available to my family."

~

During the 1970s and 1980s, the Brigham's relationship with HCHP gave Braunwald an early taste of managed care and the need for greater efficiency—but it was only a taste, compared to what ensued in the next decade. In the early to mid-1980s, hospitals were full and hospitalizations leisurely. For example, a patient undergoing a routine cardiac catheterization would be admitted two days before the procedure, and stay two days afterward. (By the mid-1990s, a patient undergoing the same procedure would routinely be admitted and discharged on the same day.) There was little real competition among hospitals, most of which were financially healthy because they could demand payments that covered whatever their costs might be.

But during the 1980s, Medicare started paying for hospitalizations on a DRG (Diagnosis-Related Group) basis—that is, a fixed amount for the entire hospitalization. And health maintenance organizations such as HCHP and those started by insurance companies began to send nurse case managers into hospitals, to make sure their patients were not staying longer than absolutely necessary. (These HMOs were paying hospitals by the day, at that time.) Hospitals became institutions where seriously ill patients received treatment, but then were discharged to home, a nursing-care facility, or a rehabilitation center for their convalescence. The result was that length of stay started to decrease. At the Brigham, Massachusetts General Hospital, and other institutions with excellent reputations, the same numbers of patients were being admitted each year, but their stays were much shorter—and so the daily census fell. Entire floors lay empty, and staff was idle.

Empty beds unnerve hospital administrators. In the late 1980s they began to vie for increased market share by offering HMOs lower rates. These discounted rates were often below their "fully loaded" costs—that is, costs per bed-day to which overhead expenses had been allocated. On the other hand, the discounted rates were higher than the "variable" costs—that is, the incremental costs of caring for an additional patient for that day. These variable costs included the personnel, the food, the medications, the laundry used by the patient, and so on—but not the overhead costs of the utilities like electricity, the administration, the security guards, the hospital equipment. When a hospital had a patient lying in a bed and was getting paid something more than the variable costs, it was better off than it would have been if the bed were empty. On the other hand, if hospitals filled their beds with patients reimbursed at the discounted rates that they were offering HMOs, they would eventually go out of business.

Fortunately for hospital administrators of that era, Medicare business had become quite profitable. Once hospitals got used to the concept of DRGs, they found that they could shorten length of stay, discharge patients to home or to a nonacute facility, and fill the bed with another patient who would bring in another DRG payment. Medicare profits allowed hospitals to fill other beds with HMO patients who were reimbursed at lower rates—that is, if the hospitals could find those patients. And through most of the 1980s they could.

As the 1990s began, however, the managed-care experience in California gave the rest of the country a preview of coming attractions. Hospitals that could not fill their beds were closing, and HMOs were offering physicians contracts in which they would have fixed budgets to cover all the healthcare costs for a population; the system was known as capitation. HCHP had shown Braunwald and others at the Brigham that capitation was compatible with good healthcare, and even compatible with full occupancy for the Brigham. But as the length of hospitalizations fell, beds and then entire floors lay empty. As the occupancy rate fell, administrators at the Brigham and other hospitals became increasingly concerned.

It was a time of enormous transition in the way healthcare was delivered, and Braunwald's department was being affected along with everyone else. Braunwald had to become involved; he could not have sat on the sidelines even if he'd wanted to.

In the winter of 1992–1993, the dean of Harvard Medical School, Daniel Tosteson, called together leadership representatives from each of the five large Harvard teaching hospitals: the Brigham, Massachusetts General Hospital, Beth Israel, Children's Hospital, and New England Deaconess Hospital. Each hospital sent the chairman of its board of trustees, its CEO, and one physician leader. Braunwald was the physician selected by Brigham CEO Dick Nesson. The other Brigham representative was John McArthur, chair of the Brigham's board and dean of Harvard Business School.

A series of meetings were held in Harvard's Countway Library; Braunwald described them as "awkward." A Washington law firm was brought in to review the legal ramifications of any affiliation among the five hospitals, but as Braunwald later recalled, "People had trouble following what they said, and didn't know where this was leading." Within two to three meetings, it seemed clear to many of the attendees that a deeper affiliation among all of them was unlikely. Some attendees expressed concern about being asked to foot the bill for a share of the consultants' fees without prior discussion. When that issue was raised, Braunwald realized how skeptical he felt that the five Harvard hospitals would be able to collaborate on the bigger challenges before them.

The three Brigham representatives talked after one session, and agreed that these meetings were going nowhere. McArthur said he was going to talk to his counterpart at Mass General, Ferdinand ("Moose") Colloredo-Mansfield, a prominent real-estate developer, to see whether a two-way collaboration might work.

McArthur and Colloredo-Mansfield had a positive meeting, and McArthur then told Tosteson that Mass General and the Brigham were pulling out. The Harvard-wide collaboration was dead, and the Brigham team began meeting with the three Mass General leaders: Colloredo-Mansfield, CEO J. Robert Buchanan, and Gerald Austen, the chairman of surgery, who thirty years before had shared an office at the NIH with Nina Braunwald.

As 1993 progressed, pressure on the Brigham and Mass General leaders to do something mounted. An increasing number of hospital beds lay empty, and both hospitals closed patient units and laid off personnel. Instead of their historic 85–90 percent occupancy, they were running 60–65 percent full. "The fear was intense," Braunwald recalled. "The idea was prevalent among this very tightly knit group that academic medicine, as we knew and treasured it, was heading for the rocks."

They were so pessimistic that one of their goals was to preserve at least one great teaching hospital for Harvard Medical School— even if that meant consolidating Mass General and the Brigham. Faced with such dire fears, they did not obsess long over details. They had six meetings of three hours each, and then a weekend retreat at Babson College, in nearby Wellesley.

The long relationship between Austen and Braunwald was an important part of the chemistry. The two physician-leaders knew that each was fiercely loyal to his hospital, but also scrupulously honest. They had known each other so long, and in so many ways, that they could be candid and realistic with each other. This enabled them to agree to disagree on some issues, and defer making decisions on them, rather than have the negotiations founder. At the end of the retreat, the six shook hands. Someone brought a bottle of champagne, and they toasted the agreement to integrate the two hospitals through a parent company, Partners HealthCare System.

When Nesson and Buchanan announced the merger the next week, it was front-page news—and a shock to the physicians and other personnel at both hospitals. The secret had been so closely held that hardly anyone outside the small group at the meetings was aware of the possibility that the two hospitals might merge. Indeed, most of them learned of the formation of Partners from reading the *Boston Globe* on December 8, 1993: "The merger of the two historic rivals, the most momentous development in a flurry of consolidations of hospitals in Massachusetts and elsewhere, is intended to reduce costs and avoid duplicating services in anticipation of national health care reform. Officials at both hospitals felt that a combined and streamlined institution would be better positioned to bid for contracts with health care purchasing groups under the managed competition scheme proposed by President Clinton, according to hospital officials familiar with the discussions."[6]

The article went on to note that more than two million people in Massachusetts belonged to HMOs, which were bargaining for discounts at hospitals and trying to eliminate unnecessary medical care, with the likely end result being the shrinking of hospitals. It quoted a respected healthcare consultant, Ann Thornburg, as saying, "Some people think we will lose 30 to 50 percent of our beds in the next few years."

The formation of Partners made sense to objective observers of the healthcare system—but it infuriated other stakeholders inside and outside the new organization. At the Brigham, Nesson and Braunwald announced the merger to the other chairs of departments, a small group of division chiefs, other physician and administrative leaders, and then made a larger joint presentation to the general hospital community. Braunwald told the physicians that he was supportive of the merger, and that it was the right thing to do in the face of an impending tsunami in healthcare, especially in overbedded Massachusetts.

Nevertheless, physicians at the Brigham and at Mass General were upset that they had been left out of the negotiations, and drew little consolation from the argument that if the merger had been the subject of a broad discussion, dozens of reasons not to go forward would have come up, obscuring the strategic imperatives that supported the bold move. The physicians also worried that they would lose their jobs as consolidation occurred. The expectation was that fewer specialists were going to be needed in the future in any case, and the merger would accelerate the exodus of specialists from the Brigham and Mass General. At one grim meeting at the Brigham, physicians joked: "Look to the left of you, and look to the right of you—one of you will be gone in two years."

Informal bets were made on which of the counterparts at the two institutions would survive in a consolidated hospital. The chief of one Brigham department sat at lunch after the announcement was made, and recounted how, as a child, he and his friends had played a game in which they would take two M&M candies and press them against each other until one of them cracked. They would continue this process until they found the strongest M&M in their bag of candy. He said that this was what was about to begin at Partners—and that when he was compared with his counterpart at MGH, "I'm going to be the M&M that cracks."

Outside Partners, there was anger mixed with embarrassment.

The *Boston Globe* article announcing the merger pointed out that Mass General and the Brigham had "proceeded independently from an effort by Dr. Daniel Tosteson, dean of the Harvard Medical School, to organize the five flagship Harvard hospitals into a unified system." Tosteson had been traveling in Europe, and learned of the formation of Partners just as he returned, on the night before it was announced. He declined to comment to the *Globe,* but his unhappiness was far from secret.

Mitch Rabkin, MD, the president of Beth Israel, was incredulous. The *Globe* quoted him as saying he was unaware of any specific deal: "I would be surprised if they came out with an announcement of a merger that had not been discussed with the dean and the other institutions." David Weiner, the president of Children's Hospital, also indicated that he was unfamiliar with the agreement.

A day later, the shock was beginning to wear off, and the goals and implications of the new relationship were undergoing serious examination. J. Robert Buchanan, the CEO of Mass General, said that the two hospitals expected major cost reductions from their combined $1.2 billion operating budgets. He was quoted as saying "We're pretty sure we've got to save 20 percent at a minimum, and our ambitions go well beyond that."[7] Buchanan said those savings could be reached within two to three years, through administrative consolidation.

Outside observers commented that the formation of Partners signaled the beginning of a wave of consolidation likely to affect all academic and community institutions. After taking a day to reflect, Dean Tosteson said: "I consider this the first in a series of constructive rearrangements." When asked how many Harvard hospitals would be left in three or four years, Tosteson shrugged, and answered in French, "Je ne sais pas."[8]

Braunwald described the change as part of the redesign of

healthcare, and was ready to sound upbeat about taking on the challenge. "We have an overabundance of specialists nationally— particularly in Boston. Merged programs should be able to shrink, yet maintain high-quality care."[9] He called the day of the announcement one of real excitement for him.

The honeymoon did not last long. The next day, buried on page fifty of the *Boston Globe,* was a story about how Mass General was proceeding with its plans to launch an obstetrical unit—even though the Brigham was the region's leader in obstetrical care.[10] The unit was to be led by six physicians who had left the Brigham just a couple of months before. Two of them had been asked by the Brigham's new chief of obstetrics and gynecology to take smaller roles, and, rather than step down, they had accepted offers to move across town to Mass General, taking some of their colleagues and patients with them.

The Brigham obstetricians who made these moves and the Mass General leaders who recruited them did so without any knowledge of the Partners discussions. Mass General had recruited them as part of a long-planned effort to grow its program in women's health, in part because hospital leadership understood that women made many of the healthcare decisions for families, and that those decisions would become increasingly important in the managed-care era. Now that the formation of Partners was under way, Mass General was giving the former Brigham obstetricians reassurance that it would honor its commitment to them. But the situation was an early embarrassment for the leaders who had negotiated the Partners deal.

The announcement that Mass General would proceed with its plans to open an obstetrics service was a sign that integration of the hospitals' clinical services would not come easily. On the following day, the *Boston Globe* ran an article on cultural differences between the two hospitals, one in which Braunwald figured prominently. Based on interviews with more than a dozen "cogno-scenti," the article speculated about the future:

> Subtle but real differences . . . could provoke fireworks and bruise egos as the two giants move together into 21st-century medicine.
> . . . Some say, tradition is such at "The General" that any doctor worth his—or more rarely, her—salt can be a director of some-thing, resulting in a mishmash of semi-autonomous kingdoms that would give Bismarck the horrors.
>
> This autonomy is fueled by the fact that many MGH doctors, some of whom are part-timers, are still paid the old-fashioned way, on a fee-for-service basis directly from patients and insurers. This means less hospital control and more take-home pay, but less paid time in which to pursue research.
>
> Quite the opposite holds true at Brigham and Women's, which was formed in 1980 when the Peter Bent Brigham, the Robert Breck Brigham and the Boston Hospital for Women merged. The Brigham, most observers agree, is a no-nonsense hierarchy domi-nated by its powerful chief of medicine, Dr. Eugene Braunwald. At the Brigham, doctors are typically full-time employees on salary, allowing the hospital more discretion and the doctors more secu-rity, if occasionally less income.
>
> The smart money, insiders say, is on Braunwald to have the up-per hand, which is denied by both him and his MGH counterpart, Dr. John Potts, chief of medicine. MGH also has a powerful chief of surgery, Dr. W. Gerald Austen, like Braunwald a prime mover behind the merger.[11]

This *Globe* article, and its implication that Braunwald was the dominant chairman of medicine and Austen the dominant chair-man of surgery, did little to ease tensions between the two new "partner" hospitals.

As it turned out, there was virtually no consolidation of clinical services in the early years of Partners, for two reasons. First, the political strife surrounding any discussion of consolidation was intense. Second, consolidation turned out to be unnecessary, because the number of patients coming to the two hospitals began to increase. By coincidence, patient volumes at Mass General and the Brigham reached a low point in December 1993, when the Partners merger was announced. The volume remained at about that same level for six months, and then started to climb. Over the next several years, both hospitals needed to reopen the floors they had closed, and then build new inpatient and outpatient facilities, both on their main campuses and in new facilities in the suburbs. Clinical consolidation was put on the back burner, because it was difficult to make the case for cost reductions through integration when the programs at both hospitals were full to overflowing.

Why did volumes increase? Several factors played a role. Consultants' doom-and-gloom predictions about an impending decrease in hospital beds were actually correct: small hospitals in Boston and the rest of Massachusetts were closing, and many of their patients came to the Partners hospitals. Of course, the reputations of both the Brigham and Mass General continued to grow, in part because of advances by their researchers—but that process had been ongoing for decades. In a newer strategy, both hospitals expanded their numbers of primary-care physicians, and Partners started a network that included community-based physicians, both primary-care and specialist.

That network was led by Ellen Zane, the former CEO of Quincy Hospital (in Quincy, Massachusetts), who was already known as a highly effective manager. By the year 2000, this network would include more than a thousand primary-care physicians. The "glue" for this network lay in the contracts that Partners was negotiating with health insurance plans, and referral of patients to the Brigham and Mass General was never mandated. Yet these new relationships and the new physicians based at the two hospitals undoubtedly helped to increase the number of referrals. A quarter-century later, the integrated academic healthcare system that Braunwald had envisioned in his "Future Shock" article was emerging.

Instead of taking on the brutal work of consolidating clinical programs, the Brigham and Mass General had to focus on handling the increased volume of patients and on improving the efficiency and quality of care, which were the targets of incentives built into the contracts. The fact that Partners did *not* try to force consolidation among clinical services at the Brigham and MGH was later described as a reason this merger succeeded, while others during the same period did not. Mergers between Geisinger Health System and Hershey Medical Center, and between Stanford and the University of California San Francisco, were created but soon fell apart. At the press conference announcing the dissolution of the UCSF-Stanford merger, a reporter asked Lee Goldman, who had left the Brigham to become chairman of medicine at UCSF, whether the breakup of that merger would be costly. Goldman replied, "Have you ever seen a divorce that wasn't more expensive than the wedding?"[12]

Meanwhile, in Boston, Beth Israel's leadership had concluded that the hospital could not be successful without forming its own partnerships. In 1996, Beth Israel merged with New England Deaconess Hospital to form Caregroup Healthcare System, which began to build its own community-based network similar to that of Partners. The Beth Israel–Deaconess merger was soon troubled by physician discontent, as the two hospitals began to integrate their campuses, which were only one block apart. The merger ultimately endured, but many physicians left, including most of the leaders who had negotiated the merger.

The Partners merger was likewise riven by internal tensions. At a peacemaking dinner that was scheduled after the *Globe* published its article on cultural differences, Braunwald addressed physician leaders from both hospitals. He preached a combination of "macro-collaboration and micro-competition." He emphasized the need for physicians at the Brigham and Mass General to work together in conducting research and improving patient care. But he said it was only natural—indeed, healthy—for them to compete for referrals on the basis of excellent service and patient care. He said that they should compete in trying to recruit the best house staff, but should never run down the other institution as they did so. That advice became the ground rules for relationships within Partners.

~

The early 1990s brought two painful personal losses for Braunwald. His mother, Claire, was in her mid-eighties and becoming increasingly frail. She was still living in her home in Queens, and Braunwald and his daughters, now adults in their thirties, went to New York frequently to do what they could to keep her independent. They knew that her time was growing short.

What Braunwald could not imagine, however, was that he would lose his mother and his wife within a six-week period in 1992. Nina was sixty-four and increasingly disabled by metastatic breast cancer, and Claire's health was worsening. Braunwald felt tortured—he could not be in two places at once. In May 1992, at age eighty-six, Claire died of aspiration pneumonia, and Nina succumbed on August 5.

"You can't see the moon if the sun shines very bright," Braunwald said, reflecting on that period. Preoccupied with the impending loss of his wife, he felt that he never had the chance to properly mourn the loss of his mother. In any case, he was not one to grieve publicly. He found ways to honor Nina and Claire as the years passed, but returned to work with little delay. One of his textbooks had its next edition postponed by a year, but otherwise he plunged back into the work of running his department.

Harvard rules dictate that department chairs retire from their administrative roles no later than the first of July following their sixty-sixth birthday. This policy meant that Braunwald had to step down from his role as chairman of the Brigham's Department of Medicine on June 30, 1996. Although Nesson asked him to stay on a year-to-year basis, Braunwald felt it was time to make the change. Some major positions in the department needed to be filled, and he thought it would be unwise to fill them and then turn the department over to his successor.

"And the truth is, I was very much caught up in Partners fever," he recalled. He was fully aware of political tensions and dysfunction within Partners, but continued to believe in the potential synergies of the overall system, especially on the academic side. He was, after all, someone who had given a decade of his life to advancing the concept of a Brigham–Beth Israel merger and the formation of a Harvard Medical Center in Boston's Longwood area. He thought that Mass General and the Brigham had a better chance of succeeding in forming a real partnership, and that the potential result could be spectacular. The development of Partners might have greater impact on medicine than running the Brigham's Department of Medicine. He was ready to enter the fray.

Braunwald stepped into a newly created position at Partners: chief academic officer and vice president for academic programs. The current leaders of Partners, Dick Nesson and Sam Thier, let Braunwald propose his own job description, since the concept of a chief academic officer at a hospital or healthcare system was a new one at the time. After a long discussion, they agreed on the outlines of a set of responsibilities that included defining institutional policies for training and research.

One of Braunwald's major tasks was leading the process through which Partners-based candidates were evaluated before being formally nominated for a professorship at Harvard Medical School. "With all of the politics at Harvard, those things are largely laid aside when it comes to appointing a full professor," he said. "There may be fierce competition in our academic world, even spiteful behavior, but when it comes to voting to evaluate someone for promotion, faculty usually checks those issues at the door. I felt it would help the integration across the Brigham and MGH if people began to appreciate what people in the sister institution had accomplished."

In contrast, Braunwald's other major responsibility—bringing together physicians and researchers across Partners—was far from pleasant. He created a Partners Research Committee to seek opportunities for collaboration, and set up a framework for the integration of Brigham and Mass General training programs that ranged from occasional electives at the "sister" institution to complete merger. In neurology, for example, residents could rotate freely between the two hospitals.

"I would get two chairmen of small departments to talk about having a single residency. And I would find that they *really* did not want to work together. What united them was the shared goal of pushing back against anything that meant a loss of their autonomy. They would say, 'No—the programs are totally different; one is five years, the other is four. How could you even suggest a merger?'"

Nevertheless, Braunwald was someone who was difficult to fend off, at least completely or indefinitely. During his seven years in this role, thirty-two training programs came together, with deeper levels of integration or complete merger. Most of those merged programs became unequivocally the most prestigious in the country. As one neurology resident said in a 2010 interview: "Before, applicants were tortured by whether you try to get into the Brigham or MGH, or perhaps one or two other good places. After the Brigham and MGH merged their neurology programs, there was no longer any question of where you wanted to go."

: 11 :

Research in Evolution

When deeply immersed in administrative responsibilities, most physicians in academic medicine reduce their direct involvement in research, or stop altogether. They move into the roles of supporter, facilitator, and observer for the research of others. But throughout his years as chairman of a department of medicine, Braunwald was always reluctant to step back too far from research—he enjoyed the thinking, the meticulous preparation, and the bright young people. Just the smell of the dog labs would lift his spirits.

In 1971, just a few months before he moved to Boston, he had published what he would always consider his single most important paper—the "Factors Paper"—with Peter Maroko and other researchers. Although the research had been performed in dogs, not human beings, the demonstration that the size of a myocardial infarction could be modified by interventions over the next few hours had obvious implications for clinical medicine. At that time, the "state of the art" of treatment for heart attacks consisted of putting patients to bed in a coronary care unit, resuscitating them if they had cardiac arrests, and otherwise hoping for the best. The findings in the Factors Paper meant that this era was coming to an end. It was time for the biomedical-research community to explore the ability of various medications, procedures, and operations to change the course of disease for actual patients.

Braunwald understood the challenge and the opportunity, and he was not going to sit on the sidelines as this new phase of medical history began—especially in the case of acute myocardial infarction or closely related topics like heart failure. His research group might not be able to dominate an area the way they had dominated hypertrophic cardiomyopathy when he was at the NIH, but Braunwald was determined to remain a player. He was going to continue to run a laboratory where young protégés could be groomed to be researchers on the cutting edge.

It was a time when people at the top of academic medicine began talking about Quadruple Threats: Triple Threats who were also excellent administrators. Braunwald was willing to delegate significant responsibility to key lieutenants in some areas (for example, teaching and patient care to Marshall Wolf; finance to Lee Goldman), and narrow his focus in cardiovascular research more than he would have liked. But he was determined to maintain excellence in the research that he did. He did not want to just turn out publications so other researchers knew he was alive. He wanted to continue to try to address questions that might be "game changers" for medicine.

He had brought Maroko and another young researcher, Steven Vatner, with him from San Diego to Boston, and had set them up in their own laboratories. For the next few years, most of the papers Braunwald published included one or both of them as fellow authors. Then, around 1976, publications began to emerge with a new generation of physician-researchers, including Robert Kloner, David Hillis, Marc Pfeffer, and many others. Throughout his twenty-four years as chairman of the Brigham's Department of Medicine, he always maintained an NIH-supported research group that published a steady stream of papers, albeit at a lower rate than when he had been at the NIH. After he stepped down from his department chairmanship, his research productivity surged, as he began devoting the majority of his time to research (see Figure 22).

The flow of Braunwald papers never stopped through these decades, but fundamental changes occurred in the nature of the

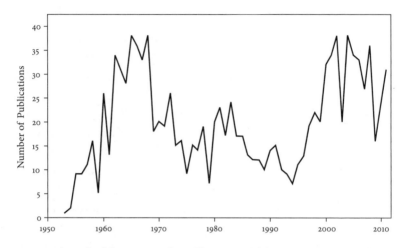

22. Number of publications authored by Braunwald per year. *Courtesy of McKinsey and Company.*

research. When Braunwald had first arrived at Stanley Sarnoff's NIH laboratory in 1955, for example, he and his colleagues studied the factors affecting myocardial oxygen consumption—a scientific question to be addressed in laboratory models. By the early 1970s, the question concerned the factors that might change infarct size in dogs in a laboratory. As the 1970s and 1980s unfolded, the investigations focused on treatments that could extend the lives of patients with myocardial infarction, or reduce the impact of heart failure on their quality of life—or perhaps prevent their infarctions from occurring at all.

As the issues changed, the nature of research and the makeup of research groups had to evolve, too. Braunwald began his career in small, intimate laboratories; but by the end of the century, he would be leading randomized clinical trials that were often performed in multiple institutions and multiple countries. The advances that resulted from cardiovascular research helped to drive a dramatic decline in deaths from cardiovascular disease,[1] but not without controversy, bitter lessons learned about academic fraud, and difficult decisions about conflicts of interest. Braunwald's research immersed him fully in the good, the bad, and the ugly associated with this progress.

～

In 1971, Braunwald was asked to write an editorial commenting on the rapid spread of coronary artery bypass graft (CABG) surgery, which had been developed just four years earlier at the Cleveland Clinic. The invitation did not come from a prestigious peer-reviewed research journal, like *Circulation,* which published the Maroko Factors Paper that same year. The editorial would appear instead in *Hospital Practice,* which was a "throw-away," a magazine that was sent to physicians around the country without charge. The costs of publication were completely covered by advertising revenue. Physicians would get such magazines in their mail, and throw them away, perhaps after flipping through them to see if there were any articles of interest to them.

There were many such throw-aways in that era, but *Hospital Practice* was widely considered the best. The illustrations were particularly well done, and *Hospital Practice* frequently published reviews of medical topics that were aimed not at describing the cutting edge of research, but at addressing the issues most relevant to clinicians who were taking care of patients. In short, *Hospital Practice* was useful to practicing doctors and to medical students learning their craft. Researchers might look down their noses at throw-aways, but Braunwald knew that tens of thousands of physicians actually might read something in them.

So Braunwald said yes to *Hospital Practice,* and wrote an editorial entitled "Direct coronary revascularization: A plea not to let the genie escape from the bottle."[2] CABG was only a few years old, but its potential benefits were so impressive that he and Nina had given up their work on the carotid sinus stimulator. Nina was performing CABGs herself, and the impact on patients who had been debilitated by angina symptoms was obvious.

But Braunwald also knew that important questions about CABG should be answered before it spread too widely—and answering these questions would require a new type of research. Braunwald summarized early experience with CABG as follows: "It is clear that this operation: (1) delivers substantial quantities of blood to previously ischemic myocardium through a graft that remains patent for at least two to three years; (2) can be accomplished with a relatively low mortality (less than 10 percent in properly selected patients) by a skilled, experienced, surgical team; and (3) results in relief of anginal symptoms in a large majority of patients." But, Braunwald noted, use of CABG was already being extended to other populations beyond patients with incapacitating angina, including the very sick (such as those with acute myocardial infarction), as well as the mildly sick (such as patients with minimal symptoms of heart disease).

Braunwald went on to express "uneasiness" with the rapid spread of CABG, since so few data on its impact were available, beyond the success stories of individual patients. He worried that physicians might be pressured to perform coronary angiography on *all* patients who might have coronary atherosclerosis, and might send those patients to surgery without clear evidence that this strategy would lead to better outcomes. "In short, is the genie even now escaping from the bottle, and will he all too soon control us? In fact, has he already escaped?"

The term "evidence-based medicine" would not become commonplace in medicine for another few decades, but Braunwald went on to call for randomized trials that would rigorously answer important questions, such as how the survival rates and symptoms compared in operated and nonoperated patients, and the impact of surgery in patients with relatively mild disease. His editorial did not mention concern about the costs of care; he was focused solely on the uncertainty about the impact of surgery on patients' outcomes.

In this editorial, Braunwald called for experiments to evaluate coronary artery bypass graft surgery that were designed with the same discipline that characterized laboratory research—namely, randomized clinical trials. Braunwald could see that the time had come for such experiments, and not just for bypass surgery. Several medications for cardiovascular disease had recently become available or were under study. Along with bypass surgery, these treatments offered theoretical benefits, but they all posed real risks. The question of whether the benefits of these treatments outweighed the risks was not going to be answered in a dog research laboratory.

In his article, Braunwald was posing the same basic question that Glenn Morrow had raised so forcefully a decade before, when he'd asked Braunwald whether a patient with aortic valve disease would be better or worse off with surgery. Braunwald had had to concede that he did not know. Now that cardiac surgery had become a real option for treating the most common cause of death among Americans, the question was obviously of great clinical importance, and Braunwald suddenly understood the work that needed to be done. His editorial in *Hospital Practice* had a similar impact for many physicians and researchers. The logic was difficult to refute: it was time for carefully designed trials of CABG and other treatment strategies.

〜

Although Braunwald had not performed randomized human trials himself before coming to Boston, he could see the imperative and the opportunity. In 1962, Congress had amended the Federal Food, Drug, and Cosmetic Act (Kefauver-Harris Amendment) to add a requirement: manufacturers now had to demonstrate the effectiveness of their products through well-designed studies, in order to get approval for their marketing.[3] The new regulation meant that pharmaceutical companies had to sponsor trials that evaluated their new drugs versus older agents or a placebo. And this meant randomized trials involving, in the early days, hundreds of patients; later, they would involve thousands or sometimes even tens of thousands of patients. These trials required funding for researchers, often over periods of several years. Such funding could help to support faculty in departments of medicine like his.

Braunwald's first direct experience with clinical trials began in 1978, with the initiation of the MILIS (Multicenter Investigation for the Limitation of Infarct Size) trial, an NIH-sponsored study of the impact of a beta blocker (propranolol) and another drug, hyaluronidase, on size of myocardial infarctions and prognosis.[4] The study enrolled 269 patients with myocardial infarction at five different hospitals. Despite encouraging data from animal experiments, neither medication seemed to help MILIS patients with heart attacks. "In the most superficial way, the trial was a bust," Braunwald later said, possibly because the medications were administered too late after the onset of the myocardial infarction.

But there was a silver lining to the cloud. In the course of putting together the MILIS study, Braunwald assembled dozens of researchers from several academic medical centers. And to entice them, he not only had to supply grant funding, but also needed to give them a piece of the intellectual pie. Various collaborators analyzed different questions using data collected through the trial. One substudy led by James Muller, then a young assistant professor at Harvard working with Braunwald, showed that heart attacks occurred most frequently in the morning.[5] This observation was repeatedly confirmed, and led Muller to propose the important concept that heart attacks are caused by rupture of unstable (so-called vulnerable) plaques—and *that* insight led to decades of research exploring what triggers heart attacks. Other "substudies" represented more modest advances, but they collectively constituted important progress in physicians' understanding of the natural history, diagnosis, and treatment of myocardial infarction. Claude Lenfant, the director of the National Heart, Lung, and Blood Institute (NHLBI), which had funded MILIS, declared that even though the overall results were negative, the government had gotten plenty of return for its investment in the trial.

Braunwald quickly realized that much of the brutal work of performing a large clinical trial consisted of assembling a group of colleagues who could work well together, and who could be trusted to perform the study with integrity, discipline, and rigor—trusted by him, and trusted by the world. Having done this once for MILIS, Braunwald did not want to start from scratch each time the chance to do a major clinical trial arose. So as the MILIS trial came to an end, he continued to work with many of the same researchers in other studies.

The number of research collaborators needed for important studies rose as the years went by, mostly because the number of patients required for important clinical trials was increasing. Why? Each successive advance against a disease raised the bar against which future innovations had to prove themselves, and researchers needed bigger study populations in order to have a good chance of detecting incremental benefit. On one hand, the clinical stakes were lower; complications rates were sufficiently low that an effective new drug would make a difference for only two or three out of a hundred patients. On the other hand, the clinical challenge itself and the financial stakes were higher. The development of a new drug was now a billion-dollar investment for pharmaceutical companies, and a sizable proportion of that investment, approximately one-third, went toward funding the clinical trials to prove the drug's effectiveness.

Such an investment was one that companies did not make casually. There was, of course, the risk that the new drug or device might not actually help patients; indeed, it might even make patients worse. (Over the years, numerous trials have been stopped because it became clear that patients receiving the new treatment were more likely to get an unexpected side effect, such as liver dysfunction or excessive bleeding.) The manufacturers were willing to make the enormous gamble of testing their products in a trial only if they really believed that the products were effective, beneficial, and safe. And if they were going to make that gamble, they wanted to do everything possible to ensure that a successful trial would be credible—that it would convince the U.S. Food and Drug Administration (FDA) to approve their drug, and induce physicians to prescribe it.

Understandably, the manufacturers who were considering funding these big trials wanted them to be led by researchers who were respected. They wanted leading physician-scientists who understood the cutting edge of medical research, and who could get genuinely excited about a potential new advance. They wanted people who had the organizational skills to run a research group that came together for a particular study and that recorded data in the same disciplined way. They wanted people who could design analyses of data that would be credible when the results of a trial were presented to the medical profession and submitted to medical journals. They wanted researchers like Braunwald. And when the questions and interventions were related to cardiovascular disease, they often went to Braunwald first.

~

This evolution and the expansion of the scale of medical research were accompanied by growing pains. Such pains affected Braunwald directly and deeply in 1981, through a research fraud incident that became known as the "Darsee affair."⁶ A young researcher in Braunwald's lab was found to be falsifying data in animal experiments. The day-to-day laboratory supervisor, cardiologist Robert Kloner, along with Braunwald, reviewed Darsee's laboratory books, and initially believed Darsee's statement that the episode had been one isolated incident in which he had "cracked" under pressure. Over the next few months, however, investigations revealed an extensive pattern of research fraud extending back through his resident and student years at Emory University and even to his undergraduate days at Notre Dame.⁷

The revelation that John Darsee had committed research fraud not just once, but repeatedly over the years, at Notre Dame, Emory, and then Harvard, came as a shock to the many faculty members who had been so impressed with him at those institutions. At Emory, he had been selected as chief resident in medicine—an indication of the hospital leadership's respect and trust. When he was seeking an appointment at Harvard, one professor at Emory wrote a recommendation saying, "In ten years of working with medical students, house officers, and cardiology trainees, both in my basic science laboratory (Physiology) and on clinical research projects (Cardiology Service), I have not encountered anyone with more curiosity, enthusiasm, or potential for developing into an excellent investigator." Another senior faculty member wrote: "Few medical trainees . . . have the amazing self-discipline and drive that John possesses. . . . John is better suited for a career in academic medicine than anyone that I have seen in the cardiology training program at Emory University in the past few years."⁸

Braunwald would later recall that Darsee "worked prodigiously, ninety to a hundred hours per week; he contributed good ideas about the research in which he was engaged, read avidly, was excellent with his hands, a good experimental surgeon, and a fine physiologist with a flair for applying electronics in the laboratory.

. . . Moreover, [Darsee] was pleasant, neat, and personable; he was a positive influence."[9] He was, in short, a rising star, someone who was often referred to as the "Golden Boy" by others at the Brigham.

He was extraordinarily productive in his research—so productive that eventually some of his coworkers became suspicious. In the spring of 1981, other researchers in the Cardiac Research Laboratory observed him as he took a series of recordings obtained minutes apart on one instrumented dog, and labeled them as obtained at intervals of twenty-four hours, seventy-two hours, one week, and two weeks. On May 22, 1981, Braunwald learned of the accusations, and immediately met with Darsee to discuss them.

Darsee admitted his guilt, apologized profusely, and insisted that it was an isolated event. Darsee said he was under pressure to meet a deadline for submitting abstracts for a research meeting, and could not find the tracings from the actual experiment, because he had moved to a different room in the laboratory. He said he was inappropriately "reproducing" data that had been previously obtained legitimately.

Braunwald immediately withdrew a proposed appointment for Darsee at Harvard, and informed the leadership of Harvard Medical School and the Brigham of the event. Darsee's NIH funding was also terminated. But Braunwald chose not to fire Darsee at that point—a decision that would later be second-guessed by critics. Instead, Kloner and Braunwald began the time-consuming process of reviewing data from experiments carried out by Darsee since his arrival at the Brigham. Initially, they found no further evidence of fraud, and while they carried out their review, they allowed Darsee to continue working, under close observation, on the "Models Study"—a multicenter randomized dog study funded by the NHLBI to study myocardial infarction size.

For several months, Braunwald believed that Darsee's story might be true—that he had had one appalling but isolated lapse in judgment. The detailed data in Darsee's laboratory notebooks matched what he had reported to them and written in his papers. But in October 1981, Braunwald and Kloner were able to review the Models Study results from the Brigham and the other three sites participating in the research. The findings horrified them.

Compared to data from the other sites, Darsee's data showed "an unexpected, perhaps unbelievably low degree of variability."[10] Some of the other investigators and the NHLBI had also noticed how perfect Darsee's data appeared to be, and were concerned. Kloner then alerted the other investigators to his and Braunwald's concerns about the validity of Darsee's results. Further analysis showed a marked difference in the variability of results obtained from Darsee before and after May 22—the date when his fabrication of data was discovered and the close observation of his work began. Prior to May 22, the data were difficult to accept as real; afterward, the data were believable.

Confronted with the suspicious data from the Models Study, Darsee denied any wrongdoing, but was unable to produce the original printouts on which the data recorded in his laboratory notebook were purportedly based. Braunwald and Kloner were now fairly certain that Darsee's fraud was not limited to the one instance in May 1981 when he had been caught in the act. As it turned out, these incidents were the tip of an iceberg, and dozens of other instances of probable data fabrication were identified from Darsee's work at the Brigham, at Emory, and even at Notre Dame. The smoking gun was found by Kloner and Braunwald when they reexamined preserved tissues from animals and detected no evidence of radioactivity in the hearts of dogs that Darsee claimed he injected with radioisotopes prior to May 22. The experiments had never been performed.

Separate investigations were conducted by Harvard Medical School and by a committee created by the NHLBI.[11] Neither found evidence of data fabrication by anyone other than Darsee. Nevertheless, the NHLBI report included criticisms of Braunwald and Kloner, calling their initial investigation of Darsee "insufficiently rigorous." The NHLBI report also expressed concern about "a hurried pace and emphasis on productivity" in the lab.[12]

Darsee never admitted explicitly that he had committed any acts of fraud, but did cease denying responsibility, saying simply that he had "no recollection" of committing them. In a retraction of articles he had written while at Emory, he wrote, "I am deeply sorry for allowing these inaccuracies and falsehoods to be published in the Journal and apologize to the editorial board and readers."[13]

This was not the first time that concerns had been raised about the integrity of data collected by a Braunwald protégé. In a 2009 interview, Burton Sobel recalled the time in the mid-1960s when a reviewer questioned the veracity of data in a paper he had written with Braunwald, based on their research at the NIH. The paper concluded that the mitochondria in the cells of failing hearts functioned normally, but the reviewer was an advocate of the theory that mitochondrial dysfunction was an important factor in heart failure. The reviewer wrote the editor of the journal asserting that Sobel's data could not be valid, and that an investigation should be launched.

The editor contacted Braunwald, who was the senior author on the paper, and Braunwald phoned Sobel, who at this point was back at the Brigham as a senior resident. As Sobel recalled, Braunwald started the conversation by saying, "I need to talk to you about something," and then described the reviewer's accusations. Full of anxiety, Sobel asked what they should do, and Braunwald said, "We have to verify that the data are absolutely solid." (In describing this conversation in the 2009 interview, Sobel emphasized that Braunwald had used the word "we" repeatedly.) Braunwald said that he knew Albert Lehninger, the famous chairman of biochemistry at Johns Hopkins. He would make a date for Sobel to visit Lehninger and go over the raw data.

"I was petrified," Sobel recalled. "I was a resident in medicine, who was supposed to be taking care of patients. The data were all at the NIH in a box someplace, and I had to go see Lehninger and defend my integrity." But Sobel found the study data, which had been recorded on long rolls of paper with his handwritten notes. He bundled them up, and paid a visit to Lehninger.

"We went over the data for ten hours. And he said, 'This is beautiful.'" Lehninger called Braunwald to assure him that the data were impeccable, and Braunwald passed the information on to the journal editor, who published the paper.[14] Sobel had been full of dread, but now could relax. Decades later, he emphasized that Braunwald's first instinct was to support him, and was still appreciative that Braunwald had constantly used the word "we" in that first phone call.

This time, however, the outcome was markedly different. The Darsee affair attracted great attention, not only because of Braunwald's prominence, but also because it occurred after a series of other high-profile fraud and plagiarism incidents that were shaking public confidence in science. *Time* magazine's coverage noted "a growing number of 'disappointing events' in laboratories around the country," with embarrassing incidents of scientific fraud at Yale, Cornell, and Boston University.[15] Controversy touched the laboratories of Nobel Laureate David Baltimore and the NIH's star HIV researcher, Robert Gallo. *Time*'s analysis attributed the trend to tremendous pressure to "publish or perish," exacerbated by intense competition for grant funding.

Suddenly, Braunwald's prodigious rate of production of research publications became a focus of criticism instead of respect. Critics asked whether anyone could really take responsibility for so many projects, keep track of the work of so many trainee-investigators, ensure the validity of contributions by so many co-authors, and do so while handling complex management responsibilities like running two departments of medicine. And they asked whether the pressure-cooker environment of modern academics—and Braunwald's laboratory in particular—had contributed to Darsee's tendencies to commit fraud.

As the dust settled, it became clear that the incident was not just about Darsee or just about Braunwald. Darsee's record ultimately revealed that he had committed extensive fraud and must have had profound psychological problems long before he arrived in Boston. The Darsee incident in Braunwald's laboratory was recognized as an example of a chronic threat that required prevention, detection, and rapid response.

For years, Braunwald himself made little public comment on the Darsee affair. But around a decade after it occurred, he was asked to write about the lessons learned from the experience; the query came from some editors who were assembling a book on research fraud. In the chapter he wrote, Braunwald reviewed the events of the Darsee affair, and reflected on their implications. He recalled how difficult it had been to detect Darsee's fraud and then uncover conclusive evidence of a pattern of data fabrication.[16]

Braunwald had always prided himself on near-obsessive meticulousness. He checked all the references in manuscripts, and enjoyed detecting even minute errors in numbers and grammar. He had been accused of "micro-management" of his laboratory. He and Kloner had routinely reviewed Darsee's tracings and graphs at laboratory meetings at least once a week. Nevertheless, even though Darsee was performing research in the presence of Kloner and others during work hours, much of his data fabrication occurred after everyone else had left for the day. Ultimately, only resourceful detective work was able to prove the fraud—after it had occurred and after the damage had been done.

Fraud by someone as intelligent and determined as Darsee is no doubt impossible to prevent completely. So Braunwald's discussion of the case focused on the lessons he had learned about how suspected fraud might be better handled. A bitter lesson had been that the transition from mentor to investigator can probably never be perfectly effective. Most important, he wrote, is that "when a trainee or student is involved in alleged misconduct, the trainer or teacher, while playing an integral role in the investigation, should not become one of the decision-makers." Such an investigation requires a group, preferably from outside the institution, whose only motivation is to expose the truth, as in any criminal investigation. Otherwise, the mentor's relationship with the accused might color the pace and direction of the investigation.

Braunwald listed a second major lesson: "I now believe that once a single act of blatant scientific dishonesty is discovered, the burden must shift from finding other evidence of misconduct to proving that the scientist's other data were produced honestly." To Braunwald, the distinction between these two perspectives was subtle but crucial. After the May 22, 1981, revelation of research fraud, he had approached his investigation of Darsee's other data with a presumption of innocence; he and Kloner were looking for other evidence of misconduct. In retrospect, he concluded that they should have *assumed* a more pervasive pattern of fraud, and approached the investigation as one that needed to prove all other data were valid. That would have led them more quickly to a reexamination of the original tissue samples from animals supposedly studied by Darsee.

As a result of the Darsee affair, rigorous guidelines for addressing incidents of apparent research fraud were developed at Harvard and other universities. Arduous new processes were imposed at many research laboratories, such as the requirement that every data point be verified by two or more people. Yet subsequent occurrences of research fraud suggest that no policies or guidelines can provide complete protection against the actions of another John Darsee, or could even have stopped Darsee himself.

Braunwald concluded his comments on the Darsee case with a warning: attempts to prevent all research fraud might damage the culture of science. "Only a rigid system requiring a researcher's superiors to supervise personally the conduct and recording of every aspect of each experiment could effectively prevent all deliberate fraud. The most creative minds will not thrive in such an environment, and the most promising young people might actually be deterred from embarking on a scientific career in an atmosphere of suspicion. Second only to absolute truth, science requires an atmosphere of openness, trust, and collegiality."[17]

~

Ironically, as the Darsee incident was unfolding, the type of research that Darsee was doing in Braunwald's laboratory was being eclipsed in importance by other forms of investigation. The major questions for cardiology in general and for coronary artery disease in particular were "ready for prime time"—that is, ready for trials in real live patients, not just dogs. A series of randomized trials on coronary artery bypass graft surgery were published in the early 1980s, helping to address the questions raised by Braunwald in his essay "Don't let the genie out of the bottle—again."[18]

Braunwald was aware of the enormous influence—indeed, the occasional definitive impact—of these large-scale human clinical trials. Despite the "negative findings" of the MILIS study, he could see that a new era was beginning in research, and he needed to adapt. "With a heavy heart, in 1984 I closed my dog laboratory, and I made the leap into human trials. We had been talking about infarct limitation for thirteen years, and now it was time to put up or shut up."

Two exciting new interventions for treatment of myocardial infarction came along in the late 1970s and early 1980s, and they demanded rigorous experimentation to define their appropriate use. These interventions were thrombolytic agents ("clot-busting" medications that could dissolve blood clots, or thrombi, occluding coronary arteries and causing heart attacks) and coronary angioplasty (in which balloons on the tips of catheters could be used to dilate narrowings or to open occlusions in coronary arteries). With funding from the National Heart, Lung, and Blood Institute, Braunwald began assembling a multicenter research group to assess the impact of intravenous streptokinase and other thrombolytic agents in the treatment of acute myocardial infarction. The initial group included thirteen clinical sites, a data-coordinating center, a drug distribution center, and core laboratories for radiographic, radionuclear, electrocardiographic, coagulation, and pathological studies. All were part of the Thrombolysis in Myocardial Infarction trial, which became known as TIMI.

The first TIMI trial was a comparison of two different thrombolytic treatments for myocardial infarction. The main study results showed that tissue plasminogen activator (a compound created by the developing biotech giant Genentech) was almost twice as effective at opening occluded coronary arteries as the older but less expensive medication streptokinase.[19] This study led to twenty-six other research papers, with twenty-three different first authors.[20] Some of the TIMI authors were based at the Brigham and at Beth Israel, but most were not.

When this initial TIMI study was finished, Braunwald kept the nucleus of researchers together for another highly influential randomized trial of three different strategies for caring for patients after myocardial infarction (conservative, immediate invasive, and delayed invasive). That study was followed by dozens of other TIMI investigations, most of which had nothing to do with thrombolysis (the "T" in TIMI), and many of which were not directly related to myocardial infarction (the "MI"). TIMI became an actual research "brand": when a study had the TIMI name in it, journal editors and readers knew that this paper was going to be rigorously done by well-respected researchers.

Braunwald had built a network of collaborators—a new type of entity that was called an Academic Research Organization (ARO). This term differentiated TIMI and other AROs from Contract Research Organizations (CROs), which were for-profit companies created to perform clinical trials for the pharmaceutical and device industries. CROs were effective and efficient, but they did not carry with them the respect of a Eugene Braunwald or of highly regarded researchers such as those involved in TIMI. CROs would organize and perform clinical trials for any issue on which the CRO believed it could turn a profit. AROs needed to produce a financial margin, too, so they could invest in young researchers.

But AROs also sought trials that would include research in addition to the main study question, so that the academics involved would be able to discover new knowledge and thereby advance their careers. Hence, AROs would not accept every trial proposed by a pharmaceutical company. And when pharmaceutical companies had *really* important issues that needed to be addressed, such as the impact of a new drug that might be a true game-changer, they tended to seek out AROs.

With Braunwald as chairman, TIMI became an academic and business success. It placed Braunwald in the middle of a network of many outstanding cardiovascular researchers. Hundreds of young cardiology researchers around the world realized that if they worked on TIMI trials, they would have funding and the chance to be an author or coauthor on research papers, some of which would document important advances.

Braunwald knew how to negotiate contracts for clinical trials that allowed TIMI to create win-win situations for other researchers. For example, a pharmaceutical company might come to him to plan a trial of a new drug involving 20,000 patients. The overall costs of the trial might be $200 million. Braunwald would also request an additional 3 percent to measure new biomarkers for detection of myocardial damage or for the prediction of future risk. Measurement of these biomarkers might not be absolutely necessary to the manufacturer seeking approval from the FDA if its product was highly effective. But, Braunwald would point out, the markers might prove useful in identifying which patients were most likely to benefit from the treatment—a good hedge for the manufacturer's bet.

～

Braunwald endured his share of disappointment and frustration during these years, but there were also instances in which everything would come together—his interest in a medical issue, his ability to design and execute research, his knack for attracting and mentoring young talent, his effectiveness in working with the wider world. An example was the fifteen years of research with the husband-and-wife team of Marc and Janice Pfeffer that culminated in the publication of the Survival and Ventricular Enlargement (SAVE) trial, a journey that captured the bench-to-bedside paradigm.

During the late 1970s, Braunwald had begun working with the Pfeffers to study the effects of myocardial infarction and high blood pressure in rats. The Pfeffers were meticulous researchers who had developed an approach to performing cardiac catheterization on rats, a procedure that is delicate when performed in human beings and even more so when performed in small animals such as rats. With their miniature-catheterization laboratory, the Pfeffers and Braunwald began creating models for myocardial infarction in rats and then, in the 1980s, exploring the effects of the drug captopril on rats.[21]

Captopril was the first of a class of medications called angiotensin converting enzyme (ACE) inhibitors. These drugs dilate the body's arteries and reduce the pressure against which the heart must pump (among other effects). The Pfeffers and Braunwald first described the impact of captopril on rats with high blood pressure, and then on the remodeling of the rat heart after myocardial infarction.[22] The findings were so encouraging that they made the leap from rats to human beings. In 1988, they published a study of fifty-nine patients with myocardial infarction who were randomly assigned to receive either captopril or a placebo. Over the next year, the patients who received captopril had better exercise capacity and less enlargement of their hearts.[23]

Based on these relatively few data, published in 1988, Braunwald and the Pfeffers were able to persuade the manufacturer of captopril (Bristol-Myers Squibb) to fund a major multicenter randomized trial of 2,231 patients with acute myocardial infarction. At 112 different hospitals in the United States and Canada, patients were randomly assigned to receive captopril or a placebo; neither they nor the researchers knew which patients were receiving the active drug. When the SAVE trial was published, in 1992, it showed that captopril led to a drop in mortality of 19 percent.[24] The SAVE results were rapidly confirmed by other investigators and led to the use of ACE inhibitors almost routinely in many patients following a heart attack. Braunwald and the Pfeffers had taken a concept from animal research to human testing, and then to a major trial that had changed the standard of patient care.

During the late 1980s, while the SAVE trial was getting under way, Braunwald saw an opportunity to enter a hot new area: clinical trials of statins, the new cholesterol-lowering medications. Cholesterol and prevention of heart disease had not previously been areas of interest for Braunwald—indeed, they were barely mentioned during his medical training. But cholesterol began its evolution into a national preoccupation in 1961, when researchers conducting a long-term epidemiological study in Framingham, Massachusetts, described the way coronary disease and high blood pressure related to high cholesterol levels.[25]

In that paper, the Framingham researchers coined the term "risk factor"—and suggested that heart disease might be preventable. They thus laid the groundwork for laboratory research, drug development, and a series of clinical trials that made prevention of heart disease a cultural obsession in the United States, a hugely successful business for the pharmaceutical industry, and a major cause of the decline in cardiac mortality over the next half-century. Prevention of coronary artery disease also became an important focus for a generation of researchers, eventually including Eugene Braunwald.

The first major randomized trial of a treatment for high cholesterol was started just a few years after the 1961 Framingham Study was released. Researchers organized by the World Health Organization compared a cholesterol-lowering drug called clofibrate with a placebo in 15,745 men in three European cities—Edinburgh, Budapest, and Prague. The study participants were followed for an average of 5.3 years, during which the subjects who received clofibrate had a 9 percent reduction in cholesterol levels, and a 20 percent reduction in coronary heart disease events such as cardiac death, myocardial infarction, and new diagnoses of angina. There was an important disappointment, however: the overall death rate from cardiac *and* noncardiac causes was higher in the group that received clofibrate. Clofibrate seemed to be lowering the cardiac death rate, but raising the risk of dying a noncardiac death—hardly the bargain the public was seeking.[26]

Cholesterol treatment became a more viable strategy with the 1984 publication of the Lipid Research Clinics Coronary Primary Prevention Trial (LRC-CPPT). This study evaluated the impact of a drug called cholestyramine in 3,806 healthy middle-aged men with marked cholesterol elevations. Cholestyramine is a medication that lowers cholesterol without ever entering the body. It is a resin that binds bile (secreted by the liver) into the upper small intestine, and prevents it from being reabsorbed farther downstream. The patient's liver then has to work overtime to make more bile—and does so by metabolizing cholesterol, thus lowering cholesterol levels.

Cholesterol levels fell 13 percent among the men in the Lipid Research Clinics study who took cholestyramine during the 7.4-year follow-up period. With that cholesterol decline came a 24 percent decline in definite coronary heart disease death, and a 19 percent reduction in nonfatal myocardial infarction. The risk of dying from any cause was only slightly reduced in the cholestyramine group, and that difference was not statistically significant—but at least there was no suggestion that cholestyramine was *raising* the overall death rate.[27]

The LRC trial strengthened the case for lowering cholesterol, but doing so via widespread use of cholestyramine was impractical. It tastes terrible, and causes constipation and many other gastrointestinal side effects. It comes as a powder that does not really dissolve in water, and patients often say that taking cholestyramine is like drinking sand dissolved in orange juice. In the Lipid Research Clinics study, 68% of patients reported at least one gastrointestinal side effect, and the average daily dose taken was only about 14 grams per day, even though 24 grams per day were prescribed. A joke at the time was: "What's the point of living longer if you feel like you want to die the entire time?"

A better idea was on the horizon, though. As the LRC trial was getting under way in the mid-1970s, scientists at the U.S. drug company Merck made several trips back and forth to Japan.[28] They went to learn about research by Akira Endo, a scientist at the Japanese company Sankyo. Endo was working to create a drug that would interfere with the manufacture of cholesterol by blocking an enzyme within the liver called HMG-CoA. Endo and his team had spent years testing more than 6,000 microbes, seeking one that might produce an inhibitor of HMG-CoA. He finally found a compound that worked: mevastatin, a compound produced by the fungus *Penicillium citrinum*. It was the first member of the "statin" class that proved safe and effective for lowering cholesterol levels, and it was virtually free of side effects in most patients.[29]

Merck soon isolated its own statin from a fungus—lovastatin (later marketed as Mevacor)—and then developed a synthetically derived compound that was more powerful: simvastatin (Zocor). Bristol-Myers Squibb developed its own statin, called pravastatin (Pravachol), and soon large randomized trials were under way to test their effects.

These trials took years to perform; after all, the researchers were testing the effects of the drugs in patients who were medically stable, and deaths and cardiac events like myocardial infarctions accumulated only slowly over time. The first of these studies to be reported was the 4S trial—the Scandinavian Simvastatin Survival Study, which was published in 1994. This trial was a "secondary prevention" study, as it focused on 4,444 patients who had known coronary disease. In this higher-risk population, simvastatin was compared with a placebo over a median follow-up period of 5.4 years. The patients who received simvastatin had a 30 percent reduction in their risk of dying, and the side effects were minimal.[30]

One year later, the West of Scotland Coronary Prevention Study (WOSCOPS) was published, demonstrating the benefits of pravastatin in people without known histories of myocardial infarction. About 5 percent of the subjects had symptoms suggestive of angina, and they all had elevated cholesterol levels (average 272 milligrams per deciliter, or mg/dL). Pravastatin led to a 22 percent reduction in risk of dying from any cause, and an even greater reduction in risk of cardiac death.[31]

Braunwald was not involved in these first trials of statins, but he had his ear to the ground, and learned about them as they were planned. While at the NIH, he had had some exposure to patients with lipid abnormalities: "The Institute threw me into a sea of fat," as he put it. Within the first month of his arrival in 1955, he had been put on the lipid service under the leading cholesterol researcher of the time, Donald Fredrickson.[32] He had rubbed shoulders constantly with the leaders of the Lipid Research Clinics trial, and was a coauthor on one research study showing that treatment of lipid abnormalities with a rather extreme low-fat diet and clofibrate in six patients led to improvement in maximum blood flow to their extremities, suggesting that their atherosclerotic plaques had shrunk in size and that their arteries had become more healthy.[33] It was one of the earliest demonstrations of clinical benefit from cholesterol treatment.

After his stays at the NIH, Braunwald had turned his attention in other directions, and was not among the researchers who led those first statin trials. But as the SAVE trial was just getting started, Braunwald heard about the new statin that had been developed by Bristol-Myers Squibb. The new drug was pravastatin (Pravachol), and Braunwald immediately began to propose research trials for it to Bristol-Myers Squibb. The company was a bit reluctant to write another enormous check to Braunwald and his colleagues, so Braunwald had to use some creativity.

"Let's do a two-fer," Braunwald said. "Let's do a two-by-two design, with pravastatin versus placebo and captopril versus placebo. We could do studies of two products for the price of one clinical trial."

Braunwald was proposing a type of study design that was quite new at the time: the 2-by-2 factorial design. This design was being used in a study of the impact of aspirin and carotene in U.S. physicians, started in 1982 by researchers in Braunwald's department at the Brigham. The design was so new and innovative that in 1985 the Brigham researchers wrote an article about its ability to increase the efficiency of research.[34]

It was perhaps *too* new for Bristol-Myers Squibb, and Braunwald could not sell the idea to the company's executives. They wanted to wait until their drug was further along in its development. They also told Braunwald that he had to make proposals about pravastatin research to a different committee within the company, rather than to the executives who were overseeing captopril.

Braunwald was not about to give up. He knew that the 4S trial was under way, and expected that it was going to be a blockbuster that demonstrated the benefits of Merck's simvastatin. In fact, it did so.[35] He told Bristol-Myers Squibb that it needed to do something other than play catch-up.

Braunwald's approach was to broaden the target population for statins. He foresaw that these drugs had tremendous potential to reduce coronary heart disease, and that they were likely to spread well beyond the patients with very high cholesterol levels in which they had been studied to date—just as coronary artery bypass graft surgery had spread rapidly in the 1970s. Braunwald had written his famous 1971 editorial urging rigorous study of the impact of surgery before the technique was allowed to spread, and he felt the same way about the spread of statins. And in such rigorous study, he saw an opportunity to answer an important medical question, while getting into this area of investigation for the sake of his own research colleagues. He made a forceful argument to Bristol-Myers Squibb.

"The real question is not what we should do for people who have total cholesterols of 300 or more, who have had a heart attack. There's no way that they're not going to benefit from statins, because the Lipid Research Clinics had in a sense proven the lipid hypothesis of atherosclerosis in 1984. Since simvastatin reduced LDL cholesterol by 40 percent, there was no way it wasn't going to be beneficial. But the 4S trial examined only a very small fraction of the population. The more important question for medicine is what we should do with all these people with coronary heart disease who have *average* cholesterol levels."

Bristol-Myers Squibb bought the argument, and agreed to fund a major trial.

Braunwald set up the Cholesterol and Recurrent Events (CARE) trial, working with a Brigham lipid expert named Frank Sacks, and with Marc Pfeffer. Like Braunwald, Pfeffer had not been a cholesterol researcher, but was rapidly learning how to manage international multicenter randomized trials through his work on the SAVE trial. They teamed with many of the same researchers and hospitals that were participating in SAVE, but their focus was a different patient population. They enrolled people with coronary disease who had cholesterol levels that were considered normal at that time (below 240 mg/dL).

The 4,159 patients were randomly assigned to take pravastatin (40 mg/day) or a placebo, and were then followed for five years. The impact: a 24 percent reduction in risk of fatal coronary events or nonfatal heart attacks (from 13.2 percent to 10.2 percent). Similar reductions were seen in the rates of bypass surgery, angioplasty, and stroke. Mortality rates were not significantly reduced.[36]

"We felt very good about that," Braunwald commented. "But then we said—if low is good, is lower even better? That's where the PROVE-IT trial came in."

"PROVE-IT-TIMI 22" stood for the Pravastatin or Atorvastatin Evaluation and Infection Therapy trial, a multicenter investigation that was designed to compare the standard approach to treatment (reducing LDL cholesterol to about 100 mg/dL) with a more aggressive approach (reducing LDL to about 65 mg/dL). Braunwald and Christopher Cannon, one of his younger colleagues, led the trial. Two different statins were used: pravastatin for the 100 mg/dL goal, and the more powerful atorvastatin (Lipitor) for the 65 mg/dL goal. The patients had recently been admitted to the hospital for coronary artery disease, but had been sufficiently stabilized to be enrolled in a long-term study.

After eighteen to thirty-six months of follow-up, there was a significant 16 percent reduction in cardiovascular events in the patients randomized to aggressive LDL reduction with atorvastatin.[37] Braunwald and his colleagues had thus expanded the number of patients who could be expected to benefit from statin therapy by demonstrating, in CARE, that treatment was beneficial for patients with normal cholesterol levels; and then, in PROVE-IT, expanding the role of statins yet again by pushing the target for LDL reduction to a new low. The guidelines for use of statins to reduce risk for heart disease had to be rewritten every few years during this period, and these trials were among the major reasons.

As with prior clinical trials, Braunwald used the CARE study to generate data for several other research projects, including one analysis that showed that patients who have lower levels of the marker of inflammation C-reactive protein (CRP) after statin therapy had a better prognosis than patients with higher CRP levels—regardless of their LDL cholesterol level.[38] This finding set the stage for the JUPITER trial (Justification for the Use of Statins in Primary Prevention: An Intervention Trial Evaluating Rosuvastatin), a trial that enrolled 17,802 people and showed that a very powerful statin, known as rosuvastatin, could reduce cardiac events and restore normal cholesterol levels, if the individuals had elevated CRP levels.[39]

Braunwald was not an author of the JUPITER trial, but he took considerable pleasure from the fact that the leader was his protégé Paul Ridker, who was subsequently named the Eugene Braunwald Professor of Medicine at Harvard Medical School. And Braunwald enjoyed pointing out that one of his earliest papers, published a half-century earlier, had described how elevated CRP levels were a poor prognostic factor for patients with heart failure.[40]

Braunwald himself continued to play a leadership role into his eighties, in studies of new medications for lowering LDL ("bad") cholesterol and for reducing heart disease risk by raising HDL ("good") cholesterol.[41] At the American Heart Association meetings in November 2010, early research results were presented by Christopher Cannon, Braunwald's co-investigator on the PROVE-IT study, for anacetrapib, a drug that more than doubled HDL while lowering LDL 40 percent in patients already on a statin.

～

In 2003, when he was seventy-four years old, Braunwald stepped down from his post as chief academic officer at Partners. By this time, he had remarried and was enjoying a new and happy phase of family life. He had met his second wife, Elaine Smith, when she was chief operating officer at the Brigham, and she had developed warm relationships with Braunwald's three daughters. Those daughters had settled in the Boston area, and were producing a growing number of grandchildren. Rena Stark, the nanny who had cared for those three daughters when Eugene and Nina Braun-wald were at the NIH, lived nearby, and remained an integral member of the extended family. Braunwald appreciated his good fortune in having two generations of family around him at this stage of his life.

Braunwald now wanted to leave administrative work, and de-vote most of his professional time to his academic life—as a re-searcher, editor, and author. Yet because of the respect he com-manded and his reputation as a master tactician, he was called upon frequently when knotty issues arose at Partners. That was how he came to lead a commission that imposed a strict new na-tional standard on academics' relationships with industry.

Braunwald had been a member of the Partners Committee on Conflicts of Interest—the group that developed policies and eval-uated individual cases of potential conflicts of interest. The group had been chaired by Dan Podolsky, Braunwald's successor as chief academic officer, but in 2008 Podolsky left to become president of the University of Texas Southwestern Medical Center in Dallas. At that time, Partners physicians and researchers were developing an increasing number of complex relationships with for-profit com-panies in the pharmaceutical and medical-device industries. Some of these relationships were attracting criticism in the press, among academic colleagues inside and outside Partners, and even from the federal government.

In the summer and fall of 2008, just as Podolsky was leav-ing Partners, Senator Charles E. Grassley (Republican of Iowa) launched an investigation of a prominent child psychiatrist and professor at Harvard Medical School. The psychiatrist was well-known as an expert on use of antipsychotic medications in chil-dren, and was highly regarded within the Boston community for taking care of some of the most severely ill children. But he came under attack for failing to report much of the $1.6 million in consulting fees he had received from drug manufacturers from 2000 to 2007. In addition to hiring him as a consultant, these pharmaceutical companies paid him to give lectures around the country, and sponsored his research.[42]

All of the various relationships that this professor had with pharmaceutical companies were in fact legal, and quite common among other prominent researchers at Partners, in other Harvard hospitals, and in the rest of academic medicine. But the amounts of money in this case were greater than usual, and the institutions with which he was affiliated—Mass General, Partners, and Harvard—were prominent. Those factors made the case an attractive focus for Senator Grassley and the press. Partners was also under criticism in the Boston marketplace because its contracts with local health plans brought its hospitals and physicians higher payments than those received by its local competitors.[43]

Under these circumstances, a strong response from Partners to the problem of conflicts of interest was essential. The CEO of Partners, James J. Mongan, asked Braunwald to chair the committee that would develop new policies. The recommendations of the so-called Braunwald Commission were released to the Partners community in late 2009, after several rounds of internal vetting in which Braunwald repeatedly met, often individually, with physicians whose work and incomes were going to be affected.

On January 3, 2010, the policies were described in a long article in the *New York Times* as going "further than those of any other academic medical center in restricting outside pay from drug companies."[44] The new policies capped the income that senior officials could earn while serving as outside directors for industry companies, and prohibited them from accepting stock. They forbade Partners personnel from earning payments for lectures as members of "speakers' bureaus," which were lists of experts that pharmaceutical representatives could offer to hospitals as potential speakers for their meetings. The hospital could pick an expert, and the drug company would pay the lecturer's expenses and an honorarium (say, $2,000). The lecturer would use slides prepared or approved by the drug company, which thus had control of important content for the talk.

The *Times* quoted Braunwald as saying, "We're the first to go in this deep, and we're still into it only up to our knees." He described internal Partners discussions of the new policies as a "very spirited debate"—a polite understatement, the academic term for a donnybrook, since the rules meant a substantial drop in income for many physicians. The physicians who were listed on speakers' bureaus at that time were often younger faculty, who argued that they needed the outside income to make up for lower academic salaries and Boston's higher cost of living, as they tried to raise their families and pay their mortgages. They said that if the new policies were implemented, they would consider leaving Partners for less restrictive teaching hospitals, or leaving academic medicine altogether.

In the *Times* article, Braunwald explained that the ban on speaking fees was one reason Partners wanted to take a tough position on the participation of its senior officials on company boards. He said that it would seem unfair to restrict the outside income of junior faculty without taking some action that affected Partners' senior physicians. Braunwald was aware that critics of the new policies were pointing out that he had derived considerable income throughout his career by serving as a director and scientific advisor to a range of pharmaceutical companies. His response was the last line of the *Times* article: "In all fairness, what was OK three years ago is not OK now."

The impact of the Braunwald Commission policies was far-reaching. In the *Times* article, Thomas Donaldson, a professor of business ethics at the Wharton School of the University of Pennsylvania, said: "It strikes me as a breath of fresh air in a room that's getting progressively more stale. I hope this will set a standard for others—hospitals, medical schools." Other institutions, including Harvard Medical School, reviewed their policies, and many revised their approach to match or even exceed those of the Braunwald Commission.

The participation of Mass General and Brigham physicians in speakers' bureaus came to an end in 2010, and when the *Boston Globe* published information on physicians who were receiving payments from industry, Mass General and Brigham doctors were conspicuously absent.[45] The article credited the new Partners policies, and noted that one—but only one—physician had resigned from the Brigham medical staff because of them. That physician was not a researcher. The threatened exodus of young Partners investigators whose incomes were reduced by the Braunwald Commission's policies did not materialize.

In the six decades that followed Braunwald's first research fellowship, the philosophical outlook for medical research evolved from descriptive to experimental, from observational to hypothesis testing. As that change occurred, the costs of advancing medical knowledge increased, so that cutting-edge research usually required major funding from the NIH and/or industry. Also changed were the institutions within which research was conducted and researchers were groomed.

Braunwald moved from the NIH to UCSD in 1968 in part because he sensed that the future of medical research was going to be more fertile at academic medical centers, and that he would have more impact as chairman of a department of medicine. In the years that followed, Braunwald noted what he called "divisionalization" due to "the subspecialization of medical knowledge and the accompanying need for advanced specialized training, especially that involving laboratory and procedural technologies." Also, as departments of medicine grew in size, they became cumbersome to administer efficiently.[46]

As early as 1982, Braunwald saw the risk that some specialty divisions would become so big—and financially prosperous—that they would want to secede from their departments and stand on their own.[47] For example, cardiologists might leave a department of medicine and take with them the profits from reading EKGs and performing other procedures. Then cardiologists might either form their own independent departments, or combine in "institutes" with other specialists involved in the care of cardiovascular disease—specialists such as cardiac surgeons, anesthesiologists, and radiologists. Funds would not be available to subsidize divisions that were compensated more poorly, such as psychiatry or infectious disease.

As the 1990s began, Braunwald could see advantages for research and patient care if clinicians were organized "horizontally" around categories of patient disease, such as cardiovascular conditions or cancers, but he was reluctant to endorse this approach. He was, after all, sitting atop one of the dominant "vertical" organizational structures, a department of medicine. He expressed concern that new trends might fragment the care of patients with multiple conditions, and argued that departments of medicine had an important role in the integration of patient care, in education, and in research.

"Internal medicine may be likened to a wide river. As more information is developed about a specific category of illnesses (for example, infectious or neoplastic disorders) or about diseases affecting a particular organ system, a separate stream branches off from this river. We now find ourselves at a point where many of these branches are far apart." Braunwald somewhat optimistically predicted that those streams would be coming back together, and that the traditional, broadly based organizational structures of medicine would play a leadership role in that reunification.[48]

He was partly right; the streams had been diverging for some time. Earlier in his career, the highlight of the year for researchers like him, Jean Wilson, Donald Seldin, and Edmund Sonnenblick had come each spring, when researchers would meet in Atlantic City for several days to hear papers presented at meetings of the "Tri-Societies": the American Federation for Clinical Research, the American Society for Clinical Investigation, and the Association of American Physicians. At these meetings, friendships were renewed, and academics caught up with the cutting edge of science in a wide range of fields.

But the impact of these broadly based scientific research societies faded away in the 1980s, losing "market share" to specialty societies. Braunwald and other cardiovascular researchers increasingly presented their most important research at the more heavily attended November meetings of the American Heart Association and at the spring meetings of the American College of Cardiology. The number of research abstracts submitted for the Tri-Society meetings started to fall in 1985, and the decline was rapid. By 1992 the number of abstracts had decreased by nearly half, and attendance fell by a similar amount by 1996.[49] One essay asked whether the famous Spring Meetings were dying.[50] The answer was yes.

Would the same fate befall that other broadly based organizational structure in academic medicine, the department of medicine? As the twenty-first century began, Braunwald and others saw another path emerge: the development of centers or institutes that cut across traditional organization structures, bringing together clinicians for clinical purposes or researchers for investigations that transcended any one specialty. In research, an example was the Harvard Stem Cell Institute, which allows researchers from several Harvard schools and many departments who are interested in stem cell science to collaborate on studies that frequently focus on diseases well outside their specialty training. Another was the Broad Institute of MIT and Harvard, which brings together scientists from multiple institutions, departments, and backgrounds for research that is often funded with the institute's substantial endowment.

The complexity of the new research world was not daunting to Braunwald. "Large successful businesses have long ago adopted matrix organizations," he wrote. "However, as medical schools, universities, and [academic medical centers] inevitably undergo continued reorganization, and both administration and faculty become more preoccupied with these organizational matters, it must remain clear that the details of the organization are only a means—albeit often an important one—to achieve an end, which remains excellence in carrying out the tripartite mission. This must remain the central goal of individual medical schools, and indeed of the entire academic medical enterprise."[51]

: 12 :

Textbooks and Education in Evolution

For young Eugene Braunwald, the sense that writing and editing medical textbooks were noble activities began to emerge late at night in 1953, when he was an intern at Mount Sinai Hospital. He would often go to the hospital's library after his last new patient had been "worked up" and his other work was done. On those library visits, he would frequently see his first professional role model, the cardiologist Charles Friedberg, working on his classic textbook, *Diseases of the Heart*.[1] Braunwald, the young intern, introduced himself to the great professor, and occasionally they would chat briefly. Friedberg's book was a key resource for Braunwald and every other physician interested in cardiology in that era.[2] A 1972 article in the *Journal of the American Medical Association* read, "For cardiology, Dr. Friedberg's conspicuous success in maintaining uniform excellence while covering the entire field provides the stratospheric standard against which other single-authored texts can continue to be judged."[3]

As it turned out, Friedberg was the last American to write a single-authored textbook of cardiology. The reason: knowledge in cardiology and virtually every other major field of medicine was expanding too quickly for any one individual to master or write about quickly enough. The new model for textbooks would be one in which editors sought numerous experts to write chapters on specific topics, and tried to impose a consistent style and philosophy on the submitted materials.

In the old model, textbooks were just one person's perspective—and in the case of *Diseases of the Heart,* that person was a magnificent clinician, a critical thinker with a keen analytic mind that could separate the wheat from the chaff. Friedberg's descriptions of the symptoms and signs of cardiovascular disease were framed in eloquent, almost lyrical prose that was treasured by his colleagues. He sought to convey to readers what he heard as he listened to patient's stories, and what he witnessed as he examined them. And that perspective is exactly what his readers were seeking. Physicians and trainees, including Braunwald, would sit down and read Friedberg's entire text, chapter by chapter, page by page —hoping thereby to become as much as possible like Friedberg himself.

In the new model, however, only very determined readers might go through an entire textbook. Most physicians would simply look up topics and read sections of chapters, as patients with specific conditions came under their care. They were not trying to become Tinsley Harrison when they sat down with *Principles of Internal Medicine;* they were trying to become modern physicians by mastering specific topics as they encountered patients with those diseases.

But at the time of Friedberg's death (he was killed in a traffic accident in 1972), the age of the single-author medical textbook had not yet ended. During the late 1960s, Friedberg and Braunwald had become friends after appearing on several cardiology panels; and shortly after Friedberg died, a senior vice president from the publisher W. B. Saunders called Braunwald to ask if he would take over the uncompleted fourth edition. Friedberg's wife, Gertrude, a respected playwright and the editor of the book, had suggested Braunwald.

Braunwald had idolized Friedberg and was deeply saddened by his death. He was touched by Gertrude Friedberg's suggestion, and sorely tempted to accept the job. He asked the publisher to send him the material that Friedberg had already written. But when he read over the drafts, Braunwald saw that he could not do a good job of finishing such a personalized work. It would be a mishmash of styles.

In addition, it was 1972 and Braunwald had just arrived in Boston. His hands were full with his work in the Brigham and its Department of Medicine. He told W. B. Saunders that he could not commit to working on this or any cardiology textbook for six years, when he could take a full-year sabbatical for the project. After some deliberation, the editorial board of W. B. Saunders told Braunwald that it was willing to wait.

~

Braunwald was intrigued by the idea of launching a cardiology textbook in part because he so enjoyed his experience as an editor of *Harrison's*, which had introduced him to a new phase as an educator. He took pleasure in teaching medical students in classrooms, in the laboratory, and on hospital wards, but those were relatively casual educational experiences; he enjoyed such instruction because it kept his thinking sharp. Being prepared to respond to questions from students forced him to master topics thoroughly.

As an author and editor of textbooks, however, he was becoming an educator on a different scale. He needed to think much more systematically about the various ranges of information that had to be mastered by physicians in training and in different types of practice. What the generalist needed to know about cardiology was different from what the cardiologist needed to know. And Braunwald had to think about how the material could be most effectively mastered. In short, he had to learn about how students and physicians learn.

The *Harrison's* team of editors took that work seriously—but they also did it in style. Before the work on a new edition began, they would have a ten-day meeting at a luxurious place chosen by the editor-in-chief (a position that rotated after Tinsley Harrison retired). The first meeting that Braunwald attended was in 1968 (shortly after his arrival at UCSD) at Reid's Palace Hotel, the legendary Orient Express hotel on Madeira, off the coast of Portugal.

At the meetings, every chapter would be carefully evaluated. Each editor was responsible for reviewing the section of another editor, and the shared expectation was that the process would be rigorous and brutally honest. The key question was how each chapter could be improved for the next edition. The editors would argue intensely about how many pages could be allotted for each topic. Braunwald found himself taking passionate stands: "Wait a minute! I'm not going to write a chapter on congestive heart failure in six pages. That's absurd. It's got to be seven!"

"That sort of 'group grope' was new to me, and I think it was new at the time," Braunwald recalled. "But the result was an intense discussion of every single major subject in internal medicine." At those meetings, Braunwald got lessons in endocrinology from George Thorn, infectious disease from Ivan Bennett, neurology from Raymond Adams, and so on. Adams was notorious for ignoring agreements on page limits, and for submitting chapters that were as long as he deemed necessary to cover the topic. Two other new editors joined: Kurt Isselbacher, a gastroenterologist from Mass General, and Robert Petersdorf, an infectious-disease expert based at the University of Washington in Seattle. "It was the best journal club in the world, maybe in history," Braunwald said.

Harrison's quickly became an important part of Braunwald's professional life, one that was synergistic with his other responsibilities. It was yet another way in which he learned who did good work and who was a rising star in a particular area—and thus might be someone he wanted to recruit to UCSD or, later, to the Brigham. The breadth of the content in *Harrison's* resonated with his youthful aspirations to be a master clinician like Isidore Snapper and Charles Friedberg. While chairman of the Department of

Medicine at the Brigham, Braunwald routinely had every *Harrison's* chapter for which he was the editor reviewed by a resident and another faculty physician, to ensure that the material was current and aimed correctly at its target audience. And residents and faculty members were generally thrilled to be asked to perform those reviews, because the request suggested that Braunwald valued their perspectives.

Braunwald served as an editor for twelve editions (longer than any editor in the history of the book), and was editor-in-chief for the eleventh and the fifteenth editions. While he was editor-in-chief, he held planning meetings in Salzburg, Austria, and timed them to coincide with the annual summer music festival so he could get a heavy dose of opera. Over the years, he recruited several other editors, including Jean Wilson, the University of Texas Southwestern endocrinologist whom he had come to know at the NIH (and an equally devoted lover of opera), as well as Anthony Fauci—a noted NIH immunologist who was to become the ranking expert on HIV-AIDS. Braunwald himself wrote dozens of chapters, and continued to serve as an author even after stepping down as an editor.

Braunwald met Tinsley Harrison only once. Prior to Braunwald's joining the editors, the title of the book had been *Principles of Internal Medicine,* but it was renamed *Harrison's Principles of Internal Medicine* when Harrison retired. A party was held to celebrate the release of the sixth edition, the first on which Braunwald served as an editor and the first to bear the new title.

Harrison sat at the long conference table and paged through the new edition, which would enshrine his name in the minds of medical trainees for generations to come. A gruff man, he was quiet for some time. "Nothing has changed," he said finally. "It's still *principles* of internal medicine and *details* of neurology." Harrison was jabbing at Raymond Adams for getting longer chapters on neurology topics into the book by ignoring the page limits.

~

Eventually, of course, Harrison was proved wrong: *Harrison's* was in fact changing, just like its readership. Research began to produce clinical trials that compared one treatment strategy to another. The results of those clinical trials were synthesized by expert panels into guidelines, and those guidelines were distilled into algorithms and quality measures. Some of the editors rebelled at the increasing number of flowcharts summarizing what decisions should be made in the care of patients with specific syndromes. "We're writing a textbook, not a cookbook," they protested.

The editors struggled to keep the book compact enough to be published in one volume, in part to discipline themselves to keep distilling the material down to the most important 2,500 pages or so. They obsessed about issues such as the thickness of the paper: if it was too thin, colored illustrations would bleed through to the other side. And they had the textbook equivalent of emergencies when important new diseases like AIDS appeared—for which they threw page limits out the window and let author Anthony Fauci write as much as he wanted (forty-one pages).

By the 1970s, *Harrison's* was reputed to be the most widely read textbook of medicine in the world. It trained more students and residents and served as a trusted reference to more practicing physicians than any other book. In the 1990s, Braunwald saw that sales outside the United States were continuing to rise rapidly, and that letters were coming from overseas readers. He and the other editors realized that they should include more material that was relevant to a global readership. Chapters on nutrition and tropical diseases were added or expanded.

With the turn of the new century and the emergence of the Internet, American medical students and trainees seemed to stop buying textbooks and medical journals, and increasingly began to use online resources such as UpToDate. The relatively brief topical discussions in these Web-based resources had not been reviewed by several layers of experts, but they were more timely—and they were free to users who worked at a hospital or school with an institutional license.

Braunwald did not waste too much time decrying the shorter attention span of modern trainees or their reluctance to pay for intellectual content. Instead, he pushed for a more compact version of *Harrison's* called *Harrison's Manual of Medicine,* which in the United States sold even better than the full-length textbook. In 1998, he became a founder and the first editor-in-chief of *Harrison's Online,* which provided Internet-based access to the book's content, as well as timely updates.

Although Braunwald understood that something fundamental was changing in the way young people acquired information, he did not feel pessimistic about the impact of this change on clinicians and researchers. "I think the young people that I've seen are as good as or better than they were at any time in the past," he said in a 2010 interview. "The best ones are still very interested in mechanisms."

He also saw a continuing role for textbooks, ideally in combination with online resources. "There's a problem with information overload, with the twenty-four-hour news cycle in medicine. But the big changes in medicine don't occur overnight. The insights build from small studies to bigger studies to even bigger clinical trials. Then the insights get synthesized in textbooks, and then the guidelines are written, and have tremendous impact on clinical practice. The guidelines tend to lag behind the texts."

An example of this sequence is the adoption of beta blockers after acute myocardial infarction. This class of drugs was developed in 1962, and researchers including Braunwald soon found that these agents decreased myocardial oxygen consumption and were useful for treating angina. In 1982, the results of the Beta Blocker–Heart Attack Trial (BHAT) were published, showing that mortality among patients with myocardial infarction was reduced from 9.8 percent to 7.2 percent if they received a beta blocker instead of a placebo.[4] The effect was so dramatic that the trial was stopped nine months early. Subsequent data suggested that the relative reduction in mortality with beta blockers might be as high as 40 percent, and that these benefits applied even to patients with relative contraindications to beta blockers, such as obstructive lung disease.

The process through which beta blockers became routine treatment after myocardial infarction played out over a quarter-century. In 1996, the American College of Cardiology and the American Heart Association issued guidelines recommending adoption of beta blockers as part of routine care. In subsequent years, quality metrics for health plans and hospitals on their use of beta blockers after myocardial infarction were publicly reported, and financial incentives provided further encouragement for improvement. Finally, in 2007, the most widely used quality measure for use of beta blockers after myocardial infarction was retired, for the very best of reasons: almost every institution achieved a perfect score, or nearly so.[5]

Although it took twenty-five years for the implications of the BHAT trial to play out, the major thrust of its findings made its way into textbooks in considerably less time. As early as 1984, at least one textbook—*Heart Disease*—carried recommendations for use of beta blockers after acute myocardial infarction, based on

BHAT and other trials, anticipating the guideline recommendations from the American College of Cardiology and the American Heart Association by twelve years.

Those early recommendations for use of beta blockers were made by the two authors of the chapter on treatment of acute myocardial infarction. They could not wait for a carefully selected panel of experts to ponder the evidence and issue guidelines; they had a textbook deadline to meet, and they had to give their best advice to readers on an everyday issue of obvious clinical importance. So they did, and in this instance, the recommendations to use beta blockers after myocardial infarctions stood the test of time. The authors of that chapter were Burton Sobel and Eugene Braunwald.[6]

⁓

After Braunwald turned down the opportunity to take over Charles Friedberg's *Diseases of the Heart* in 1972, the idea of doing his own cardiology textbook lingered in his mind. At that time, the authoritative textbook for cardiologists was *The Heart,* edited by J. Willis Hurst, the long-standing chairman of the Department of Medicine at Emory University Hospital. When *The Heart* made its debut, in 1966, it was the first comprehensive, multiauthor cardiology textbook.

The Heart was a direct result of the growing realization that cardiology had become too big and was moving too quickly for single-author textbooks. In Hurst's description of how the book was conceived, he described a 1962 conversation with Paul Wood, a famous English cardiologist whose book *Diseases of the Heart and Circulation* was highly respected. Wood described his frustration at his inability to complete the next edition of his book: "By the time I write the last chapter, the first chapter will be out of date."[7]

Hurst realized that his old mentor from Massachusetts General Hospital, Paul Dudley White, had decided not to write a fifth edition of his book, *Heart Disease,* for much the same reason. The only remaining comprehensive cardiology textbook was Charles Friedberg's *Diseases of the Heart,* and Hurst wrote, "I sensed that he too would have trouble continuing to write a single-authored book. This was obviously true, because cardiovascular research was beginning to bring many new insights to every area of cardiology and no single person could hope to master them all."

So Hurst began work on a multiauthor book, assigning numerous chapters to Emory faculty, but also inviting contributions from authors elsewhere who were expert in specific fields. From the outset, Hurst understood that he was trying to meet the needs of two different types of readers. "I have always believed that there are two types of reading. The *quick read* is used by physicians who wish to look up information that is needed immediately. Reading about the criteria required to diagnose hypertrophic cardiomyopathy is an example of the *quick read.* The *long read* is used when physicians want to understand certain aspects of a disease process. This type of reading is done in a more leisurely fashion without a feeling of urgency. Reading about and understanding the evolution of an atherosclerotic plaque is an example of the *long read.*"[8]

The Heart was an immediate success, and Braunwald wrote chapters on hypertrophic cardiomyopathy in the 1970, 1974, and 1978 editions. But, as good as it was, Braunwald wondered whether he couldn't do better. He talked to trainees at the Brigham about the book, and was surprised to find that they were even less satisfied with it than he was. Braunwald was using it for quick reads— looking up information on specific topics, and finding references for research papers that supported the key points. In the days before Internet search engines, the identification of such source material was an invaluable function of textbooks for academics like Braunwald. It was a major reason for buying new editions as they came out.

But for someone learning about a disease, someone needing to do what Hurst called "the long read," *The Heart* was not as well suited as the single-author texts it was replacing. Information about a clinical condition like myocardial infarction might be scattered across several chapters, each by a different author. The index could steer a reader to the various places in the book, and a reader like Braunwald could find what he needed quite quickly. But relative novices needed something closer to what Friedberg had provided: a text by one excellent clinician laying out how to think about a disease.

Braunwald wondered if there wasn't a middle ground between the encyclopedic book by Hurst and the single-author text by Charles Friedberg. He talked to senior executives at W. B. Saunders, the publishers who had approached him about taking over Friedberg's book. They liked the idea, but were not happy about waiting years for it, as Braunwald suggested. After all, Friedberg's third edition of *Diseases of the Heart* was already four years old, and for a major publishing house to go without a current cardiology text for a dozen years was far from ideal.

Ultimately, however, Saunders was willing to wait for Braunwald to put in six years as chairman of the Department of Medicine at the Brigham, and then take a sabbatical year to deliver the first edition of *Heart Disease*. Saunders was in competition with McGraw-Hill, which published *Harrison's Principles of Internal Medicine* and Hurst's book *The Heart*. Saunders's medical textbook *(Cecil-Loeb Textbook of Medicine)* was in second place behind *Harrison's*, and a Braunwald cardiology textbook seemed like its best shot at having a front-runner.

Braunwald had his hands full with Brigham hospital and Department of Medicine business during the 1972–1978 period, but he was planning *Heart Disease* the entire time. He asked colleagues to write specific chapters, and on July 1, 1978, he began a one-year sabbatical to work on the book. Marshall Wolf assumed Braunwald's leadership role in the Brigham's Department of Medicine, and Braunwald worked at his home in Weston, Massachusetts, except for occasional visits to the office.

Braunwald was also coordinating a new edition of *Harrison's* that year, and he struggled to keep the projects separate in his mind. He was editing manuscripts on various topics written by a range of authors, with different target audiences in mind. He used two rooms in his home for the work: one was the *Harrison's* room; the other, the *Heart Disease* room. All the correspondence and drafts for each book stayed in the proper room.

Braunwald wrote or coauthored more than half of the first edition of *Heart Disease,* because he wanted to capture some of the "long read" strengths of a single-author textbook like Friedberg's. He wanted every reader who sought to master a cardiology topic to be able to do so by sitting down and reading the right chapter.

Braunwald had learned this approach from working on *Harrison's.* Max Wintrobe had written virtually all of the hematology material in that book; George Thorn, the endocrinology; Raymond Adams, the neurology; and so on. Braunwald wanted the same consistency, broad perspectives, and clear streams of thought in his cardiology book.

Each day, Braunwald would begin work in the *Heart Disease* room at about 7:00 A.M., take a break for lunch, then work on *Harrison's* in the afternoon ("to clear my mind"), and return to the more intense work on *Heart Disease* after dinner. He worked nonstop for about sixteen hours a day, for six and a half days each week, throughout an entire year. He would write by hand on pads of lined yellow paper, and would list articles that he would ask his research assistant to photocopy at the Harvard Medical School library. Each morning, a taxi would pick up his drafts and requests for articles, and bring them to Mary Jackson, his secretary at the Brigham. (Fax machines were not yet available.) At 6:00 P.M., another taxi would bring his typed manuscript pages and photocopied articles back to Weston.

Braunwald lived like a hermit during that sabbatical year, surrounded by pads of paper, manuscript drafts, and piles of photocopied articles. On many days, he did not shave. He took no vacation and accepted no invitations to speak anywhere. His research program went into hibernation. But he finished the manuscript of the book within hours of the June 30, 1979, deadline. Its release was timed to coincide with the November meeting of the American Heart Association.

Heart Disease was an immediate success. The review published in the *New England Journal of Medicine* said:

> Braunwald's new book will assume a position as the model textbook of contemporary cardiovascular medicine because it couples an excellent description of basic cardiovascular physiology and pharmacology with a thorough discussion and elegant presentation of the clinical aspects of cardiovascular diseases. . . . Dr. Braunwald wrote or contributed to approximately half the chapters. This approach ensures continuity, allowing the reader to benefit from the expertise of various authors within a consistent style. . . .
>
> This is an excellent textbook of cardiovascular diseases. For the immediate future it will serve as the "gold standard" for others in the field. Anyone with a serious interest in the diagnosis and treatment of cardiovascular disorders will want a copy.[9]

Other reviews were equally positive, and the sales rewarded W. B. Saunders for its patience. In later years, Braunwald brought in other colleagues as coeditors, and eventually he followed the model of Tinsley Harrison—stepping aside as an editor of the book. His colleagues and W. B. Saunders (now Elsevier) incorporated his name into the title, which became *Braunwald's Heart Disease.* Even after Braunwald was no longer an editor for the textbook, he authored several chapters and remained the editor for its online updates, which included frequent focused reviews: five-page articles delving into topics with material that was not available at the time the textbook was published. He would solicit these reviews from colleagues, and often worked with the writers to summarize late-breaking clinical trials.

~

By the end of the first decade of the twenty-first century, Braunwald had stepped down from his role as editor of *Heart Disease* and an editor of *Harrison's,* but not because he was retiring. He wanted to be where the action was, and adapt to the new ways in which clinicians learned. He wanted to turn textbooks into living systems.

He encouraged the development of companion books to go with the "mother ship" textbook—volumes such as the pocket manual version of *Harrison's,* a cardiac nursing companion book for *Heart Disease,* and a book focusing on treatment options in cardiology.[10] And he devoted increasing amounts of his own time to the online updates and supplementary materials.

"What I'm trying to do now is integrate the whole thing," he said in a 2010 interview. "I think that should be done electronically, so that if you want to look up atrial fibrillation, you can get eight looks at atrial fibrillation. I don't know whether this is a dream that I can see through, but I'm interested in a system that begins with a mother book, that goes out electronically, and that branches out into all matters cardiovascular."

Braunwald was in fact trying to create a learning system for someone like himself, someone who wanted to begin to master a topic by reading a good chapter in a textbook, and then stay up to date by having access to the latest material via the Internet. And such a person would want to be able to look at the topic from different directions, such as the nursing perspective, the pathologist's perspective, the surgeon's perspective—just as he himself had thrived as a researcher by examining issues from the perspectives of colleagues with different types of expertise. When Braunwald began to formulate the idea of such a system for learning, and estimated the work that it involved, he decided to stop being the editor of *Heart Disease,* comfortable that the book itself was in the capable hands of his successors.

⌣

In an interview in 2000, Braunwald described going to a community hospital emergency department for a personal medical problem. "I saw an opened copy of *Harrison's* on the emergency physician's desk. I found it to be reassuring."

In that interview, Braunwald went on to comment on an unexpected source of gratification from his work on textbooks: "I receive letters, usually from India or Pakistan, in which the writer has picked up a mistake. They may write something like, 'On page 1147 on the nineteenth line you say this . . . Professor, with deep respect, I think you are wrong.' And these letter writers are always correct! It might be a typo or even a serious error, but it means that people around the world are really reading the book, and this is a great responsibility."[11]

: 13 :

The Still Years

In the summer of 2009, shortly before he turned eighty, Eugene Braunwald was greeted by one of his former trainees, who asked how he was doing. "I'm in my 'Still Years,'" he said. "Do you know what that means?"

His former trainee said that he did not. Braunwald continued, "It's that point in life when people run into you, and they ask, 'Are you *still* working full time? Are you *still* doing research? Are you *still* traveling to meetings around the world? Are you *still* drawing a salary? Are you *still* editing? And sometimes they ask, 'Are you *still* enjoying it?'"

The answer to each of those questions was yes. The cardiology prodigy who had been the youngest person in the room for so many years was now virtually always the oldest—but he was *still* in the room, and, when he was, he was somehow *still* the dominant presence. He was working about sixty hours a week, versus the ninety or so he had put in almost every week during the previous six decades. He was in the process of stepping back from some of his roles, such as leadership of the TIMI Study Group, but he remained deeply involved in the conception, planning, and execution of major clinical trials.

In some ways, it had become the very best of times for Braunwald the researcher. He was free of administrative headaches, such as the need to allocate space and resources. He did not have to write grants or worry about supporting dozens of young faculty. He could focus virtually all of his professional energy on research, on trying to answer the questions that he believed most important.

He was helping to design a huge study of a drug that could dramatically raise HDL ("good" cholesterol) and reduce LDL ("bad" cholesterol). He was chairing worldwide trials of anti-inflammatory drugs and anticoagulant drugs in patients recovering from myocardial infarction and arrhythmias. He was branching out into research on antidiabetes drugs, in the largest trial thus far conducted on diabetic patients who also had coronary heart disease.

Braunwald's prior achievements had led to extraordinary acclaim. He had won every major award from the national and many international cardiology societies; he was one of the only three cardiologists ever elected to the National Academy of Sciences; and he had won twenty honorary degrees from distinguished universities around the world. If he'd wished to do so, he could have traveled somewhere every week to give a Grand Rounds, accept an award, be fêted at a dinner. Some trips still seemed worth making, such as the chance to meet the pope in 2012. But, in general, pomp and circumstance made him restless.

He seemed to draw his greatest satisfaction from the sustained "returns" from his investments in people and programs. At that moment, in the summer of 2009, the director of the National Heart, Lung, and Blood Institute (NHLBI)—the place where his adventures in research had truly begun—was one of his former trainees, Elizabeth "Betsy" Nabel, MD. In 2012, that role would be taken by *another* of his former trainees, Gary H. Gibbons, MD. Physicians and scientists who had been his faculty or trainees were everywhere one looked, in medicine and beyond.

From his own experiences and those of his family, he knew all too well how easily people's lives can be thrown into turmoil, preventing them from reaching their potential. He thus took pride in having worked at so many fine institutions and made them even better, and in having helped to launch so many outstanding careers. The institutions themselves were thriving—the NIH, the departments of medicine at San Diego, Beth Israel, and the Brigham, Partners HealthCare System—and they were often thriving under the leadership of his former trainees. His two beloved textbooks were likewise still dominant in their fields.

Those programs, those people, and those books continued to keep him busy, curious, even excited. In its trials, TIMI often recruited 15,000 to 20,000 patients from about a thousand sites in forty countries. When Betsy Nabel was leading the NHLBI, she had asked him to develop and chair a network of academic centers that would conduct trials of new treatments for heart failure. He had quickly accepted, because the work reminded him of the creation of TIMI and because it allowed him to remain on the cutting edge of heart failure research, one of his original passions from his NIH days. He continued to write and publish and edit, in textbooks and prestigious journals. So much good research was coming to fruition that he was author or coauthor of about twenty papers per year.

Even when he was not an official member of the research team, Braunwald remained in demand for his judgment and advice. In discussions of clinical medicine, research, or medical politics, the phrase "I talked to Gene Braunwald, and here's what he had to say . . ." continued to make people pause and listen.

When asked to reflect on his career, Braunwald mused about the role of chance and of the generosity shown by so many people—the Whites, the English farmers who had taken him and his brother in during Operation Pied Piper; his Aunt Rose, who had sponsored his family's entry into the United States; Robert Berliner; Glenn Morrow; and on and on. If any of them had not stepped forward to help when they did, who knew how his life would have turned out?

He commented on his amazement at the magnitude of the

changes that had occurred in the six decades since his first exposure to medicine. "In 1951, cardiovascular mortality in the United States was more than twice what it is today. Acute rheumatic fever was very common, and most large cities in the country had special 'Rheumatic Fever Hospitals.' Now a new case of acute rheumatic fever is a great rarity.

"The only noninvasive cardiac imaging available was chest roentgenography or fluoroscopy. Today we have two- and three-dimensional echocardiography, computed tomography, magnetic resonance imaging, and positron emission tomography, making diagnostic cardiac catheterization unnecessary in many instances.

"Coronary care units, cardiac resuscitation, clinical trials, coronary risk factors, and pacemakers had never been heard of. There were no effective drugs to treat hypertension, hypercholesterolemia—no oral diuretics or effective anti-arrhythmics. And the advances that have occurred in treating cancer, neurological diseases, and many other conditions have been equally astounding.

"I feel so lucky to have had a ringside seat during the sixty years in which all of these developments have occurred. And a couple of times I've even been fortunate enough to get into the ring, especially in cardiology."

~

After all the years, all the research papers, all the scientific meetings, all the committees, all the hirings and firings, Braunwald came back over and over to the special importance of caring for patients. His comments still reflected the perspectives of the twenty-year-old medical student who, in 1949, after years of uncertainty, could not believe his good fortune to be sitting across from a patient—*his* patient—in the Thursday Night Cardiology Clinic at Bellevue Hospital. After his earlier experiences, he could never cease to feel that it was a privilege to take care of patients.

He never seriously considered a job as dean of a medical school, even though he had been offered such positions a half-dozen times over the years, and even though that role was considered by many the pinnacle of academic medicine. Braunwald wanted to stay at the Department of Medicine level, where he could be closer to patient care. He wanted to be actively involved in training medical students and residents in clinical medicine, and in conducting research that could lead to improved patient care.

When Braunwald had been chairman of the Brigham's Department of Medicine, he had welcomed the new interns each summer with a thirty-minute talk during their orientation. Many of those interns had come to the Brigham because they wanted to become famous researchers like him, but that first talk by Braunwald was always about patient care. He would tell the interns that they had much to learn from everyone in the hospital—from radiologists, from nurses, from pharmacists.

But then he would say that one important characteristic separated internal-medicine trainees from other staff. "Don't ever forget that there is a qualitative difference between your relationship to the patient and theirs. You are going to find yourself working in an ICU, dealing with a critically ill patient. You'll get called away to deal with another emergency, and when you come back, there might be a different nurse, because there has been a shift change. Don't be angry or resentful that others have come and gone as the shift has changed. That person lying in the bed is *your* patient, and you should take pride in being there for him until he is stable."

Braunwald's perspective was that of the former "Osler Marine," someone who had trained at Johns Hopkins in the era when residents were on call for the entire year. As medical knowledge had progressed, more physicians had become involved in the care of complex patients, and their commitment was often circumscribed. The number of consecutive hours that a medical trainee could work was limited, and most hospitals now employed "hospitalists"—doctors who assumed the care of hospitalized patients from their primary-care physicians. These changes gave Braunwald pause, because they interfered with the concept of the doctor-patient relationship in which he had been trained. But he had adjusted.

"Sure, I've wondered about that fundamental question of what is happening to our profession," he said in a 2010 interview. "What do I think of the eighty-hour workweek? What do I think of 'shift medicine'? What do I think of hospitalists? I'm concerned that with the move to 'shift medicine,' the continuity of care, which is a fundamental principle of good medical practice, seems to be dying on the vine."

Braunwald said that initially he'd been opposed to the idea of hospitalists. But then he had visited his former colleague and close friend Lee Goldman, when Goldman was chairman of the Department of Medicine at the University of California, San Francisco, where the hospitalist concept was first developed. "I realized that my initial reaction was a conservative one, because I'm rooted in the 1950s and the 1960s, when approaches and values were different. Now I think that what we can do diagnostically and therapeutically is so powerful that the concept of the physician in that famous Norman Rockwell painting, just sitting by the bedside of a very ill patient, is out of date. We can do so much better than that now. And, yes, I guess there is a place for hospitalists."

Asked to name the medical professionals he most admired, Braunwald repeatedly mentioned Donald Seldin, his role model as an inspiring department chairman and researcher who had built a great program at the University of Texas Southwestern out of next to nothing. In October 2010, Braunwald was invited to attend Seldin's ninetieth birthday party, but was already committed to participating in a research symposium in Lisbon. He sent Seldin a handwritten note with his regrets, saying, "When I began to understand what you were doing, I changed my career goals and decided to become a chairman of medicine in institutions that would let me use the 'Seldin Model.' This gave me great joy for twenty-eight years!"

Braunwald spoke wistfully about his parents, who had been robbed of their comfortable lives when the Nazis seized Vienna in 1938. Long after their deaths, he could not stop thinking about how they had sacrificed endlessly to give him and his brother opportunities. They had never completely shed their bitterness over what had happened to them, he said, but they had pushed on. He drew satisfaction from the pride he had brought them, but expressed regret that he had worked so hard and traveled so much that he was not immersed more in the lives of his three daughters, Karen, Allison, and Jill, as they grew up.

He talked proudly of his daughters and their accomplishments. Karen had become a clinical psychologist and the chief clinical officer at a mental-health facility; Allison, an associate professor of medicine, a diabetologist, and head of clinical research at the Joslin Diabetes Center, a Harvard Medical School affiliate; and Jill, a busy and respected healthcare attorney. He was amazed at his good luck that all three lived close by, that he genuinely liked his sons-in-law, that he was now "surrounded" by them and their families, including seven grandchildren.

～

In a conversation in February 2013, Braunwald described an amazing development in his life at home: he had been manipulated into becoming a football fan. The manipulator behind this transition was his wife, Elaine, whom Braunwald often credited with bringing his family much closer together. Elaine started inviting Braunwald's daughters and their families over on Sunday afternoons, when the New England Patriots were playing on television. Braunwald would put down his work and join them.

"So I started sitting down with the boys [his sons-in-law] to watch the game. I just wanted to be with the family, but I started to find the game interesting. I stayed longer and longer—I'd even have a beer!"

By the end of that season, Braunwald would sit with his family and watch most of a game. He was no longer the restless young man who, as a high school student, would force himself to study thirteen hours every Saturday and Sunday—who would be called downstairs when his relatives came to visit, make pleasantries for seven or eight minutes, and then drift back upstairs to his books.

Many factors led to that change, but none as important as the influence of his wife, Elaine. Braunwald was very aware of his good fortune to be sharing this period of his life with her, someone widely known among friends and colleagues for her intelligence, warmth, and sensitivity. She had once used those qualities effectively as a senior administrator in several teaching hospitals, including the Brigham, but now she was using them to weave the social fabric of Braunwald's multigenerational family. Daughters, sons-in-law, grandchildren, Rena Stark (the former nanny)—Elaine understood how to manage the happy chaos of a modern family, and integrate Braunwald into it.

They were enjoying a shared life outside the family, too. Elaine knew a great deal about medicine, but also had many nonmedical interests and community involvements. While she understood and was a reliable sounding board for Braunwald's professional activities, she had widened his horizons. "Elaine has opened my eyes to a world that I knew was out there but had never entered," he said. They enjoyed foreign travel, and when they went to their favorite destination, Salzburg, they would make an obligatory stop in Vienna to see the house at Number 4 Zelinkagasse, where he had lived as a boy.

~

When Braunwald was asked whom he admired most among historical figures in medicine, he reached back several centuries, and cited William Harvey (1578–1657) as "one of my true heroes." Harvey, an English physician, was the first to describe the circulation of the blood, from the heart to the arteries to the tissue, then into the veins and back to the heart. "It was a breakthrough in thinking," Braunwald believed, "but the breakthrough goes beyond his specific insight into the circulation. He made a lot of observations, and realized that the traditional concept about the movement of blood was simply wrong. The liver could not be generating all the blood that the heart was pumping, as then believed. Harvey then came up with a theory, and he did a beautiful series of experiments. He severed the carotid artery of a rabbit and it bled, yielding much more blood than could have been in the arterial tree. Where did all that blood come from? It had to come from the venous circulation. It was a brilliant piece of thinking and probably the first hypothesis-driven research in the life sciences. The ultimate impact of this experiment and the concept of hypothesis-driven research on humankind can't be overestimated."

Braunwald remained very interested in the training of future generations of investigators, the intellectual heirs of William Harvey. In 2008, Braunwald—in collaboration with Eduardo Marbán, a distinguished cardiovascular researcher—wrote of the challenges facing young clinicians who might seek to do what they had done: combine clinical work with research. They described the difficulty of getting funding, and the temptation of greater income obtainable through private practice as a clinician. They noted the long duration of training that one required in order to become a clinician—a period that would increase if one devoted time to research.

Despite these barriers, Braunwald and Marbán wrote that opportunities for the clinician-investigator had never been greater. They argued that major questions were of interest to both clinicians and researchers (questions such as: How can we repair in-

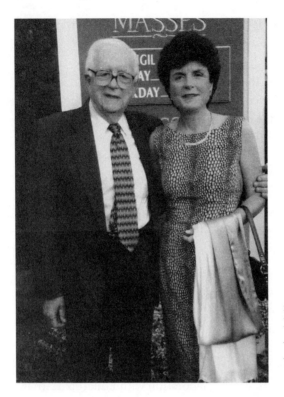

23. Eugene and Elaine Braunwald. *Photo courtesy of Eugene Braunwald.*

jured organs?), demonstrating that the gap between researcher's bench and patient's bedside had become narrower than ever. They pointed out that clinical work and research made complementary demands but offered complementary rewards. "On the wards, one has to know at least a little about almost everything to function effectively. The goal in investigation is, instead, to know everything there is to know about a focused problem. . . . Caring effectively for an ill patient brings immediate gratification; investigation offers long-term rewards and lasting impact, but on a long-term time scale."

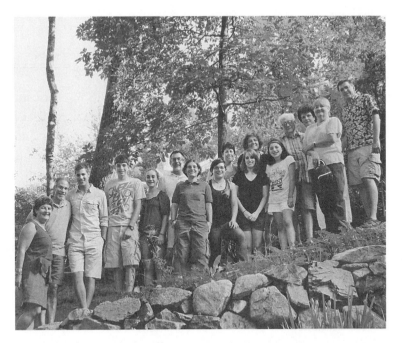

24. Three generations of Braunwalds. *Photo courtesy of Eugene Braunwald.*

Braunwald and Marbán cited two paths for the potential clinician-investigator: the MD-PhD program, and the MD with postgraduate research, a path in which a physician pursues at least two years of postgraduate research. They offered very specific tactical advice, including:

Choose the right environment. Training in a noninsular, collaborative environment is often a key to success.

Select the right mentor, someone who is willing and able to devote the time necessary to fulfill this important role. An investigator with a "big name" is not necessarily a good mentor.

Don't become the slave of a single technique.

Don't shun industry support.

Don't limit your relations to a single company.

Never underestimate the power of the written or the spoken word.[1]

Their advice was striking for its idealistic and even romantic attitude toward research. They suggested that potential clinician-investigators should ask themselves, "Are you truly curious and passionate about finding the answer to a significant question?" If so, they said, "Nothing can quite equal the joy of finding something entirely new, and then applying that discovery to effect changes in medical practice." They urged potential clinician-investigators to "ask a bold question . . . work on a problem about which you can feel passionate." They concluded that "no career is nobler; no profession is more rewarding."

Braunwald's own career had focused on several questions, but at least one—how to reduce mortality after myocardial infarction —had remained an obsession for more than half a century. He had begun working on that question at the NIH in the 1950s, and was still engaged on clinical trials on the topic in the 2010s. Tremendous progress had been made, but the problem persisted, and Braunwald was still at work. He had participated in laboratory studies, animal experiments, multinational clinical trials, observational studies of cardiac markers, risk stratification analyses, epidemiological investigations, and cost-effectiveness studies—all aimed at providing insight into how to reduce mortality in the wake of myocardial infarction. He employed different tools for different times and different nuances of the challenge. And he never got bored of the topic. He had recently become strongly interested in the potential of regenerative medicine to "completely change the game of treating myocardial infarction."

Of all his research experiences, the one he cherished the most was his work on SAVE, the trial that first showed the benefits of administering the ACE inhibitor captopril to patients soon after acute myocardial infarction.[2] He loved SAVE because it began where he had begun: in the animal laboratory. His colleagues Janice and Marc Pfeffer would produce myocardial infarctions in rats, and then administer the drug, which reduced damage to the left ventricle and improved the chances of survival.

"You make an observation, get an idea, and develop a hypothesis. You test it in an animal model and it works brilliantly, better than you expected," he said, describing the overall arc of the SAVE story. "You take it to patients with large myocardial infarcts, and study them via cardiac catheterization. The drug worked hemodynamically, not by salvaging myocardium but by preventing changes in the shape of the ventricle. We followed these patients for several years and observed a reduction in death! It was then confirmed repeatedly elsewhere.

"So this was a home run, and it was a wonderful experience for me and for Marc and Janice Pfeffer. We formed a very tight relationship."

It was indeed a home run—a home run in which Braunwald and the Pfeffers had carved the bat and stitched the ball. It was also the type of home run that causes the fences to be moved farther away from home plate for the next batter. Mortality from myocardial infarction falls, and the next therapeutic challenge has an even greater challenge to show its worth.

Braunwald found that trend energizing, rather than discouraging. He was especially excited about two trials testing new strategies for reducing patients' risk of myocardial infarction. He and his TIMI colleague David Morrow were studying a new agent that might make blood clot prevention more effective; and he and TIMI were working with colleagues at Oxford University to study a compound that might increase the level of "good" cholesterol. "This could be a real game-changer."

~

That ability to imagine changing the game, to become thrilled about the potential impact of an innovation, to feel the surge of energy and interest generated by some new data or a new idea—those things remained the same.

"I am as excited about what I'm doing now as I have ever been about any of my previous work, including valvular heart disease, where I started, and hypertrophic cardiomyopathy—my great adventure in the 1960s. The possibility of having a large positive impact on the millions of patients with atherosclerosis, myocardial infarction, and heart failure is an enormously powerful driver.

"It's not very hard to write papers that get published in good journals, but it's immensely difficult to develop treatments that will help people and change medical practice. To think that somewhere, thousands of miles away, somebody whom I've never met and never will meet is living longer and better because he is receiving an ACE inhibitor following a myocardial infarction—now that's gratifying.

"I would like to remain involved in clinical research and continue to try to have some impact for the better. I know that's asking a lot, but how many people in their eighties get the chance to even dream of this? I'm very, very lucky."

Appendix

Notes

Index

Appendix

Impact on the Field

In 2000, as the European Society of Cardiology approached its fiftieth birthday, the editors of its journal asked all the living winners of the Nobel Prize in Physiology or Medicine this question: Who has contributed the most to the practice of cardiology in recent years? Only one name was suggested by every respondent: Eugene Braunwald. In their tribute to Braunwald, the editors wrote that his "contribution has, and continues to be, on all fronts. He is first and foremost an outstanding doctor. His research contributions in the field of heart failure, ischaemic heart disease, and more recently clinical trials have been unique. However, it may well be that his principal contribution is in the world of teaching. His textbook *Heart Disease* has been an inspiration for doctors learning the importance of the science of cardiology and a unique source of knowledge and reference in the field."[1]

Braunwald, in his response, recalled the toll exacted by rheumatic heart disease, heart failure, and coronary artery disease when he'd been a medical student in the 1950s, and reflected on the challenges that lay ahead.[2] He did not directly allude to his own research. After all, he knew that advances in science often require the efforts of hundreds, even thousands of people—some actively collaborating, and others criticizing or competing. He frequently invoked a metaphor for medical progress—many streams, sometimes separating, sometimes coming together.

Braunwald's work was more than just another stream feeding into the river of cardiology, however. For almost six decades, he was among the most prolific and influential cardiology researchers in the world—an unusually long period of leadership in any field. Braunwald's list of research publications begins in 1954, with a paper on measurement of pressures in the chambers of the human heart and the aorta. That paper was followed by more than 1,200 additional scientific papers.

For most academics, 100 publications is a benchmark signifying a productive career. The difference between 1,200 and 100 publications does not mean that Braunwald worked twelve times as hard or twelve times as long as other researchers. Examination of his career and those of other prodigiously productive leaders in medicine reveals that some researchers work in ways qualitatively different from the methods of others.

First and foremost, research leaders set out to address important and enduring questions. For example, Braunwald began working in the 1950s on the question of how to reduce the death rate from heart attacks. In the ensuing decades, he attacked this issue from a range of angles. He used different research methods in different eras, but the basic question was always the same. He collaborated with colleagues from various fields—basic scientists, cardiac catheterization specialists, epidemiologists, biostatisticians, and so on. He used their different perspectives and skills to shine new light on the questions that obsessed him.

Such research leaders have had sufficient good fortune and success that they can aim for a goal beyond sustaining a career. Their goal is to have an impact—on scientific knowledge, on other researchers, and on the health of patients, including patients they have never met and patients who are not yet born.

~

How does one quantify something that is inherently unquantifiable—namely, the impact of an individual's work? In recent years, analytic tools have emerged from the social sciences that provide insight into the influence of scientific leaders. These tools have roots in library and social-networking science, and help to reveal how a scientist's contributions are being used by others.

The first generation of these tools came along in the 1960s, when a young librarian named Eugene Garfield began to wonder if "footnotes" (citations) in scientific papers might provide a measure of the impact of prior publications. The logic was that a research paper that influenced many subsequent researchers would be cited in their publications. The greater the number of citations, the greater the impact of the article. In contrast, a research paper that was rarely or never cited by other researchers was unlikely to be important.

Garfield began laboriously tracking footnotes generated by research papers—and thus began mapping networks of connections within fields of scientific knowledge.[3] He published the *Scientific Citation Index*, which catalogued research articles and the publications that had cited them. In the pre-Internet era, the *Scientific Citation Index* was an enormous set of volumes that sat in the library, rarely consulted, but occasionally useful to researchers writing a paper.

It was a brilliant idea that quickly became unworkable. There was simply too much new information, too many new articles, and too many new journals—in part because Braunwald's generation of researchers were creating so much new knowledge and generating so many publications. Garfield realized that not all journals were created equal, and that he needed to focus his *Index* on the journals that mattered most.

But how to decide which journals had the greatest impact? His solution was a simple equation: divide the number of citations that were generated by the journal's articles over a two-year period by the number of articles it published during that time.[4] The best journals would be those that published the articles that generated the most citations per article—and thus had the most impact.

This "journal impact factor" was developed in the 1970s,[5] at which point Braunwald was already well known for research published in articles in prestigious medical journals such as the *New England Journal of Medicine, Circulation, Circulation Research,* and the *Journal of Clinical Investigation.* When the impact factor for these journals was quantified, it confirmed a "virtuous cycle" that surprised no one: respected experts like Braunwald published their research in respected journals, which enhanced their status by publishing articles by respected authors like Braunwald (after subjecting the manuscripts to rigorous review, of course). The combination of respected authors and respected journals led to more citations, which increased the impact factors and further enhanced the reputations of the authors and the journals.

This system persisted, and grew in prominence, in the absence of a better mechanism for assessing the impact of scientific journals. Yet not everyone was happy with it, since it had well-recognized potential liabilities.[6] Some critics thought that the journal impact factor created a "club" of elite researchers. Researchers who considered themselves outsiders complained that the most prestigious journals sometimes overlooked their most important work.

Enter the "h-index," introduced in 2005 and named after its inventor, Jorge Hirsch.[7] Hirsch, a physicist at the University of California, San Diego, proposed theories on low-temperature superconductors that challenged the conventional wisdom. He was convinced that his ideas were correct, and he believed that his work was slowly finding its audience even though his papers were often rejected by the most prestigious journals. Like-minded researchers eventually found them, and were citing his research in their papers.

Hirsch wanted to shift attention from the journals in which papers are published to the work itself—and thus to its authors. So he came up with the h-index, which focuses not on *where* the articles were published, but on *how many times* other researchers have cited the work. To calculate the h-index for a researcher, you take all the papers that an author has ever published, and find out the number of times each article has been cited in subsequent papers. (Electronic databases available on the Internet make such data readily accessible.) The papers are then ranked in descending order according to the number of times they have been cited. The h-index is the number (n) of articles that an author has published which have been cited at least the same number of times (n) in other papers.

For example, a researcher might have published one hundred articles in his or her career, and, of these papers, thirty-eight have been cited in other publications at least thirty-eight times. But the thirty-ninth paper has been cited only thirty-seven times. That author's h-index is thus 38. With the passage of time, if that thirty-ninth paper gets cited twice more, his or her h-index would rise to 39.

In the years after its description, this relatively simple index and variants upon it became widely used in academia, where universities must decide whether or not to hire researchers or promote them to tenure. The h-index provides a tool to evaluate and choose among researchers that is more objective than flipping a coin. Even academics not on the job market are interested in their h-index, which offers insight into whether their work is being used.

The h-index is not perfect, of course. A brilliant researcher might publish two hugely important papers before dying young, leaving behind an h-index frozen at 2 for eternity. Conversely, the h-index is kind to older researchers, since earlier papers have a longer time to accumulate citations. And, like any system, the h-index can be gamed. Researchers can be vigorous self-citers, or enlist their colleagues to cite their work repeatedly. In fact, several medical journals ask authors to cite other articles previously published in their pages in an attempt to raise their impact factor; nevertheless, such tactics do not appear to be sufficient to create major changes in either journal impact factors or individual researcher h-indices.

Analysis of Eugene Braunwald's publications provides some quantitative insights into the nature of his role in medical research. As already noted, Braunwald was extraordinarily prolific throughout an unusually long research career. For most researchers, averaging four to five publications per year is impressive. Braunwald averaged twenty papers per year, most of which focused on cardiovascular medicine.

As noted in Chapter 11, his rate of publications was always high but not necessarily constant (Figure 22). The 1960s and the first decade of the twenty-first century were the most productive periods for Braunwald: during each of these decades, he published close to 300 publications, most of which focused on cardiovascular medicine. During the 1970s, 1980s, and 1990s, he averaged just fourteen to sixteen papers per year. During those middle decades, Braunwald was deeply involved with administrative responsibilities, serving as chairman of departments of medicine, first at the University of California, San Diego, and then at Boston's Peter Bent Brigham Hospital (later Brigham and Women's Hospital), and for nine years also at Beth Israel Hospital.

Braunwald's list of publications is unusual not just for its length, but also for the status of the journals in which the papers appeared and the frequency with which they have been cited by other authors. In a 2012 analysis of his publications and those of other leading researchers, 10 percent of Braunwald's papers appeared in the top general medical journals (the *New England Journal of Medicine,* the *Journal of the American Medical Association,* and the *Lancet*), and 37 percent were published in the top cardiology journals (such as *Circulation,* the *European Heart Journal,* the *Journal of the American College of Cardiology,* and, prior to 1983, the *American Journal of Cardiology*). Only two other cardiology researchers who focused on coronary artery disease, heart failure, and other topics that have been Braunwald's main interests had comparable success rates at key medical journals, and these younger researchers lagged Braunwald by about 150 published papers as of 2012. Overall, Braunwald had more publications in top general medical and cardiology journals than any of the more than 42,000 authors in the PubMed database.

As of 2012, Braunwald's articles had been cited more than 136,000 times in other scientific papers, and his h-index was 187— meaning that he had 187 articles with 187 or more citations. An informal rule of thumb is that an h-index greater than 45 indicates that the author is a national leader in his or her field; a 2011 analysis of the publications of ten winners of the Nobel Prize in Physiology or Medicine in the prior ten years found that they had an average h-index of 62 ± 24 (mean ± standard deviation) with a range from 22 to 93.[8] (This analysis included publications only up to the year before the individuals won the Nobel Prize—a condition designed to eliminate any "halo" effect of publicity surrounding the award.)

Braunwald's unusually high h-index reflects, in part, the fact that research papers on major clinical trials tend to be cited more often than basic-science reports, and that many of his papers in recent years were clinical trials or substudies of such trials. Collectively, however, the impact of Braunwald's work as measured by citations was increasing with time. The number of Braunwald citations per year was 2,000–3,000 in the 1990s, but averaged more than 5,000 per year from 2005 to 2012.

Only part of the nature of the work by Braunwald and other scientific leaders with comparable h-indices can be captured in their number of research papers, the rate at which the papers have been published, and the frequency with which they have been cited by other authors. Social-networking science provides some new methods for analyzing researchers' impact that go beyond these contributions at the level of the individual. For example, a researcher can bring new energy and ideas to a field by collaborating with colleagues in other disciplines on an important question (for example, How do we reduce the death rate from heart attacks?). By working at the interface of different fields, researchers can spur innovation—and influence the research of many more people around them. In other words, "networking" research leaders not only do good work within their own research groups, but also raise the performance of others around them.

This "network" effect is apparent in analysis of the long list of Braunwald's research coauthors. These coauthors come from a wide range of fields: basic scientists, researchers who do experiments on animals, cardiac catheterization specialists, experts in international multicenter randomized trials, epidemiologists, biostatisticians, economists, and more. Many of these individuals had never previously collaborated with one another on a research paper—but the one characteristic they share is that they wrote papers with Eugene Braunwald. Their interests intersected around the questions in which Braunwald was interested. He was often the "connector."

Braunwald's role among researchers in cardiology is evident from the following analysis performed on PubMed publication data from the first five decades of his academic career. During that period, a total of 6,339 authors published four or more papers in top journals (as identified earlier in this appendix) on heart failure, coronary artery disease, and a few other key areas of cardiology. Of these 6,339 researchers, Braunwald had worked directly (that is, coauthored a paper) with 396, or 6 percent. Braunwald's

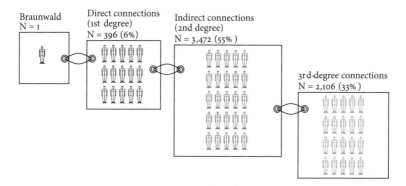

25. Percentage of authors in the coauthor cardiology network with direct, second-degree, or third-degree ties to Braunwald. Based on the results of a PubMed search in the *New England Journal of Medicine,* the *Journal of the American Medical Association,* the *Lancet, Circulation,* the *European Heart Journal,* the *Journal of the American College of Cardiology,* and the *American Journal of Cardiology* (pre-1983), using selected MeSH terms ("heart failure," "coronary artery disease," "acute coronary syndrome," "myocardial infarction"), 1960–present. The search resulted in 6,339 authors with four or more publications. *Courtesy of McKinsey and Company; PubMed; UCINET.*

universe of indirect or second-degree connections was 3,472, or 55 percent—that is, 55 percent of the authors had not worked directly with Braunwald, but had worked directly with one of the 396 researchers who had been Braunwald coauthors. Another 33 percent of the authors had worked with these 3,472 authors, and thus were third-degree connections. In short, Braunwald was just two phone calls removed from nearly two-thirds of the researchers who contributed to these fields during the past half-century, and three phone calls removed from almost all the rest (see Figure 25).

Similar analyses of the "connectedness" of other leading researchers suggest that Braunwald is unusual in this regard. The likely explanation is that Braunwald focused his career on clinical issues that are sometimes explored in animals or basic-science laboratories, but are also sometimes studied in large clinical trials, which can involve hundreds of coauthors on multiple continents. As he pursued these clinical issues, Braunwald naturally fell into collaborations with a high number and percentage of other researchers with a wide variety of expertise.

This connector function can be quantified in terms of variables called "betweenness" and "status." "Betweenness" measures the significance of a scientist to the information flow within, and the integrity of, the whole social network of researchers in a field. On this measure, Braunwald (as well as other scientists) accumulated "betweenness points" when researchers wrote papers with him, but not directly with each other. The more central researchers are to the action, the higher their "betweenness" ranks.

Figure 26 is a computer-generated graphic display of authorship and coauthorship relationships among investigators who have written papers on hemodynamics (the flow of blood within the body, and the factors that affect that flow). In this depiction, each individual researcher is a "node." Braunwald emerges in the center of the network because he published often, and was a coauthor to so many of the other researchers in the field. Other researchers have relatively high betweenness scores, but Braunwald is pulled to the center of this figure because of his central role among so many researchers.

Braunwald also scores high on a metric that social-networking scientists call "status." Status reflects the extent to which a person is "sought" by others as a coauthor, and the strength of collaborative ties. Authors with high authority in a field are identified by having repeated publications. Repeated professional relationships with high-status authors elevate one's own status.

When "betweenness" and "status" ratings of cardiovascular researchers are calculated decade by decade since 1960, Braunwald is the only one who ranked in the top ten in one or the other or

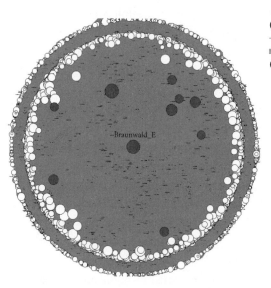

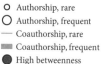

○ Authorship, rare
○ Authorship, frequent
— Coauthorship, rare
▬ Coauthorship, frequent
● High betweenness

26. Hemodynamic authors, 1960–present: betweenness. *Courtesy of McKinsey and Company; PubMed; Visone.*

both, in all five decades. Some younger investigators have been in the top ten for three decades in a row, and if they remain scientifically productive at high levels for another twenty years, they might match Braunwald's durability. But no researcher of Braunwald's generation achieved so much impact on research, as measured by these tools—and then maintained it for so long.

For Braunwald to have achieved this record, good health was necessary but not sufficient. He had to maintain his research interests during decades when he was the management leader for departments of medicine, which are businesses with huge budgets, staffed by physicians with substantial egos. And he had to be flexible—he had to evolve as an investigator as the nature of research changed.

When Braunwald entered research, laboratories consisted of

only a few people: the chief and his or her followers. The number of authors on a paper might be just one, and usually no more than four. In contrast, to answer the pressing questions of the 1990s and beyond, researchers like Braunwald often assembled the equivalent of multinational corporations, with hundreds of researchers spread out over several continents. Braunwald's papers reflect this trend: his mean number of coauthors was three on the papers he published in the 1960s, rose to four in the 1970s and 1980s, and jumped to eight in the 1990s and to nine in the 2000s.

Bigger is not necessarily better, though. Of Braunwald's eleven most widely cited papers, half had ten or fewer coauthors. Two of those papers introduced important concepts of how the heart responds to the damage associated with heart attacks, and were written with just one other author. One paper, which introduced a framework for classifying patients with unstable angina, had only a single author: Braunwald himself.

Notes

Introduction

1 Oscar Handlin, *The Uprooted: The Epic Story of the Great Migrations That Made the American People* (Boston: Little, Brown, 1951).

1. Flight from Europe

1 Carl Zuckmayer, *A Part of Myself,* trans. Richard and Clara Winston (New York: Harcourt, Brace, Jovanovich, 1970).

2 W. R. Roberts, "Eugene Braunwald, MD: A conversation with the editor," *American Journal of Cardiology* 82 (1998): 93–108.

3 Ibid., 95.

4 David Palmer, "Evacuation of children from London on 1st September 1939, as written by Eileen Wright," www.bbc.co.uk/ww2peopleswar/stories/97/a5147697.shtml (accessed 3/18/2012).

5 Eric R. Kandel, "Autobiography," nobelprize.org/nobel_prizes/medicine/laureates/2000/kandel-autobio.html (accessed 3/18/2012).

2. An American Education

1 Ilana Abramovitch and Sean Galvin, eds., *Jews of Brooklyn* (Waltham, MA: Brandeis University Press, 2001), 2.

2 Kenneth T. Jackson and John B. Manbeck, *The Neighborhoods of Brooklyn* (New Haven: Yale University Press, 1998), xvii.

3 Abramovitch and Galvin, *Jews of Brooklyn,* 2.

4 Ibid., 6.

5 Ibid.

6 Malcolm Gladwell, *Outliers: The Story of Success* (New York: Little, Brown, 2008), 151–158.

7 "Eugene Kleiner: Obituary," *Economist,* December 4, 2003.

3. Medical Education and Training

1 Edward C. Halperin, "The Jewish problem in U.S. medical education, 1920–1955," *Journal of the History of Medicine* 56 (2001): 140–167.

2 Kenneth M. Ludmerer, *Time to Heal: American Medical Education, from the Turn of the Century to the Era of Managed Care* (New York: Oxford University Press, 1999), 64.

3 Leon Sokoloff, "The rise and decline of the Jewish quota in medical school admissions," *Bulletin of the New York Academy of Medicine* 68 (1992): 497–518.

4 Howard E. Wilson et al., *A Study of Policies, Procedures, and Practices in Admissions to Medical Schools in New York State* (Albany: University of the State of New York, 1952), 33.

5 Halperin, "The Jewish Problem," 166. In the current New York State code (Education Laws), this is Title 1, Article 7, Section 313; see public.leginfo .state.ny.us. The passage in the current law has been expanded: "without regard to race, color, sex, religion, creed, marital status, age, sexual orientation as defined in section two hundred ninety-two of the executive law, or national origin."

6 Stephen L. Johnson, *The History of Cardiac Surgery, 1896–1955* (Baltimore: Johns Hopkins Press, 1970), 3.

7 Elliot Cutler and Samuel A. Levine, "Cardiotomy and valvulotomy for mitral stenosis: Experimental observations and clinical notes concerning an operated case with recovery," *Boston Medical and Surgical Journal* 188 (1923): 1023–1027.

8 Elliot Cutler and Claude S. Beck, "The present status of the surgical procedures in chronic valvular disease of the heart," *Archives of Surgery* 18 (1929): 403–416.

9 Werner Forssmann, *Experiments on Myself: Memoirs of a Surgeon in Germany* (New York: St. Martin's, 1975).

10 Wilson, *A Study of Policies,* 27.

11 "Dr. George E. Schreiner interviewed by Agnes Fogo and Kim Solez, Great Falls, Virginia, June 27, 1997," *International Society of Nephrology Video Legacy Project.* cybernephrology.ualberta.ca/ISN/VLP/Trans/Schreiner.htm (accessed 3/18/2012).

12 George E. Schreiner, interview with author, 1998.

13 I. Snapper, *Isidore Snapper's Notes for Memoirs, 1889–1973: The Autobiographical Recollections of "the Champion of Bedside Medicine,"* ed. M. J. van Lieburg (Rotterdam: Erasmus, 2004). Snapper's first name is sometimes spelled "Isadore."

14 Jean Medawar and David Pyke, *Hitler's Gift: The True Story of the Scientists Expelled by the Nazi Regime* (New York: Arcade, 2000), 148.

15 Tinsley R. Harrison et al., *Principles of Internal Medicine* (New York: Blakiston, 1950).

16 Ibid., 1250.

17 Ibid., 1273.

18 Ibid., 1266.

19 Ibid., 1342.

4. *Internship and Research at Mount Sinai and Bellevue*

1 Jonathan W. Uhr, interview with author, January 11, 2010.

2 Eugene Braunwald and Jonathan W. Uhr, "Chylothorax," *Journal of the Mount Sinai Hospital* 21 (1954): 62–79.

3 Eugene Braunwald et al., "The hemodynamics of the left side of the heart as studied by simultaneous left atrial, left ventricular, and aortic pressures; particular reference to mitral stenosis," *Circulation* 12 (1955): 69–81. R. A. Bader et al., "Hemodynamics at rest and during exercise in normal pregnancy as studied by cardiac catheterization," *Journal of Clinical Investigation* 34 (1955): 1524–1536. Eugene Braunwald et al., "Timing of electrical and mechanical events of the left side of the human heart," *Journal of Applied Physiology* 8 (1955): 309–314.

4 William Theodore De Bary, *Living Legacies at Columbia* (New York: Columbia University Press), 238.

5 Allen B. Weisse, *Heart to Heart: The Twentieth Century Battle against Cardiac Disease—An Oral History* (New Brunswick, NJ: Rutgers University Press, 2002), 34.

6 Ibid., 35.

7 Eugene Braunwald et al., "Time relationship of dynamic events in the cardiac chambers, pulmonary artery and aorta in man," *Circulation Research* 4 (1956): 100–107. Eugene Braunwald et al., "Estimation of the volume of a circulatory model by the Hamilton and Bradley methods at varying flow volume ratios," *Journal of Applied Physiology* 12 (1958): 445–446.

5. *Clinical Associate at the NIH*

1 Office of NIH History, "A Short History of the NIH," history.nih.gov/exhibits/history/index.html (accessed 3/18/2012).

2 E. T. Lanahan, *A Salute to the Past: A History of the National Heart, Lung, and Blood Institute* (Bethesda, MD: National Institutes of Health, 1987), 12.

3   Stanley J. Sarnoff et al., "Performance characteristics and oxygen debt in a nonfailing, metabolically supported, isolated heart preparation," *American Journal of Physiology* 192 (1958): 141–147. Stanley J. Sarnoff et al., "Hemodynamic determinants of oxygen con sumption of the heart with special reference to the tension-time index," *American Journal of Physiology* 192 (1958): 148–156. Eugene Braunwald et al., "Hemodynamic determinants of coronary flow: Effect of changes in aortic pressure and cardiac output on the relationship between myocardial oxygen consumption and coronary flow," *American Journal of Physiology* 192 (1958): 157–163.

4   Eugene Braunwald and A. Glenn Morrow, "A method for the detection and estimation of aortic regurgitant flow in man," *Circulation* 17 (1958): 505–511.

5   Eugene Braunwald et al., "Hemodynamic effects of quantitatively varied experimental mitral regurgitation," *Circulation* 5 (1957): 539–545. George H. Welch et al., "Hemodynamic effects of quantitatively varied experimental aortic regurgitation," *Circulation* 5 (1957): 546–551.

6   Braunwald and Morrow, "A method for the detection and estimation of aortic regurgitant flow."

7   John Ross, Jr., Eugene Braunwald, and Andrew G. Morrow, "Transseptal left atrial puncture: New technique for the measurement of left atrial pressure in man," *American Journal of Cardiology* 3 (1959): 653–655.

6. Johns Hopkins Hospital

1   Alan Mason Chesney, *The Johns Hopkins Hospital and the Johns Hopkins University School of Medicine: A Chronicle*, vol. 1: *Early Years, 1867–1893* (Baltimore: Johns Hopkins Press, 1943).

2   Ibid. *The History of Johns Hopkins Medicine*, www.hopkinsmedicine.org/About/history (accessed 3/20/2012).

3   Chesney, *The Johns Hopkins Hospital*, 63.

4   A. McGehee Harvey, *Adventures in Medical Research: A Century of Discovery at Johns Hopkins* (Baltimore: Johns Hopkins University Press, 1974), 4.

5   Ibid., 6.

6   Thomas B. Turner, *Heritage of Excellence: The Johns Hopkins Medical Institutions, 1914–1947* (Baltimore: Johns Hopkins University Press, 1974).

7   R. H. Shyrock, "The unique influence of the Johns Hopkins University on American Medicine," *Acta Historica Scientiarum Naturalium et Medicinalium* (Copenhagen: Ejnar Munksgaard, 1953).

8   Abraham Flexner, "Medical Education in the United States and Canada," *Carnegie Foundation Bulletin* 4 (1910): 12.

9   Harvey Cushing, *The Life of Sir William Osler* (Oxford: Clarendon, 1925).

10 Gerald Imber, *Genius on the Edge: The Bizarre Double Life of Dr. William Stewart Halsted* (New York: Kaplan, 2010).

11 Ibid. William G. MacCallum, *William Stewart Halsted, Surgeon* (Baltimore: Johns Hopkins Press, 1930).

12 Howard Markel, *An Anatomy of Addiction: Sigmund Freud, William Halsted, and the Miracle Drug Cocaine* (New York: Pantheon, 2011).

13 Chesney, *The Johns Hopkins Hospital,* 193.

14 Ibid., 203.

15 Ibid., 218.

16 "Women—or the Female Factor: About Johns Hopkins Medicine," www.hopkinsmedicine.org/about/history/history6.html (accessed 2/4/2013).

17 "A Timeline of Women at Hopkins," *Johns Hopkins Magazine,* www.jhu.edu/jhumag/1107web/women2.html (accessed 2/4/2013).

18 Burton Sobel, interview with author, December 18, 2009.

7. The "Golden Years" at the NIH

1   James A. Shannon, "The National Institutes of Health: Some critical years, 1955–1957," *Science* 237 (1987): 865–868.

2   Ibid., 867.

3   Stanhope Bayne-Jones, *The Advancement of Medical Research and Education through the Department of Health, Education, and Welfare: Final Report of the Secretary's Consultants on Medical Research and Education* (Washington, DC: Government Printing Office, 1958).

4   Shannon, "The National Institutes of Health," 865.

5   W. Gerald Austen, interview with author, April 6, 2010.

6   Braunwald-Morrow Mitral Heart Valve, available online at nih.pastperfect-online.com/37870cgi/mweb.exe?request=record;id=387C5 FAA-25D0-4846-A527-191280794604;type=101 (accessed 4/2/2012).

7   Nina S. Braunwald et al., "Complete replacement of the mitral valve: Successful clinical application of a flexible polyurethane prosthesis," *Journal of Thoracic and Cardiovascular Surgery* 40 (1960): 1–11.

8   John Ross and Eugene Braunwald, "Aortic stenosis," *Circulation* 38, Supplement V (1968): 61–67.

9   Ibid., V-66.

10   Raphael Rosenhek et al., "Natural history of very severe aortic stenosis," *Circulation* 121 (2010): 151–156.

11   Eugene Braunwald et al., "Effects of mitral-valve replacement on the pulmonary vascular dynamics of patients with pulmonary hypertension," *New England Journal of Medicine* 273 (1965): 509–514.

12   Clarence G. Lasby, *Eisenhower's Heart Attack: How Ike Beat Heart Disease and Held on to the Presidency* (Lawrence: University Press of Kansas, 1997).

13   Samuel A. Levine, "Carotid sinus massage: New diagnostic test for angina pectoris," *Journal of the American Medical Association* 182 (1962): 1332–1334.

14   Eugene Braunwald et al., "Relief of angina pectoris by electrical stimulation of the carotid sinus," *New England Journal of Medicine* 227 (1967): 1278–1283.

15   Andrew Glenn Morrow and Eugene Braunwald, "Functional aortic stenosis: A malformation characterized by resistance to left ventricular outflow without anatomic obstruction," *Circulation* 20 (1959): 181–189.

16   Russell C. Brock, "Functional obstruction of the left ventricle (acquired aortic subvalvular stenosis)," *Guy's Hospital Reports* 106 (1957): 221–238. Bernard A. Bercu et al., "Pseudoaortic stenosis produced by ventricular hypertrophy," *American Journal of Medicine* 85 (1958): 814–818.

17   Eugene Braunwald, "Hypertrophic cardiomyopathy: The early years," *Journal of Cardiovascular Translational Research* 2 (2009): 341–348.

18   Brock, "Functional obstruction of the left ventricle."

19   Eugene Braunwald et al., "Idiopathic hypertrophic subaortic stenosis: Clinical, hemodynamic and angiographic manifestations," *American Journal of Medicine* 29 (1960): 924–945.

20   Eugene Braunwald, "Adventures in cardiovascular research," *Circulation* 120 (2009): 170–180.

21   Eugene Braunwald et al., "Idiopathic hypertrophic subaortic stenosis, I: A description of the disease based upon an analysis of 64 patients," *Circulation* 30 (1964): IV3–IV119. Andrew Glenn Morrow et al., "Idiopathic hypertrophic subaortic stenosis, II: Operative treatment and the results of pre- and postoperative hemodynamic evaluation," *Circulation* 30 (1964): IV120–IV151.

22   Eugene Braunwald et al., "The circulatory response of patients with idiopathic hypertrophic subaortic stenosis to nitroglycerin and to the Valsalva maneuver," *Circulation* 29 (1964): 422–431. Dean Mason et al., "Effects of changes in body position on the severity of obstruction to left ventricu-

lar outflow in idiopathic hypertrophic subaortic stenosis," *Circulation* 33 (1966): 374–382. Edwin C. Brockenbrough et al., "A hemodynamic technique for the detection of hypertrophic subaortic stenosis," *Circulation* 23 (1961): 189–194. Eugene Braunwald and Paul A. Ebert, "Hemodynamic alternations in idiopathic subaortic stenosis induced by sympathomimetic drugs," *American Journal of Cardiology* 10 (1962): 489–495. Donald C. Harrison et al., "Effects of beta-adrenergic blockade on the circulation with particular reference to observations in patients with hypertrophic subaortic stenosis," *Circulation* 29 (1964): 84–98. Lawrence S. Cohen and Eugene Braunwald, "Amelioration of angina pectoris in idiopathic hypertrophic subaortic stenosis with beta-adrenergic blockade," *Circulation* 35 (1967): 847–851.

23 Brockenbrough et al., "A hemodynamic technique," 190.

24 Harrison et al., "Effects of beta-adrenergic blockade."

25 Morrow et al., "Idiopathic hypertrophic subaortic stenosis, II."

26 John Michael Criley, "Pressure gradients without obstruction: A new concept of 'hypertrophic subaortic stenosis,'" *Circulation* 32 (1965): 881–887.

27 Barry J. Maron et al., "The 50-year history, controversy, and clinical implications of left ventricular outflow tract obstruction in hypertrophic cardiomyopathy: From idiopathic hypertrophic subaortic stenosis to hypertrophic cardiomyopathy," *Journal of the American College of Cardiology* 54 (2009): 191–200.

28 Lawrence Cohn, interview with author, April 23, 2010.

29 J. Michael Criley and Robert J. Siegel, "Has 'obstruction' hindered our understanding of hypertrophic cardiomyopathy?" *Circulation* 72 (1985): 1148–1154.

30 Eugene Braunwald, "Edmund H. Sonnenblick," *Journal of Clinical Investigation* 118 (2008): 390.

31 Edmund H. Sonnenblick, "Force-velocity relations in mammalian heart muscle," *American Journal of Physiology* 202 (1962): 931–939.

32 Braunwald, "Edmund H. Sonnenblick," 390.

33 Edmund H. Sonnenblick et al., "The contractile properties of human heart muscle: Studies on myocardial mechanics of surgically excised papillary muscles," *Journal of Clinical Investigation* 44 (1965): 966–977. Gerald Glick et al., "Myocardial force-velocity relations in intact unanesthetized man," *Journal of Clinical Investigation* 44 (1965): 978–988. Edmund H. Sonnenblick et al., "Effects of exercise on myocardial force-velocity relations in in-

tact unanesthetized man: Relative roles of changes in heart rate, sympathetic activity, and ventricular dimensions," *Journal of Clinical Investigation* 44 (1965): 2051–2062.

34 Ibid.

35 James F. Spann, Jr., et al., "Contractile state of cardiac muscle obtained from cats with experimentally produced ventricular hypertrophy and heart failure," *Circulation Research* 21 (1967): 341–354.

36 Burton Sobel, interview with author, December 18, 2009.

37 Roland Folse and Eugene Braunwald, "Determination of fraction of left ventricular volume ejected per beat and of ventricular end-diastolic and residual volumes: Experimental and clinical observations with a precordial dilution technique," *Circulation* 25 (1962): 674–685.

38 Charles A. Chidsey et al., "Augmentation of the plasma norepinephrine response to exercise in patients with congestive heart failure," *New England Journal of Medicine* 267 (1962): 650–654.

39 Eugene Braunwald, "The heart as an endocrine organ," *American Journal of Medicine* 6 (1964): 1–4.

40 Finn Waagstein et al., "Effect of chronic beta adrenergic receptor blockade in congestive cardiomyopathy," *British Heart Journal* 37 (1975): 1022–1036.

41 John R. Hogness and Malin VanAntwerp, eds., *The Artificial Heart Program: Current Status and History* (Washington, DC: National Academy Press, 1991), 14–25.

42 Michael J. Strauss, "The political history of the artificial heart," *New England Journal of Medicine* 310 (1984): 273–278.

43 Daniel J. DiBardino, "The history and development of heart transplantation," *Texas Heart Institute Journal* 26 (1999): 198–205.

44 William C. DeVries et al., "Clinical use of the total artificial heart," *New England Journal of Medicine* 310 (1984): 273–278.

45 William C. Roberts, interview with author, January 10, 2010.

46 Richard L. Kahler et al., "Studies on digitalis, VI: Reduction of the oxygen debt after exercise with digoxin in cardiac patients without heart failure," *Circulation* 27 (1963): 397–405.

47 Jean Wilson, interview with author, January 10, 2010.

48 Henry K. Beecher, "Ethics and clinical research," *New England Journal of Medicine* 274 (1966): 1354–1360.

49 Robert D. Truog, "Patients and doctors: The evolution of a relationship," *New England Journal of Medicine* 366 (2012): 581–585.

50 David J. Rothman, *Strangers at the Bedside: A History of How Law and Bioethics Transformed Medical Decision Making* (New York: Basic Books, 1991), 72.

51 Ibid., 76.

52 Ibid., 75.

53 George A. Mashour, "Altered States: LSD and the Anesthesia Laboratory of Henry Knowles Beecher," *CSA Bulletin* (Winter 2009): 68–74.

8. Building a Medical School in San Diego

1 Eugene Braunwald, "Chronic valvular heart disease," in *Cecil-Loeb Textbook of Medicine*, 12th ed., ed. P. B. Beeson and Walsh McDermott, 615–633 (Philadelphia: W. B. Saunders, 1967).

2 L. J. Witts, "Textbook of Medicine," *British Medical Journal* 1 (1952): 748.

3 Anonymous, "Book News," *Journal of the Association of Medical Colleges* 25 (1950): 458.

4 Herbert L. Fred, "Maxwell Myer Wintrobe: New history and a new appreciation," *Texas Heart Institute Journal* 34 (2007): 328–335.

5 Abraham Flexner, *Medical Education in the United States and Canada: A Report to the Carnegie Foundation for the Advancement of Teaching*, Bulletin no. 4 (New York: Carnegie Foundation for the Advancement of Teaching, 1910), 216–217.

6 William T. Mallon and David J. Vernon, *The Handbook of Academic Medicine: How Medical Schools and Teaching Hospitals Work* (Washington: Association of American Medical Colleges, 2008).

7 Joanne Gribble, "Forty years of UCSD perspective," *San Diego Metropolitan*, web.archive.org/web/20080417234035/http://www.sandiegometro.com/2000/sep/coverstory.html (accessed 4/3/2012).

8 Martin Körbling and Zeev Estrov, "Adult stem cells for tissue repair: A new therapeutic concept?" *New England Journal of Medicine* 349 (2003): 570–582.

9 Jeffrey Kahn, "Ronald Reagan launched political career using the Berkeley campus as target," *UC Berkeley News*, June 8, 2004. www.berkeley.edu/news/media/releases/2004/06/08_reagan.shtml (accessed 4/3/2012).

10 Donald Seldin, interview with author, January 12, 2010. Errol C. Friedberg, *From Rags to Riches: The Phenomenal Rise of the University of Texas Southwestern Medical Center at Dallas* (Durham: Carolina Academic Press, 2007), 54.

11 Ibid., pp 49–69.

12 Peter R. Maroko et al., "Factors influencing infarct size following experimental coronary artery occlusions," *Circulation* 43 (1971): 67–82.

13 Robert J. Hall, "In memoriam: F. Mason Sones, Jr., MD," *Texas Heart Institute Journal* 12 (1985): 356–358.

14 William Grossman, *Cardiac Catheterization and Angiography,* 2nd ed. (Philadelphia: Lea and Febiger, 1974), 4.

15 Allen B. Weisse, *Heart to Heart: The Twentieth Century Battle against Cardiac Disease—An Oral History* (New Brunswick, NJ: Rutgers University Press, 2002), 203–220.

16 Hall, "Mason Sones," 357.

17 Weisse, *Heart to Heart,* 207.

18 Joseph L. Thomas, "The Vineberg legacy: Internal mammary artery implantation, from inception to obsolescence," *Texas Heart Institute Journal* 26 (1999): 107–113.

19 Weisse, *Heart to Heart,* 213–214.

20 Kahn, "Ronald Reagan launched political career," www.berkeley.edu/news/media/releases/2004/06/08_reagan.shtml (accessed 4/3/2012).

21 Burton Sobel, interview with author, December 18, 2009.

9. *Rebuilding the Brigham*

1 Eugene Braunwald, "Future shock in academic medicine," *New England Journal of Medicine* 286 (1972): 1031–1035.

2 John W. Gardner, *No Easy Victories* (New York: Harper and Row, 1968), 44.

3 Nicholas L. Tilney, *A Perfectly Striking Departure: Surgeons and Surgery at the Peter Bent Brigham Hospital, 1912–1980* (Sagamore Beach, MA: Science History Publications, 2006). Stephen J. Ferzoco and Michael J. Zinner, "A brief surgical history of the Peter Bent Brigham Hospital," *Archives of Surgery* 140 (2005): 326–327.

4 Tilney, *A Perfectly Striking Departure,* 13.

5 Francis D. Moore, "The Brigham in Emile Holman's day," *American Journal of Surgery* 80 (1955): 1094.

6 Joseph Dorsey, interview with author, November 21, 2010.

7 Marshall Wolf, interview with author, October 6, 2010.

8 Lewis Dexter, "Eugene C. Eppinger," *Transactions of the American Clinical and Climatological Association* 92 (1981): ii–iii.

9 Marshall Wolf, interview with author, October 6, 2010.

10 Tracy Kidder, *Mountains beyond Mountains* (New York: Random House, 2003).

11 Murray F. Brennan, "Francis D. Moore, 1913–2001," *Annals of Surgery* 235 (2002): 600–601.

12 Francis D. Moore, *The Metabolic Care of the Surgical Patient* (Philadelphia: W. B. Saunders, 1959).

10. Growth and Integration

1 Eugene Braunwald, "Annual Report of the Physician-in-Chief, 1972–1973," Brigham and Women's Hospital (Boston, 1973), 38.

2 *Transforming Patient Care: The Vision Continues* (Boston: Harvard Vanguard Medical Associates, 2009).

3 *HCHP: The First Decade—Harvard Community Health Plan Annual Report* (Boston: Harvard Community Health Plan, 1980), 3.

4 Joseph Dorsey, interview with author, November 21, 2010.

5 Ibid.

6 Daniel Golden and Charles Stein, "MGH, Brigham plan to merge. Consolidation geared to lower costs in anticipation of US health reform," *Boston Globe,* December 8, 1993, 1.

7 Richard A. Knox, "Hospitals expect merger to save millions: MGH, Brigham super-hospital deal would change face of Boston medical establishment," *Boston Globe,* December 9, 1993, 1.

8 Ibid.

9 Ibid.

10 Daniel Golden, "MGH still plans obstetrical unit," *Boston Globe,* December 9, 1993, 50.

11 Judy Foreman, "Merger will require the right blend: Hospitals' cultures may imperil unity," *Boston Globe,* December 10, 1993, 37.

12 John A. Kastor, *Mergers of Teaching Hospitals in Boston, New York, and Northern California* (Ann Arbor: University of Michigan Press, 2003).

11. Research in Evolution

1 Elizabeth G. Nabel and Eugene Braunwald, "A tale of coronary artery disease and myocardial infarction," *New England Journal of Medicine* 366 (2012): 54–63.

2   Eugene Braunwald, "Direct coronary revascularization: A plea not to let the genie escape from the bottle," *Hospital Practice* 6 (1971): 9–10.

3   U.S. Department of Health and Human Services, Food and Drug Administration: Guidance for Industry, "Providing clinical evidence of effectiveness for human drugs and biological products," May 1998. Available at www.fda .gov/downloads/Drugs/GuidanceComplianceRegulatoryInformation/ Guidances/ucm078749.pdf (accessed 2/16/2013).

4   MILIS Study Group, "Effect of Propranolol on myocardial infarct size in a randomized, blinded, multicenter trial," *New England Journal of Medicine* 311 (1984): 218–225.

5   MILIS Study Group, "Circadian variation in the frequency of onset of acute myocardial infarction," *New England Journal of Medicine* 313 (1985): 1315–1322.

6   Arnold S. Relman, "Lessons from the Darsee affair," *New England Journal of Medicine* 308: 1415–1417.

7   Eugene Braunwald, "Cardiology: The John Darsee experience," in David J. Miller and Michel Hersen, eds., *Research Fraud in the Behavioral and Biomedical Sciences* (New York: John Wiley, 1992), 55–79. Barbara J. Culliton, "Coping with fraud: The Darsee case," *Science* 220 (1983): 31–35.

8   Braunwald, "Cardiology: The John Darsee experience," 58.

9   Ibid., 59.

10 Ibid., 63.

11 Culliton, "Coping with fraud," 31.

12 Braunwald, "Cardiology: The John Darsee experience," 69.

13 John Darsee, "A retraction of two papers on cardiomyopathy," *New England Journal of Medicine* 308 (1983): 1419.

14 Burton E. Sobel et al., "Normal oxidative phosphorylation in mitochondria from the failing heart," *Circulation Research* 21 (1967): 355–363.

15 Claudia Wallis et al., "Fraud in a Harvard Lab," *Time,* February 28, 1983.

16 Braunwald, "Cardiology: The John Darsee experience," 75–79.

17 Ibid., 79.

18 Marvin L. Murphy et al., "Treatment of chronic stable angina: A preliminary report of survival data of the randomized Veterans Administration Cooperative Study," *New England Journal of Medicine* 297 (1977): 621–627. European Coronary Surgery Study Group, "Long-term results of prospective randomized study of coronary artery bypass surgery in stable angina pectoris," *Lancet* 2 (1982): 1173–1180. CASS Principal Investigators, "Coronary Artery Surgery Study (CASS): A randomized trial of coronary artery bypass surgery—Survival data," *Circulation* 68 (1983): 939–950. CASS Prin-

cipal Investigators, "Coronary Artery Surgery Study (CASS): A randomized trial of coronary artery bypass surgery—Quality of life in randomized subjects," *Circulation* 68 (1983): 951–960. James E. Muller, Peter H. Stone, John E. Markis, and Eugene Braunwald, "Don't let the genie out of the bottle—again," *New England Journal of Medicine* 304 (May 1981): 1294–96.

19 TIMI Study Group, "The Thrombolysis in Myocardial Infarction (TIMI) trial," *New England Journal of Medicine* 312 (1985): 932–936.

20 See www.timi.org/?p=332 (accessed 4/4/2012).

21 Marc A. Pfeffer et al., "Myocardial infarct size and ventricular function in rats," *Circulation Research* 44 (1979): 503–512.

22 Janice M. Pfeffer et al., "Regression of left ventricular hypertrophy and prevention of left ventricular dysfunction by captopril in the spontaneously hypertensive rat," *Proceedings of the National Academy of Science* 79 (1982): 3310–14. Janice M. Pfeffer et al., "Influence of chronic captopril therapy on the infarcted left ventricle of the rat," *Circulation Research* 57 (1985): 84–95.

23 Marc A. Pfeffer et al., "Effects of captopril on progressive ventricular dilation after anterior myocardial infarction," *New England Journal of Medicine* 319 (1988): 80–86.

24 Marc A. Pfeffer et al., on behalf of the SAVE Investigators, "Effect of captopril on mortality and morbidity in patients with left ventricular dysfunction after myocardial infarction: Results of the Survival and Ventricular Enlargement trial," *New England Journal of Medicine* 327 (1992): 669–677.

25 William B. Kannel et al., "Factors of risk in the development of coronary heart disease: Six-year follow-up experience—The Framingham Study," *Annals of Internal Medicine* 55 (1961): 33–50.

26 WHO Cooperative Trial Committee of Principal Investigators, "A cooperative trial in the primary prevention of ischaemic heart disease using clofibrate," *British Heart Journal* 40 (1978): 1069–1118.

27 Lipid Research Clinics Program, "The Lipid Research Clinics Coronary Primary Prevention Trial results, I: Reduction in incidence of coronary heart disease," *Journal of the American Medical Association* 251 (1984): 351–364.

28 John Simons, "The $10 billion pill," *Fortune,* January 20, 2003.

29 Akira Endo, "The discovery and development of HMG-CoA reductase inhibitors," *Journal of Lipid Research* 33 (1992): 1569–1582.

30 Scandinavian Simvastatin Survival Study Group, "Randomised trial of cholesterol lowering in 4,444 patients with coronary heart disease: The Scandinavian Simvastatin Survival Study (4S)," *Lancet* 334 (1994): 1383–1389.

31 James Shepherd et al., for the West of Scotland Coronary Prevention Study Group, "Prevention of coronary heart disease with pravastatin in men with

hypercholesterolemia," *New England Journal of Medicine* 333 (1995): 1301–1307.

32 James B. Wyngaarden, "Donald Sharp Fredrickson," in *Biographical Memoirs* (Washington, DC: National Academy of Sciences, 2006), 164–179.

33 Robert Zelis et al., "Effects of hyperlipoproteinemias and their treatment on the peripheral circulation," *Journal of Clinical Investigation* 49 (1970): 1007–1015.

34 Meir J. Stampfer et al., "The 2-by-2 factorial design: Its application to a randomized trial of aspirin and carotene in U.S. physicians," *Statistics in Medicine* 4 (1985): 111–116.

35 Scandinavian Simvastatin Survival Study Group, "The Scandinavian Simvastatin Survival Study (4S)."

36 Frank M. Sacks et al., "The effect of pravastatin on coronary events after myocardial infarction in patients with average cholesterol levels," *New England Journal of Medicine* 335 (1996): 1001–1009.

37 Christopher P. Cannon et al., "Intensive versus moderate lipid lowering with statins after acute coronary syndromes," *New England Journal of Medicine* 350 (2004): 1495–1504.

38 Paul M. Ridker et al., "C-reactive protein levels and outcomes after statin therapy," *New England Journal of Medicine* 352 (2005): 20–28.

39 Paul M. Ridker et al., "Rosuvastatin to prevent vascular events in men and women with elevated C-reactive protein," *New England Journal of Medicine* 359 (2008): 2195–2207.

40 Samuel K. Elster et al., "A study of C-reactive protein in the serum of patients with congestive heart failure," *American Heart Journal* 51 (1956): 533–541.

41 Robert M. Califf et al., "An update on the IMProved reduction of outcomes: Vytorin Efficacy International Trial (IMPROVE-IT) design," *American Heart Journal* 159 (2010): 705–759.

42 Gardner Harris and Benedict Carey, "Researchers fail to reveal full drug pay," *New York Times,* June 8, 2008.

43 Globe Spotlight Team, "A healthcare system badly out of balance," *Boston Globe,* November 16, 2008, 1.

44 Duff Wilson, "Harvard teaching hospitals cap outside pay," *New York Times,* January 3, 2010.

45 Liz Kowalczyk, "Prescription for prestige," *Boston Globe,* October 19, 2010.

46 Eugene Braunwald, "Departments, divisions, and centers in the evolution of medical schools," *American Journal of Medicine* 119 (2006): 457–462.

47 Eugene Braunwald, "The present state and future of academic cardiology,"

Circulation 66 (1982): 487–490. Eugene Braunwald, "Cardiology—Division or department?" *New England Journal of Medicine* 329 (1993): 1887–1890. Eugene Braunwald, "Subspecialists and internal medicine: A perspective," *Annals of Internal Medicine* 114 (1991): 76–78.

48 Ibid., 78.

49 Charles Seth Landefeld, "The spring meetings—Are they dying?" *New England Journal of Medicine* 328 (1993): 1645–1647. Ralph Snyderman, "The AAP and the transformation of medicine," *Journal of Clinical Investigation* 114 (2004): 1169–1173. Joel D. Howell, "A history of the American Society of Clinical Investigation," *Journal of Clinical Investigation* 119 (2009): 682–697.

50 Landefeld, "The spring meetings," 1647.

51 Braunwald, "Departments, divisions, and centers," 462.

12. Textbooks and Education in Evolution

1 Charles Friedberg, *Diseases of the Heart*, 1st ed. (Philadelphia: W. B. Saunders, 1950).

2 Nanette K. Wenger, "Charles K. Friedberg," *Clinical Cardiology,* 9 (1986): 356–359.

3 David H. Spodick, Book forum, *Journal of the American Medical Association* 221 (1972): 306.

4 Beta-Blocker Heart Attack Trial Research Group, "A randomized trial of propranolol in patients with acute myocardial infarction, I: Mortality results," *Journal of the American Medical Association* 247 (1982): 1707–1714.

5 Thomas H. Lee, "Eulogy for a quality measure," *New England Journal of Medicine* 357 (2007): 1175–1177.

6 Burton Sobel and Eugene Braunwald, "The management of acute myocardial infarction," in Braunwald, ed., *Heart Disease,* 2nd ed., 1320–1322 (Philadelphia: W. B. Sanders, 1984).

7 J. Willis Hurst, Foreword, in Valentin Fuster et al., eds., *Hurst's The Heart,* 11th ed., xxv–xxvii (New York: McGraw-Hill, 2004).

8 Ibid.

9 James T. Willerson, "*Heart Disease:* A textbook of cardiovascular medicine," *New England Journal of Medicine* 304 (1981): 551–552.

10 Debra K. Moser and Barbara Riegel, *Cardiac Nursing: A Companion to Braunwald's Heart Disease* (Philadelphia: W. B. Saunders, 2008). Elliott Antman et al., *Cardiovascular Therapeutics: A Companion to Braunwald's Heart Disease* (Philadelphia: W. B. Saunders), 1996.

11 Allen B. Weisse, *Heart to Heart: The Twentieth Century Battle against Car-*

diac Disease—An Oral History (New Brunswick, NJ: Rutgers University Press, 2002), 322.

13. The Still Years

1 Eduardo Marbán and Eugene Braunwald, "Training the clinician investigator," *Circulation Research* 103 (2008): 771–772.
2 Marc A. Pfeffer et al., on behalf of the SAVE Investigators, "Effect of captopril on mortality and morbidity in patients with left ventricular dysfunction after myocardial infarction: Results of the Survival and Ventricular Enlargement trial," *New England Journal of Medicine* 327 (1992): 669–677.

Appendix

The analyses in this appendix were generated with support from McKinsey and Company. Certain data included here are derived from the Web of Science prepared by Thomson Reuters, Inc. (Thomson), Philadelphia, Pennsylvania, USA, copyright © Thomson Reuters 2009. All rights reserved.

1 Kim Fox, "Nobel Prize winners' prize winner: Eugene Braunwald," *European Heart Journal* 21 (2000): 1275.
2 Eugene Braunwald, "Fifty years of cardiology: Brief reflections on the past and a look into the future," *European Heart Journal* 21 (2000): 1275–1276.
3 Eugene Garfield, "Citation indexes for science," *Science* 122 (1955): 108–111. Eugene Garfield, "'Scientific Citation Index': A new dimension in indexing," *Science* 144 (1964): 649–654.
4 Eugene Garfield, "The history and meaning of the journal impact factor," *Journal of the American Medical Association* 295 (2006): 90–93.
5 Ibid.
6 Joseph Loscalzo, "Can scientific quality be quantified?" *Circulation* 123 (2011): 947–950.
7 Jorge E. Hirsch, "An index to quantify an individual's scientific research output," *Proceedings of the National Academy of Sciences* 102 (2005): 16569–16572.
8 Loscalzo, "Can scientific quality be quantified?"

Index